Interfaces of PSYCHIATRY

Interfaces of
PSYCHIATRY

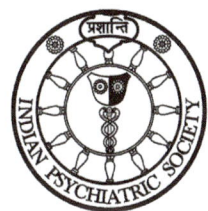

Indian Psychiatric Society Publication

Editors

Vinay Kumar MD
Consultant Psychiatrist
Manoved Mind Hospital
Patna, Bihar, India

Sandeep Grover MD
Professor
Department of Psychiatry
Postgraduate Institute of Medical Education and Research
Chandigarh, India

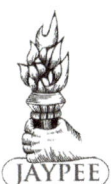

JAYPEE BROTHERS MEDICAL PUBLISHERS
The Health Sciences Publisher
New Delhi | London

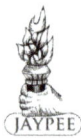 **Jaypee Brothers Medical Publishers (P) Ltd**

Headquarters

Jaypee Brothers Medical Publishers (P) Ltd
EMCA House, 23/23-B
Ansari Road, Daryaganj
New Delhi 110 002, India
Landline: +91-11-23272143, +91-11-23272703
+91-11-23282021, +91-11-23245672
Email: jaypee@jaypeebrothers.com

Corporate Office

Jaypee Brothers Medical Publishers (P) Ltd
4838/24, Ansari Road, Daryaganj
New Delhi 110 002, India
Phone: +91-11-43574357
Fax: +91-11-43574314
Email: jaypee@jaypeebrothers.com

Overseas Office

JP Medical Ltd
83 Victoria Street, London
SW1H 0HW (UK)
Phone: +44 20 3170 8910
Fax: +44 (0)20 3008 6180
Email: info@jpmedpub.com

Website: www.jaypeebrothers.com
Website: www.jaypeedigital.com

© 2023, Jaypee Brothers Medical Publishers and Indian Psychiatric Society

The views and opinions expressed in this book are solely those of the original contributor(s)/author(s) and do not necessarily represent those of editor(s) or publisher of the book.

All rights reserved. No part of this publication may be reproduced, stored or transmitted in any form or by any means, electronic, mechanical, photocopying, recording or otherwise, without the prior permission in writing of the publishers.

All brand names and product names used in this book are trade names, service marks, trademarks or registered trademarks of their respective owners. The publisher is not associated with any product or vendor mentioned in this book.

Medical knowledge and practice change constantly. This book is designed to provide accurate, authoritative information about the subject matter in question. However, readers are advised to check the most current information available on procedures included and check information from the manufacturer of each product to be administered, to verify the recommended dose, formula, method and duration of administration, adverse effects and contraindications. It is the responsibility of the practitioner to take all appropriate safety precautions. Neither the publisher nor the author(s)/editor(s) assume any liability for any injury and/or damage to persons or property arising from or related to use of material in this book.

This book is sold on the understanding that the publisher is not engaged in providing professional medical services. If such advice or services are required, the services of a competent medical professional should be sought.

Every effort has been made where necessary to contact holders of copyright to obtain permission to reproduce copyright material. If any have been inadvertently overlooked, the publisher will be pleased to make the necessary arrangements at the first opportunity.

Inquiries for bulk sales may be solicited at: jaypee@jaypeebrothers.com

Interfaces of Psychiatry

First Edition: 2023

ISBN: 978-93-89188-63-9

Contributors

Abhinav Tandon MD
Associate Professor
Department of Psychiatry
United Institute of Medical Sciences
Allahabad, Uttar Pradesh, India

Abhishek Ghosh MD DM (Addiction Psychiatry)
Additional Professor
Department of Psychiatry
Postgraduate Institute of Medical Education
and Research, Chandigarh, India

Adarsh Tripathi MD
Professor
Department of Psychiatry
King George's Medical University
Lucknow, Uttar Pradesh, India

Ajit Avasthi MD
Professor and Head
Department of Psychiatry
Postgraduate Institute of Medical Education
and Research, Chandigarh, India

Ajit V Bhide MD
Consultant
Department of Psychiatry
St Martha's Hospital
Bengaluru, Karnataka, India

Alka Subramanyam MD
Associate Professor
Department of Psychiatry
Topiwala National Medical College and
BYL Nair Charitable Hospital
Mumbai, Maharashtra, India

Amulya Koneru MD
Consultant
Department of Psychiatry
Asha Hospital
Hyderabad, Telangana, India

Anish Shouan MBBS MD
Psychiatry Registrar
Northern Area Mental Health Services
Melbourne, Australia

Badr Ratnakaran MD
Assistant Professor
Carilion Clinic
Virginia Tech Carilion School of Medicine
Roanoke, Virginia, USA

Biswa Ranjan Mishra MD DPM
Additional Professor
Department of Psychiatry
All India Institute of Medical Sciences
Bhubaneswar, Odisha, India

Dalton N MD
Senior Clinical Fellow
Black Country Healthcare
NHS Foundation Trust
West Midlands, UK

Debadatta Mohapatra MD
Assistant Professor
Department of Psychiatry
All India Institute of Medical Sciences
Bhubaneswar, Odisha, India

Contributors

Debasis Bhattacharya DPM MD
Former Associate Professor
Department of Psychiatry
Institute of Postgraduate Medical Education
and Research
Kolkata, West Bengal, India
Chairperson for the Creativity and Mental
Health Taskforce
Indian Psychiatric Society (IPS)

Debasish Basu MD DNB MAMS
Professor and Head
Department of Psychiatry
Postgraduate Institute of Medical Education
and Research
Chandigarh, India

Devakshi Dua MD MRCPsych
Specialty Registrar
General Adult Psychiatry
(West Midlands Deanery)
Midlands Partnership Foundation Trust
Stafford, UK

Erika Pahuja MD
Senior Trainee
Specialty Training (ST4)
North Central London General Adult and Old
Age Higher Psychiatry Training Programme
Chase Farm Hospital
London, UK

G Prasad Rao MD
Consultant Psychiatrist
Director
Schizophrenia and Psychopharmacology
Division
Asha Hospital
Hyderabad, Telangana, India

Ganesan Venkatasubramanian MD
Professor
Department of Psychiatry
National Institute of Mental Health
and Neurosciences
Bengaluru, Karnataka, India

Koushik Sinha Deb MD
Additional Professor
Department of Psychiatry
All India Institute of Medical Sciences
New Delhi, India

Mahadev Singh Sen MD
Assistant Professor
Department of Psychiatry
Institute of Human Behavior and Allied Sciences
New Delhi, India

Pavitra KS MD
Professor and Head
Department of Psychiatry
Basaveshwara Medical College and Hospital
Chitradurga, Karnataka, India
Consultant Psychiatrist
Sridhar Neuropsychiatric Centre
Shivamogga, Karnataka, India

PK Singh MD
Former Professor and Head
Department of Psychiatry
Patna Medical College
Patna, Bihar, India

Pratap Sharan MD PhD
Professor
Department of Psychiatry
All India Institute of Medical Sciences
New Delhi, India

Preethy K MD DNB DM (Addiction Psychiatry)
Assistant Professor
Department of Psychiatry
All India Institute of Medical Sciences
Jodhpur, Rajasthan, India

Rahul Bhattacharya
DPM (Ireland) MRCPsych MSc (Clinical Neuro Psychiatry)
Consultant Psychiatrist and Associate
Clinical Director
East London NHS Foundation Trust
Honorary Clinical Senior Lecturer
Barts and the London School of Medicine, UK

Contributors

Sachin Nagendrappa MD
Assistant Professor
Department of Psychiatry
St John's Medical College Hospital
Bengaluru, Karnataka, India

Sai Krishna Tikka MD
Associate Professor
Department of Psychiatry
All India Institute of Medical Sciences
Hyderabad, Telangana, India

Samir Kumar Praharaj MD
Professor and Head
Department of Psychiatry
Kasturba Medical College, Manipal
Manipal Academy of Higher Education
Manipal, Udupi, Karnataka, India

Sandeep Grover MD
Professor
Department of Psychiatry
Postgraduate Institute of Medical Education
and Research
Chandigarh, India

Sangha Mitra Godi MD
Assistant Professor
Department of Psychiatry
Central Institute of Psychiatry (CIP)
Ranchi, Jharkhand, India

Santosh K Chaturvedi MD FRCPsych
Consultant Psychiatrist
Jagadguru Kripalu Chikitsalaya
Vrindavan, Barsana, and Mangarh
Uttar Pradesh, India
Former Dean and Senior Professor of Psychiatry
National Institute of Mental Health
and Neurosciences
Bengaluru, Karnataka, India

Savita Malhotra MD PhD FAMS
Former Dean, Professor and Head
Department of Psychiatry
Postgraduate Institute of Medical Education
and Research
Chandigarh, India

Shahbaz Ali Khan MD
Professor and Head
Department of Psychiatry
Command Hospital
Lucknow, Uttar Pradesh, India

Shahul Ameen MD
Consultant Psychiatrist
St Thomas Hospital
Kottayam, Kerala, India

Shashidhara HN DPM MD
Psychiatrist Specialist Grade
National Institute of Mental Health
and Neurosciences
Bengaluru, Karnataka, India

Shinjini Choudhury
MD DM (Addiction Psychiatry)
Former Senior Resident
Department of Psychiatry
All India Institute of Medical Sciences
Rishikesh, Uttarakhand, India

Shiva Shanker Reddy MD DM
Assistant Professor
Department of Psychiatry
Viswabharathi Medical College and
General Hospital
Kurnool, Andhra Pradesh, India

Shivanand Manohar MD
Assistant Professor
Department of Psychiatry
JSS Medical College and Hospital
JSS Academy of Higher Education and Research
Mysuru, Karnataka, India

Shubh Mohan Singh MD
Professor
Department of Psychiatry
Postgraduate Institute of Medical Education
and Research
Chandigarh, India

Shubrata Kalmane MD
Professor
Department of Psychiatry
Subbaiah Institute of Medical Sciences
Shivamogga, Karnataka, India

Siddharth Sarkar MD DNB
Additional Professor
Department of Psychiatry and National Drug Dependence Treatment Centre
All India Institute of Medical Sciences
New Delhi, India

Sonia Shenoy MBBS MD
Associate Professor
Department of Psychiatry
Kasturba Medical College, Manipal
Manipal Academy of Higher Education
Manipal, Udupi, Karnataka, India

Srinivas Balachander MD
Assistant Professor
Department of Psychiatry
National Institute of Mental Health and Neurosciences
Bengaluru, Karnataka, India

Sujita Kumar Kar MBBS MD
Additional Professor
Department of Psychiatry
King George's Medical University
Lucknow, Uttar Pradesh, India

Suresh Bada Math
MD DNB PGDMLE PGDHRL PhD
Professor
Department of Psychiatry
National Institute of Mental Health and Neurosciences
Bengaluru, Karnataka, India

Sweta Singh MS (Obs & Gyne)
Additional Professor
Department of Obstetrics and Gynecology
All India Institute of Medical Sciences
Bhubaneswar, Odisha, India

Tarun Narang MD MNAMS
Associate Professor
Department of Dermatology, Venereology and Leprology
Postgraduate Institute of Medical Education and Research
Chandigarh, India

TS Sathyanarayana Rao MBBS MD
Professor
Department of Psychiatry
JSS Medical College and Hospital
JSS Academy of Higher Education and Research
Mysuru, Karnataka, India

V Sriramya
Research Officer
Asha Hospital
Hyderabad, Telangana, India

Venkataram Shivakumar MBBS
Scientist D
Department of Integrative Medicine and Wellcome Trust/DBT
National Institute of Mental Health and Neurosciences
Bengaluru, Karnataka, India

Vinay B MD PGDMLE PGDHRL
Psychiatrist Specialist Grade
National Institute of Mental Health and Neurosciences
Bengaluru, Karnataka, India

Vinay Kumar MD
Consultant Psychiatrist
Manoved Mind Hospital
Patna, Bihar, India

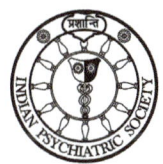

Indian Psychiatric Society

It is a matter of pleasure to write a few words for the book, *Interfaces of Psychiatry*, edited by Dr Vinay Kumar and Dr Sandeep Grover which is an important addition to the ever-evolving science. The scientific and not too scientific underpinnings of psychiatric disorders closely share with other medical disorders so much that a treatise on common factors is mandatory. We are happy that the Publication Committee of Indian Psychiatric Society (IPS) has taken the timely task of inviting some of the big names in the field. Unfortunately, the knowledge shared among various specialists with psychiatrists is poor and it is the responsibility of the mental health professionals to dispel the misconceptions among non-psychiatrists which help in dispelling the wrong notions prevailing in public and other medical fraternity. We are happy that renowned psychiatrists from India and abroad, and professionals from other specialties have taken up the task of discussing the interface between not only other physical disorders but also of humanities like mythology and we are sure those who read this book will be immensely benefited.

The lack of understanding mental health and mental illnesses among non-psychiatric physicians is one of the biggest stumbling blocks for providing holistic treatment to the needy. It is equally true about psychiatrists who lack knowledge of other medical specialties. The rise of the pandemic has only worsened the situation of everyone by more emotional problems and less understanding. The management of infections and its long-term consequences mandated all physicians to have a basic understanding of basic pathophysiology with the application of philosophy. The resources and manpower are severely crumbled. The impact on psychological well-being is immense while the need to address such problems is imminent. It is interesting that a Chapter on Interface with Law too is added.

We are sure, the readers will have an overall view of the problems and likely solutions. We congratulate all contributors and wish the Sub-Committee under the Chairmanship of Dr Anil Kakunje bring out many more such projects in future.

Long live IPS!

<table>
<tr><td align="center">**NN Raju**
President</td><td align="center">**Arabinda Brahma**
Hony General Secretary</td></tr>
</table>

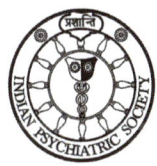

Publication Committee

It is a matter of great pleasure to write a message for a book on *Interfaces of Psychiatry* which is a unique book; the first of its kind addressing psychiatry interfaces so extensively.

It is heartening to see IPS coming up with a lot of books in psychiatry; it is not just textbooks but books on many specialty topics and niche areas. The knowledge of latest developments is paramount not just for students but also practicing psychiatrists and the additional information through publications will be very handy to learn.

Psychiatrists now have to handle varied illness related to all specialties unlike in the past when they were confined to treating mental illness mainly. We feel glad to highlight that the book on *Interfaces of Psychiatry* has more than 26 chapters covering several branches of medicine such as dermatology, neurology, gastroenterology, cardiology, rheumatology; also covers interfaces with law, mythology, anthropology, spirituality, sexuality, literature, biology, technology, and politics. Dr Vinay Kumar has worked in the Publication Committee of IPS for several years, and his knowledge and experience is immense. Dr Sandeep Grover is a teacher par excellence. The publication committee congratulates Dr Vinay Kumar and Dr Sandeep Grover for editing this book which will be released in ANCIPS 2023.

We, on behalf of the publication committee thank the IPS office bearers for their continued support and cooperation. We, also thank M/s Jaypee Brothers Medical Publishers (P) Ltd, New Delhi, India, for their efforts.

We are sure, this book will be a hugely popular and will be considered a significant contribution to the field of Psychiatry.

Long Live IPS!

Anil Kakunje	**Dipayan Sarkar**	**Mrugesh Vaishnav**
Chairperson	Convener	Advisor

Preface

A mentally healthy person is defined not merely by the absence of a mental disorder but is understood as having healthy mental well-being. Mental well-being is further understood as a state of being healthy and happy. Multiple aspects of life define happiness for different people. These include hobbies, vocation, career and profession, family, love, sleep, etc. Similarly, various aspects of human life influence the development and manifestation of mental illnesses and the management of mental disorders. However, many of these aspects are usually not included in the standard textbooks of psychiatry. Similarly, books from other specialties do not address mental health issues in detail. Accordingly, there was a need to have a book to address the problems at the interface of mental health and other aspects of life.

Psychiatry, as a specialty, interacts with arts, philosophy, literature, poetry, ethics, mythology, law, parapsychology, culture, politics, history, sociology, anthropology, religion, spirituality, biology, sexuality, technology, education, cinema, dance, music, theater, social media, etc. Keeping these in mind, this book covers chapters addressing how these aspects influence mental health, the manifestation of mental disorders, help-seeking, management of mental disorders, and prevention of mental disorders.

The book also includes chapters on the interface of psychiatry with cardiology, neurology, rheumatology, gastroenterology, dermatology, obstetrics and gynecology, and surgical specialties. These chapters provide information about psychiatric manifestations in patients with various physical illnesses and also provide information about how to manage mental morbidity in patients with various physical morbidities.

We thank President, Professor NN Raju; Hony General Secretary, Dr Arabinda Brahma; Treasurer, Dr Aleem Siddiqui; and Hony Editor, Professor Omprakash Singh for their support and encouragement in compiling this book. We thank all the authors for their contributions and for accepting our suggestions. For artistic image of front cover of this book, we are grateful to Mr Shyam Sharma, who is a Padma Shree Awardee and an artist of international repute.

We also thank Shri Jitendar P Vij (Group Chairman), Mr Ankit Vij (Managing Director), Mr MS Mani (Group President), Ms Chetna Malhotra (Senior Director–Professional Publishing, Marketing and Business Development), Ms Pooja Bhandari (Production Head) and Nikita Chauhan (Senior Development Editor), M/s Jaypee Brothers Medical Publishers (P) Ltd, New Delhi, India for all their support and help.

We hope mental health professionals will find this updated book useful.

Vinay Kumar
Sandeep Grover

Contents

1. **Interfaces of Psychiatry: An Outline** 1
   Vinay Kumar, Shahbaz Ali Khan

2. **Interface with Biology** 9
   Venkataram Shivakumar, Ganesan Venkatasubramanian

3. **Interface with Neurology** 18
   Adarsh Tripathi, Erika Pahuja, Sujita Kumar Kar

4. **Interface with Obstetrics and Gynecology** 42
   Debadatta Mohapatra, Biswa Ranjan Mishra, Sweta Singh

5. **Interface with Rheumatology** 60
   Sandeep Grover, Anish Shouan

6. **Interface with Gastroenterology** 72
   Samir Kumar Praharaj, Sonia Shenoy

7. **Interface with Medical and Surgical Specialties** 88
   Shiva Shanker Reddy, Santosh K Chaturvedi

8. **Interface with Dermatology** 99
   Shubh Mohan Singh, Tarun Narang, Dalton N

9. **Interface with Cardiology** 112
   G Prasad Rao, Amulya Koneru, V Sriramya

10. **Interface with Sexuality and Sexual Disorders** 122
    TS Sathyanarayana Rao, Abhinav Tandon, Shivanand Manohar

11. **Interface with Ethics and Culture** 136
    Savita Malhotra, Srinivas Balachander

12. **Interface with Politics** 144
    Sangha Mitra Godi, Sai Krishna Tikka

13. **Interface with History** 157
    Ajit Avasthi, Abhishek Ghosh

14. **Interface with Sociology** 166
   Shinjini Choudhury, Abhishek Ghosh, Debasish Basu

15. **Interface with Mythology** 174
   Ajit V Bhide

16. **Interface with Philosophy** 181
   Pratap Sharan

17. **Interface with Religion** 191
   Sandeep Grover, Devakshi Dua

18. **Interface with Art Therapy** 208
   Debasis Bhattacharya, Rahul Bhattacharya

19. **Interface with Law** 218
   Vinay B, Shashidhara HN, Suresh Bada Math

20. **Interface with Parapsychology** 229
   PK Singh

21. **Interface with Technology and Mental Health** 239
   Koushik Sinha Deb, Preethy K

22. **Interface with Education** 248
   Alka Subramanyam

23. **Interface with Cinema** 265
   Sachin Nagendrappa, Shubrata Kalmane

24. **Interface with Dance, Music, and Theater** 271
   Pavitra KS

25. **Interface with Anthropology** 286
   Siddharth Sarkar, Mahadev Singh Sen

26. **Interface with Social Media** 297
   Badr Ratnakaran, Shahul Ameen

Index *313*

CHAPTER 1

Interfaces of Psychiatry: An Outline

Vinay Kumar, Shahbaz Ali Khan

INTRODUCTION

Psychiatry today stands at a juncture where it touches almost all aspects of human life, interacting with philosophy, culture, religion, sociology, jurisprudence, politics, economics, and cinema among others, apart from sister medical streams. One has to appreciate the ripple effect of collective emotions on rise and fall of the Sensex to understand the impact of mind on aspects as distant as economy. Thus, it traverses various frontiers and makes significant interfaces at every front. Let us briefly look at the various interfaces before we take the jump into the ocean of knowledge that this book provides to the readers.

MEDICAL AND SURGICAL DISCIPLINES

If we look at the interface of psychiatry with biology in general, it is evident that psychiatry is now significantly integrated with other medical and surgical specialties than in the past. Psychiatric disorders are highly prevalent among medically ill patients. Studies done in our country found 38.6% of psychiatric comorbidity with depressive disorder (28.2%) being the most common psychiatric diagnosis in the outpatient medically ill.[1] The interface between psychiatry and medical specialties is very vast. It starts from the etiopathogenesis of a medical illness due to psychological and emotional problems to psychiatric consequences of medical diseases, especially those which are chronic or life-threatening, and this interface also deals with psychiatric side effects of medications and procedures, as well as drug interactions between drugs for medical treatment and psychopharmacological agents. In contrast to the few known subspecialties of psychiatry such as addiction, child, and geriatric psychiatry, some of the interfaces have developed into super specialties such as *psycho-oncology, psychonephrology, psychocardiology, psycho-ophthalmology, psychogynecology, neuropsychiatry, and psychodermatology.*

Severe Mental Illness

Another matter of concern with psychiatric illness is the high prevalence and poor outcome of physical illnesses associated with them—the issue of medical diseases in psychiatry patients. Several reviews and studies have shown that people with severe mental illness (SMI) have an excess mortality, being two or three times as high as that in the general population.[2] About 60% of this excess mortality is due to physical illness. Evidence suggests that persons with SMI are, compared to the general population, at increased risk for overweight, obesity, metabolic syndrome, diabetes mellitus, cardiovascular diseases, cancer, and even infectious diseases such as hepatitis B and C, which are much more prevalent in psychiatric patients than the general population.[3] This further underlines the need for the psychiatrist to work in close cooperation with the medical and surgical specialties and her multidimensional role in healthcare.

If we consider primary major mental illness schizophrenia as a prototype of SMI, one wonders whether schizophrenia is the evolutionary price we pay for continuing creativity? Is it the risk humans take collectively to keep creativity alive to aid future survival in an ever-changing world. As we know the only fixed thing in the universe is change. To cope up and survive in this fast-changing world, our weapon is creativity, and schizophrenia is the risk we take to toy with creativity. For every Albert Einstein who helps humanity survive, we have Eduard Einstein, a schizophrenic, or John Nash has to suffer schizophrenia to contribute with his genius creativity for the human race. Sometimes it is both; Bertrand Russel had to suffer from schizophrenia himself and so did many of his relatives. Is schizophrenia then a small price to pay for human survival through continuous creativity?.[4] A lot is happening at this interface of psychiatry and computational biological research due to the unlimited ability of computers to handle big data.

Neurology

Psychiatry and neurology are like twins, born together but got separated. One where the cause was clear and this branch picked up motor, sensory, and such clear domain abnormalities with elicitable physical signs, established etiologies, and demonstrable anatomic pathology and came to be called neurology while the more elusive and complex domain function of the brain—emotions, perception, cognition, behavior which could not be easily allocated to one brain area of Broadman or even one region had no clear etiologies or demonstrable pathologies—came under the umbrella of psychiatry. So, the more tangible and evident aspect inside the head was taken away and the more complicated, complex, nuanced functions were left for psychiatry. With relation between the mind and the brain still not very definitely understood, the Siamese twins better stay together with a clear need for this interface, for the nonphysical mind is forever dependent on the physical brain though not entirely reducible to brain.[5] Nonreductive physicalism is the most prevalent philosophy of psychiatry as of now. It is the need of the hour to encourage psychiatric training for a neurologist and potentiate the neurology training of a psychiatrist, so that both the facilities can work hand in hand, supplement each other in areas of cross-fertilization, and lead to a successful future alliance of both the branches.

Obstetrics and Gynecology

Coming to the interface of psychiatry and reproductive health, we know that psychiatric disorders are equally prevalent in both males and females. However, there exist some gender-specific differences in onset, clinical course, prognosis, treatment resistance, etc. Also, some disorders are specific to females. Women experience various stages of life starting from menarche, menstrual cycle, pregnancy, postpartum period, and menopause, which are greatly influenced by hormonal changes and impact the psychological vulnerability and, in turn, lead to the predisposition of women to certain psychiatric illnesses. While a woman passes through these times along with the transitional stages, she has to go through tremendous hormonal and psychological challenges and biological alterations, which have potential consequences in her mood, behavior, and thought processes. The interface between psychiatry and female psyche has been very sensitive. When psychiatry was blind to this interface, it ostracized women, and as science grew it understood the female biology behind psychic issues specific to the females better.

Rheumatology

An important interface that psychiatry has is with psychosomatic medicine. Rheumatoid arthritis (RA) was included as one of the seven psychosomatic disorders in the original description of "holy seven" by Alexander. Over the years with the improvement in the understanding of various rheumatological disorders, there is also an improvement in understanding about the prevalence of various psychiatric disorders in patients with rheumatic diseases, especially systemic lupus erythematosus (SLE) and RA. Available data suggest a wide range of psychiatric morbidity in patients with SLE and RA and other such immune-related disorders of the body, with depression and anxiety disorders being the most commonly reported morbidities.[6] At the interface also sits the big masquerader like chronic fatigue syndrome (CFS), which is commonly diagnosed as depression.[7] Then there are many rheumatological diseases which first present to the psychiatrist as psychiatric symptoms much before or along with other physical symptoms; a case in point is SLE.

The role of autoimmune factors in the manifestation of obsessive-compulsive disorders (OCDs) are well known. Patients with pediatric autoimmune neuropsychiatric disorders associated with streptococcal infection (PANDAS) and pediatric acute-onset neuropsychiatric syndrome (PANS) can present to the psychiatrists with features of tics, obsessive-compulsive behavior, and other neuropsychiatric symptoms.[8] Hence, when a young patient presents with first-episode psychosis/schizophrenia, catatonia, or OCD-like symptoms, a thorough physical examination needs to be conducted to look for features of SLE and other autoimmune disorders, and if required, the clinician should order diagnostic tests. There is a bidirectional relationship between various psychiatric disorders, psychosocial factors, and manifestations of rheumatological diseases. The role of autoimmunity and inflammation is well known in various psychiatric disorders, which are considered to be at the core of all rheumatological diseases. It is suggested that in patients with rheumatological diseases, alteration in the inflammatory markers impacts the brain. Chronic inflammation leads to impairment in the normal physiological stress responses and results in psychiatric symptoms. The inflammatory changes also directly influence the brain and lead to the development of psychiatric manifestations. Sleep disturbances can influence the perception of the pain, inflammatory response, and the levels of various cytokines. As we see, liaison between psychiatry and rheumatology is inescapable in the management of rheumatological diseases and the interface is bidirectional and well established, and a close cooperation between the treating physicians, the psychiatrist, and a good therapeutic alliance will go a long way in patient care in this domain.

Gastroenterology

The complex and seminal bidirectional interactions between the enteric nervous system (ENS), autonomic nervous system (ANS), central nervous system (CNS), and the hypothalamic–pituitary–adrenal (HPA) axis are evolving and throwing a new light on the gut-brain interactions where emotions and thinking affect the visceral sensitivity, gut motility, secretions, mucosal and immune functions, and gut microbiome and vice versa. In the specialty of the gastrointestinal (GI) system, research has proven that a biopsychosocial approach is the best way forward in management of the plethora of symptoms referred to as functional GI disorders (FGIDs). These are syndromes that include a set of GI symptoms that cluster together, in the absence of any structural disease. These are also called "disorders of gut–brain interaction." To emphasize this hugely important interface of psychiatry with GI system disorders, suffice it to say that there are 33 adult and 20 pediatric FGIDs, which the International Classification of Diseases (ICD) describes as somatoform disorder category.[9]

Sexuality

Sexuality is a primary instinct of human species, enabling pleasure and survival. Various biopsychosocial factors can help us understand the etiopathogenesis of sexual disorders. Race, ethnicity, religion, socioeconomic factors, interpersonal relationships, social stigma, and personality of an individual interact in complex ways to influence the sexuality of an individual. With contributions from Alfred Kinsey to Fritz Klien, the understanding of sexuality as a spectrum, and with sexual identity itself being assessed under sexual attraction, sexual behavior, sexual fantasies, emotional preference, social preference, self-identification, and homosexual/heterosexual lifestyle, sexuality has become a complex construct.[10]

Sexuality is such a fundamental aspect of life that any aberration/convolution/deviation, biological or acquired, is bound to affect the psyche significantly apart from inviting social scrutiny and stress. Apart from that, mental illness has an intricate relationship with sexuality at different levels whether in the form of increased prevalence of sexual disorders in SMI, abuse of persons with mental illness (PMI), or effect of psychotropics. Hence, sexuality is an interface that is extremely pertinent to psychiatry and psychiatrists. With the fast-changing horizons of sexuality, with rising feminism bringing down the age-old bastion of male dominance, with more power to individualism and liberalism, the traditional concept of sexuality is bound to be stressed and lead to distress and disorder (for where there is stress, there is disorder), as is wont and when things change and when societies reorganize around new constructs/domains. Higher incidences of distress, anxiety, and depression in the LGBTQI community are a case in hand. Hence, this interface becomes even more important, and psychiatry has to be ready to face this challenge.

ART, CULTURE, RELIGION, AND ETHICS

The field of psychiatry is unique in its place, as cultural values, norms, and ideals have an influence in its practice more than in any other branch of medicine. Humans are but a product of their culture and ethics, the rules governing the good and bad arise from cultural norms. Psychiatry has a very intimate interface with culture and ethics, much more than any other discipline of science due to the fact that the very concept of normalcy and deviance in behavior is intertwined with culture and social norms to a large extent. Also, the stigma and prejudice attached to psychiatric diagnosis are a baggage from eternity that we have to carry and manage. The situations where involuntary treatment may be required against the free will of the individual and the private and personal nature of divulgences made in therapeutic relationship add to the importance of ethics specific to psychiatry. Considering these special domains of psychiatry, ethics plays a crucial role in protecting the rights of the PMI as well as safeguarding psychiatry as a profession itself.

There is ample evidence that religiosity and its various dimensions influence many mental illnesses. The influence of religiosity and its dimensions has been understood concerning the development of the disorder (especially depression), with some evidence to suggest that religiosity plays a protective role in the development of depression. Contemporary research also sheds light on the association of religiosity/religious beliefs with symptoms of mental illness (i.e., symptoms with religious content and suicidality), help-seeking, pathways to care, medication adherence, treatment response, psychosocial adaptation, relapse rates, social integration, and quality of life (QoL), etc.[11]

Literature and Fine Arts

Literature and fine arts may look unscientific from a distance, but they have been part of sociocultural existence and journey. All these creative pursuits are primarily mental activities, hence the process and the products both influence mental functioning and health. Artworks and literary writings not only reflect thoughts and aesthetics but also the underlying pathology. Therapeutic effects of reading, expressive writing and viewing, listening, and creatively involving in fine arts work have been studied. The jury is still not out with robust evidence supporting as well as refuting its benefits. However, with the concept of holistic and integrative care of concept in mental illness, and the shift in focus from symptom reduction to mental well-being and QoL, these therapies have an active interface with psychiatry, especially in management and rehabilitation domain, with ever-expanding footprint and huge potential, and has been recommended as such in many guidelines. These interfaces are integral to the existence of an evolved mental healthcare system and psychiatry.

POLITICS

The interface of politics and psychiatry is a double-edged sword with both advantages and disadvantages that affect both the disciplines with rising conflict and controversy. On the positive side of this interface, the international and national political partners have started emphasizing the role of mental health by celebrating World Mental Health Day, bringing reforms in existing laws, incorporating mental health indicators to be achieved in the global sustainable goals in World Health Organization (WHO) Mental Health Action Plan, and thereby paving way to the universal coverage for mental health services and equal rights for the mental disability. However, the catastrophic effects of intrusion of political ideology into the realm of mental health have carved a strong impression in the face of history of the world politics and continue to do so. "Personal and political are different domains and the two shall never meet" is an interesting paradigm except that it is false. Politics evolves from personal, and personal is affected by political. A positive relationship between the two results in healthy ecosystem, thriving minds, and great policies to further the cause of universal mental health and its determinants, and a toxic, overbearing, ideological mix of the two or the use of psychiatry as a political tool is pure catastrophe as has been seen time and again. The branch of political psychology must remain independent and scientific for it studies the interface of political behavior and psychological processes. Realizing the importance of this interface, in 1980, the International Association on the Political Use of Psychiatry (IAPUP) was formed in order to fight against political misuse of psychiatry, and since 2005 this is renamed as Global Initiative on Psychiatry (GIP) that focuses on not only political abuse of psychiatry but also human rights monitoring throughout the world with goal of implementing humane, ethical, and effective mental health care.[12]

The mental health professionals need to be aware and alert to the interface of political history and psychiatry lest a "sluggish schizophrenia" may raise its ugly head again.

SOCIOLOGY AND PHILOSOPHY

Sociology deals with the study of groups and their collective consciousness. It is the study of social behavior or society whereas psychiatry, as per the current biomedical model, is a disorder of an individual. However, a closer look makes it inevitable to be aware of the interactions between the two. An individual lives in, to, and for a society. Therefore, societal influence on the individual is undeniable. The disciplines of psychiatry and sociology share a dynamic relationship. Before the 20th century, interaction between these fields was regarded as inconceivable. The very society which, not very long ago, banished mental illness and psychiatry and kept it away from its borders soon saw the development and predominance of sociological view to understand mental illness; the roosts had come home. The two streams again seemed to come apart with the predominance of biological psychiatry, evidence-based medicine, and psychopharmacology in the 1970s before swinging widely toward "Sociatry," egged by Emil Durkheim's social roots of suicide, before finding a comfortable balance with a well-defined interface today seeded in Engel's biopsychosocial dimension.[13]

Social psychiatry's seminal contribution to knowledge in the field of mental health and mental illness, in the form of psychosomatic medicine, abnormal illness behavior, therapeutic community, expressed emotions, and culturally bound idioms of distress, cannot be overemphasized.[14]

Regarding philosophy, the dimension has shifted from philosophy and psychiatry to philosophy of psychiatry, and the tide seems to be turning full circle from rejection of Cartesian dualism to rekindled interest in "property dualism" as the quest of mind's relation with brain searches for newer paradigm. Such is the importance of this interface of psychiatry with philosophy that the external goals of psychiatric research (e.g., deciding which research programs to fund, which research designs are ethically permissible, and how to apply research results to develop more efficacious treatments) are hugely determined by ethical and epistemological domains, which are but core branches of philosophy.

TECHNOLOGY

Talking of technology and its interface with mental health, it can be safely said that technology is intricately linked to modern human existence. Our social life is linked to our battery life, our connections are as strong as our network, and we log on and log off on life every day. The word is consumption; we consume technology and technology in return consumes us, affecting the mental health in the bargain. Also, the mental health of an individual can influence the way she uses and interfaces with technology. Technology thus is a culture tool now, to be wielded for benefit or harm, but it cannot be ignored. From its role in development of personality to psychopathology, as our childhood and adolescence are immersed in it, to its use in assessment, evaluation and treatment, technology, especially information technology, social media, and such other forms of technology have a huge interface with psychiatry. Digital phenotyping [artificial intelligence (AI)-based real-time psychological monitoring and assessment], personalized psychopharmacology (gene-based individualized drug effect and tolerability), huge growth of telemedicine and its application during the COVID-19 pandemic, and Food and Drug Administration (FDA)-approved mobile apps for substance use disorders are just a few instances of the potential of this interface between psychiatry and technology, which has been dealt in detail by the domain experts.[15]

CINEMA

Cinema not only reflects the society it is set in but also acts as a reflector to the society. From spreading awareness and changing public perception to use of cinema in psychiatry teaching programs to mental health advocacy and stigma mitigation, cinema has potential to bring about huge impact on mental health and psychiatry. Similarly the fields of art, theater, music, and dance are creative expressions of human beings and universal modes of communication of ideas and emotions. There is evidence base for their therapeutic potential in mental health, mental illness, and rehabilitation, and these disciplines have an interface with psychiatry, which is beautifully laced, dancing to glory, in tune with each other, singing in rhythm, and synced musically. This aspect has been dealt in detail too, in respective chapters.

CONCLUSION

To conclude, as we discussed in brief here, no sister specialty is complete without exploring the psychological factors; be it at prevention, treatment, or rehabilitation level, the management will have deep voids and will be grossly inadequate and often frustrating if the psyche behind the physical illness is not addressed. Such is the importance of psyche and psychiatry that a close interaction between psychiatry and all the sister specialties, and all the branches of knowledge, is the need of the hour. From the realms of madhouses, psychiatry has come to claim its rightful place in the center of medical science and man's existence itself. We believe that if mental health is an integral part of health and is an absolute human right of everyone irrespective of gender, race, culture, ethnicity, and nationality as propounded by the WHO, then the psychiatrists have to be the advocates of these rights, and be active and alert at all these interfaces outlined above.

In many ways, psychiatry is a social institution, not merely an academic/medical discipline. It is a social institution in the sense that it is embedded and intertwined with other social institutions and has an interface with all of them. This increases the moral obligation and responsibility of the psychiatrists to which they must be alive.

In this context, the interface of psychiatry is with vast and varied fields ranging from biology to culture to religion/spirituality to history to philosophy and more. Through this effort in the form of a book, a humble attempt has been made to explore the various interfaces of psychiatry and take a holistic view of the stream. In general, with the expanding boundaries, bloom in knowledge, and research challenging old concepts by the moment, there is felt need for a balancing interface which psychiatry is well poised to provide. If these interfaces are recognized and realized, it is hoped that it will finally lead to better understanding of concepts and help in collaborative decision-making. This is a humble attempt in that direction. We have collected thoughts of greats in the field on this contemporary and challenging topic to address this interface in a holistic approach to the topic.

REFERENCES

1. Kulkarni V, Chinnakali P, Kanchan T, Rao A, Shenoy M, Papanna MK. Psychiatric comorbidities among patients with select noncommunicable diseases in a coastal city of South India. Int J Prev Med. 2014;5:1139-45.

2. Citrome L, Vreeland B. Schizophrenia, obesity, and antipsychotic medications: what can we do? Postgrad Med. 2008;120:18-33.
3. Osborn DP, Levy G, Nazareth I, Petersen I, Islam A, King MB. Relative risk of cardiovascular and cancer mortality in people with severe mental illness from the United Kingdom's General Practice Research Database. Arch Gen Psychiatry. 2007;64:242-9.
4. Polimeni J, Reiss J. Evolutionary perspectives on schizophrenia. Can J Psychiatry. 2003;48:34-9.
5. Boller F, Dalla Barba G. The evolution of psychiatry and neurology. In: Jeste DV, Friedman JH (Eds). Psychiatry for Neurologists. New York: Springer; 2006. pp. 11-5.
6. Asano NM, Coriolano MD, Asano BJ, Lins OG. Psychiatric comorbidities in patients with systemic lupus erythematosus: a systematic review of the last 10 years. Rev Bras Reumatol. 2013;53(5):431-7.
7. Griffith JP, Zarrouf FA. A systematic review of chronic fatigue syndrome: don't assume it's depression. Prim Care Companion J Clin Psychiatry. 2008;10(2):120-8.
8. Lepri G, Rigante D, Bellando Randone S, Meini A, Ferrari A, Tarantino G, et al. Clinical-serological characterization and treatment outcome of a large cohort of Italian children with pediatric autoimmune neuropsychiatric disorder associated with streptococcal infection and pediatric acute neuropsychiatric syndrome. J Child Adolesc Psychopharmacol. 2019;29(8):608-14.
9. Mukhtar K, Nawaz H, Abid S. Functional gastrointestinal disorders and gut–brain axis: what does the future hold? World J Gastroenterol. 2019;25:552-66.
10. Ventriglio A, Bhugra D. Sexuality in the 21st century: sexual fluidity. East Asian Arch Psychiatry. 2019;29:30-4.
11. Braam AW, Koenig HG. Religion, spirituality, and depression in prospective studies: a systematic review. J Affect Disord. 2019;257:428-38.
12. Voren R van. The abuse of psychiatry for political purposes. In: Mental Health and Human Rights: Vision, Praxis, and Courage. Oxford, UK: Oxford University Press; 2013.
13. Engel GL. The biopsychosocial model and medical education. Who are to be the teachers? N Engl J Med. 1982;306:802-5.
14. Hooley JM, Gotlib IH. A diathesis-stress conceptualization of expressed emotion and clinical outcome. Appl Prev Psychol. 2000;9:135-51.
15. Moshe I, Terhorst Y, Opoku Asare K, Sander LB, Ferreira D, Baumeister H, et al. Predicting symptoms of depression and anxiety using smartphone and wearable data. Front Psychiatry. 2021;12:625247.

CHAPTER 2

Interface with Biology

Venkataram Shivakumar, Ganesan Venkatasubramanian

INTRODUCTION

Historical precedents for ascribing somatic (biological) underpinnings for the pathogenesis of psychiatric disorders date back to 4th century BC. The modern beginnings of biological views about psychiatric disorders perhaps started from mid 1800s with the observations by the influential psychiatrists who recognized the importance of heredity. The prevalent view of simplistic organicity to underlie the manifestations of psychiatric disorders was refined by the concept of psychobiology. Over the next decades advances in the neuroscience coupled with research techniques have emboldened the biological basis of psychiatric disorders.[1]

It has been suggested that the first wave of biological psychiatry started in the second half of the 19th century with an aim "to uncover the relation between mind and brain by doing systematic research linking neuropathology and mental disorder and by using the experimental method in animals and humans".[2] The second wave perhaps originated in the later part of the 20th century primarily due to the advances in genetics and psychopharmacology. The third wave, which started just about two decades before, is promulgated by the technological advances in neuroscience research methods coupled with exciting advances in basic science that has led the conglomeration of several -omics (e.g., genomics, proteomics, metabolomics, connectomics and similar others).[2] This overview attempts to summarize selectively (due to space limitations) certain key interfaces between biology and psychiatry. Since, it is exhaustive to list the interface with respect to all psychiatric disorders, the emphasis has been put forth on schizophrenia as an exemplar illustration to elucidate the application of these paradigmatic perspectives—increasingly, evidence to support similar applications are emerging for several other disorders as well [e.g., bipolar affective disorder, obsessive-compulsive disorder (OCD), autism, dementias, and similar others].

PARADIGM OF ABERRANT NEURODEVELOPMENT AND NEUROIMMUNOPATHOGENESIS

Neurodevelopmental model postulates the manifestations of several psychiatric disorders (e.g., schizophrenia) as a behavioral outcome of an aberration in brain development processes that begin long before the onset of clinical symptoms and are caused by a combination of genetic and environmental factors.[3,4] Gene-environment interaction especially involving genetic factors and obstetric complications have been put forth as one of the important mechanisms that increase the risk toward schizophrenia.[5] Fetal brain development is particularly vulnerable to environmental insults, and deviations from the normal course of brain development are assumed to underlie several mental disorders.

Disparate lines of evidence compellingly support the association between abnormal fetal neurodevelopment and increased risk for schizophrenia.[6,7] Fetal neurodevelopment in schizophrenia can be affected by several obstetric complications like maternal infection, preeclampsia, bleeding, gestational diabetes, rhesus incompatibility, intrauterine growth retardation.[8] All these putative obstetric risk factors of schizophrenia are linked by the common denominator of fetal hypoxia.[8-10]

Epidemiological studies have indicated that maternal infections during pregnancy increase the risk for these disorders in the offspring. Multiple lines of evidence from epidemiologic, clinical, and preclinical studies have provided evidence that gestational exposure to infection contributes to the etiology of schizophrenia.[11] Season of birth findings in schizophrenia robustly implicates birth in winter or spring months as a significant risk factor for schizophrenia; more specifically, a wealth of studies suggest that the prevalence of influenza in winter months might contribute significantly to this risk.[12] Studies on schizophrenia incidence after epidemics of influenza offer unequivocal support to increased incidence of this disorder among exposed offspring. Examination of medical records of >12,000 pregnant women revealed threefold to sevenfold increase in the risk for schizophrenia in the offspring following second-trimester respiratory infection in the mother.[13] Given the high prevalence of influenza infection, it has been estimated that about 14–21% of schizophrenia cases could have been due to maternal infection.[14]

In this context, the maternal cytokine response to infections (maternal immune activation) may play a crucial role in this association, because the induction of cytokines is a fundamental immunological event triggered by virtually any infection.[14,15]

More specifically, it has been suggested that activation of proinflammatory cytokines [with robust support for interleukin-6 (IL-6)][14,15] mediates the neurodevelopmental effects of maternal infections on the offspring. While these cytokines can modulate neuronal differentiation, survival, and dendrite growth and complexity, they have also been critically involved in the precipitation of the long-term behavioral, cognitive and pharmacological consequences of aberrant prenatal immune system activation.[16,17]

The compelling role of IL-6 in the pathogenesis of schizophrenia is emphasized by the following factors: (1) rigorous meta-analytic studies supporting significantly higher serum levels of IL-6 in schizophrenia patients that correlate with symptom severity;[18] (2) association of schizophrenia with IL-6 gene;[19] (3) potential influence on hippocampus by serum IL-6 with hippocampus being the most important brain regions implicated in schizophrenia;[20] (4) IL-6 playing a vital role in established models like "ketamine model" of schizophrenia;[21] and (5) IL-6 being implicated in fetal pathogenetic model of neurodevelopmental aberrations in schizophrenia.[15] Thus, immunopathogenesis involving IL-6 is among the comprehensive models to understand schizophrenia.

Emerging research points toward novel functions of the major histocompatibility complex (MHC) class I molecules in the central nervous system in that these molecules could play an important role in brain development as well as playing a role in the T- and B-cell maturation. MHC class I molecules and their immunoreceptors play pivotal roles during neurodevelopment by influencing neurological cell interactions and signaling. It has been suggested that MHC class I expression is not only essential for the activity-dependent synaptic rearrangements during normal neural development but also for its negative regulation of the density and function of cortical synapses during their initial establishment as reviewed in Debnath et al.[22] Recent genome-wide association studies have uncovered critical insights with respect to immunopathogenesis of schizophrenia.[23]

BRAIN PLASTICITY BASIS FOR PSYCHIATRIC DISORDERS

The paradigm of brain plasticity deficit to underlie the genesis of psychiatric disorders like schizophrenia is another key perspective.[24] Neuroplasticity, the ability of the human brain to actively grow and change itself, has been a path breaking revelation in the field of neuroscience.[25,26] Aberrant neuroplasticity has been used as a framework to understand the complex psychiatric disorders such as schizophrenia, bipolar disorder, and several others.[24] Schizophrenia is increasingly being understood as a disorder of disrupted neuroplasticity.[27,28] Interestingly, the critical genes implicated in neuroplasticity signaling with functional significance in schizophrenia are Disrupted-in-Schizophrenia 1 (DISC1),[29] Neuregulin 1 (NRG1) and ErbB4 signaling pathway,[30] dystrobrevin-binding protein 1 (dysbindin),[27,31,32] V-akt murine thymoma viral oncogene homolog 1 (AKT1),[33] brain-derived neurotrophic factor (BDNF),[34] and the N-methyl-D-aspartate (NMDA) receptor.[35] A majority of the genetic links, their molecular products, and their interactions converge toward glutamate signaling, GABA (gamma-aminobutyric acid) and its receptors, the dopamine system and the cell migration and neuronal development pathways.[27] Further, dorsolateral prefrontal cortex (DLPFC) mediated executive functions deficits that are universally reported in schizophrenia have been conceptualized as markers of deficit in neuroplasticity since neural mechanisms associated with working memory are also closely related to those governing neural plasticity.[28] These findings suggest that aberrant cortical plasticity may be an inheritable trait, and possibly a biomarker, for disorders like schizophrenia.[24]

NEUROCHEMICAL AND NEUROTRANSMITTER BASIS FOR PSYCHIATRIC DISORDERS

Several neurochemical systems interact in disorders like schizophrenia, bipolar disorder, OCD, and similar others; these involve most importantly serotonin, glutamate, and dopamine.[36]

Serotonin: Serotonergic abnormalities are documented in both schizophrenia and OCD; elevated levels of 5-HT$_2$ receptors are demonstrated in the frontal cortex in schizophrenia and lysergic acid diethylamide (LSD), a 5-HT$_2$ agonist, is a well-known psychotomimetic.[37] Moreover, serotonergic modulation of dopaminergic function provides a viable mechanism in schizophrenia.[38] Serotonergic abnormalities play a pivotal role as indicated by the differential efficacy of serotonergic reuptake inhibitors in alleviating OCD[39] over noradrenergic tricyclic antidepressants like desipramine. In addition, serotonin transporter and serotonin receptor[40,41] abnormalities are documented in OCD.

Glutamate: Glutamate abnormality, mainly NMDA receptor deficiency is one of the influential hypotheses for schizophrenia pathogenesis.[42] The phencyclidine model of schizophrenia symptoms and upregulation of glutamate receptor expression in the frontal cortex after chronic exposure to clozapine or olanzapine[43] provide further support to glutamate abnormalities in schizophrenia.

In OCD, reports from neuroimaging, genetic, and cerebrospinal fluid (CSF) studies support involvement of glutamatergic system in the pathogenesis of OCD:[44] (1) neuroimaging studies using magnetic resonance spectroscopy (MRS) consistently have demonstrated increased glutamate in caudate and frontal cortex;[45,46] (2) genes involved in glutamate transmission (SLC1A1) have been implicated in association studies;[47] (3) a CSF study examining glutamate levels has reported increased glutamate in OCD patients;[48] and (4) the glutamate antagonist riluzole is useful in treatment refractory OCD.[49]

Dopamine: The revised dopaminergic hypothesis of schizophrenia postulates a regional abnormality in the dopaminergic system and dopamine as the final common pathway in the pathophysiology of schizophrenia.[50] In its current form, the dopamine hypothesis of schizophrenia postulates hyperdopaminergic state in mesolimbic pathway resulting in psychotic symptoms and a hypodopaminergic state in the frontal cortical terminal fields of the mesocortical dopamine neurons as the basis of the "negative symptoms" of schizophrenia.[51]

Dopamine and serotonin abnormalities have been demonstrated in patients with OCD[52] and several lines of evidence from preclinical and clinical investigations implicate dopamine in the mediation of certain types of repetitive behavior.[53] Antipsychotic augmentation of treatment with serotonin reuptake inhibitors (SRIs) suggests that dopamine receptor antagonism may further reduce symptom severity in selective serotonin reuptake inhibitor (SSRI)-refractory OCD patients.[54] Similar aberrations involving neurochemical pathways have been demonstrated in other psychiatric disorders as well.

FINAL COMMON PATHWAYS: OXIDATIVE STRESS AND METABOLIC ABNORMALITIES

Oxidative stress abnormalities have been proposed to play an important role in the pathogenesis of schizophrenia.[55,56] Evidence points to the role of mitochondrial dysfunction and elevated levels of oxidative damage as potential pathogenetic mechanisms in several psychiatric disorders including schizophrenia.[57] Independent studies have provided evidence to this in the form of genetic and functional impairment in schizophrenia patients to synthesize glutathione, an antioxidant molecule.[58] Apart from glutathione and total antioxidant levels, some researchers have reported increased levels of neopterin in schizophrenia.[59] High neopterin production is associated with increased production of reactive oxygen species by stimulated immunocompetent cells and it has also been proposed that neopterin may not only be an indicator of oxidative stress resulting from immune activation, but may also contribute to the oxidative stress by modulating reactive oxygen species.[56,60] MRS imaging studies in neuroleptic-naïve schizophrenia patients have demonstrated lower phosphocreatine/total phosphorus and phosphocreatine/total ATP ratios in basal ganglia, which could be due to reduced synthesis, perhaps related to mitochondrial dysfunction.[61] The translational evidence to the oxidative damage theory has been provided by Berk et al.[62] in their randomized, multicenter, double-blind, placebo-controlled study, which demonstrated the beneficial effects of administration of antioxidants like N-acetylcysteine, a precursor of glutathione.[56] The oxidative stress abnormalities have complex relationship with the insulin signaling aberrations both at the pathogenetic as well as the pathoplastic effect of the illness as well as treatment.[63,64]

OVERARCHING PARADIGM OF EVOLUTIONARY NEUROSCIENCE

Evolutionary theories have been considered as potentially relevant to understand the genesis and persistence of schizophrenia; such evolutionary conceptualizations can be classified into one of the two categories: (1) theories that assume schizophrenia as a disadvantageous by-product of human brain evolution and (2) theories that propose evolutionary advantages that are associated with the condition; the latter theories usually focus on one of the following vehicles of selection, namely individual, kin, or group.

A clear and unequivocal hypothesis on the evolutionary basis of schizophrenia was first proposed by Huxley et al. (1964). In their hypothesis, it was postulated that schizophrenia represented a genetic polymorphism accompanied by advantageous and disadvantageous characteristics. The net result would be no positive or negative selection pressure upon the genotype. The authors speculated that reduced fecundity in schizophrenia was compensated by higher resistance to shock, allergies, and infection; however, these possibilities have been substantiated.[65]

Along the lines of models to suggest evolutionary advantages, various propositions include benefits due to territorial instincts, benefits in the domain of social behavior, resistance to infections in relatives of schizophrenia patients, group-splitting hypothesis of schizophrenia suggesting advantages as group leaders or schizophrenia could have enhanced a shaman's ability to conduct religious-based rituals; these theoretical conceptualizations attempt to unravel the "evolutionary enigma" of schizophrenia.[65,66]

A series of much debated and researched evolutionary proposition is the potential relation between exceptional ability and mental illness has been used to explain the persistence of schizophrenia genes. Historically as reviewed by Polimeni and Reiss,[65] this association dates back to Aristotle[67] and includes various eminent personalities such as Isaac Newton, Albert Einstein (with his son Eduard Einstein reported having suffered from schizophrenia),[68] John Nash, Bertrand Russell (with many of his relatives having diagnosed to have schizophrenia).[65] Studies based on records from Iceland's stable populations by Karlsson found superior academic success among relatives of schizophrenia patients.[69,70] These evolutional neuroscientific perspectives offer overarching paradigmatic conceptualizations that can facilitate understanding persisting risk for psychiatric disorders.

COMPUTATIONAL PSYCHIATRY: THE FUTURE

Increasingly, it is being realized that use of formal models of brain function to understand psychiatric disorders can potentially facilitate characterization of the mechanisms of psychopathology in a way that can be described in computational or mathematical terms;[71] these computational psychiatry approaches promise immense theoretical insights and translational implications.[71] With regards to schizophrenia, such approaches can offer critical insight toward understanding how the "abnormal" perceptions, thoughts, and behavior that are currently used to define the puzzling clinical manifestations relate to normal function and neural processes.[72] Thus, by formalizing mathematically the relationship between symptoms, environments, and neurobiology, computational psychiatry hopes to provide tools to identify the causes of particular symptoms in schizophrenia in terms of aberrant interactions of brain networks.[73] Indeed, initial applications of these computational psychiatry techniques have promised immense implications for understanding the biological basis of disorders like schizophrenia.[74,75]

SUMMARY AND CONCLUSION

To summarize, the impactful advances cutting-edge research techniques over the past two decades have immensely facilitated better understanding of the bidirectional "vectors of influence" that link genes, the brain and social behavior. This, in turn, has led to remarkable progress in biological research principles, paradigms, and processes has rendered critical insights on the pathogenesis of various psychiatric disorders.[76]

For instance, neuroimaging has revolutionized the research on understanding the biological underpinnings of several psychiatric disorders.[50] Coupled with the immense expansions on the computational techniques and resources to handle "big-data", the neuroimaging procedures have facilitated nonradioactive, noninvasive research to examine the in vivo brain aberrations in patients with psychiatric manifestations.[77] These techniques attempt to profile the "panorama" of brain dysfunction involving structural, neurohemodynamic, neurochemical as well connectivity aspects. One is hopeful that these significant advances in neuroimaging techniques will pave way for insights about the disruption of neural networks in neuropsychiatric disorders (pathoconnectomics).[78]

In tandem with vast advances in neuroimaging research, the progress in molecular biology involving genomics, proteomics, and several other related fields has been astonishing. Noteworthy among such advances is the feasibility of utilizing "stem cell models" to characterize the complex pathogenetic interactions that underlie the genesis of complex psychiatric disorders.[79] These exciting advances have generated immense hope and novel avenues for identifying biological basis for psychiatric disorders that will have potential diagnostic as well as therapeutic utility.[76]

ACKNOWLEDGMENTS

Dr Venkataram Shivakumar is supported by the Wellcome Trust-DBT India Alliance Early Career Fellowship grant (IA/CPHE/18/1/503956. This work is supported by the Department of Science and Technology (Government of India) Research Grant (DST/SJF/LSA-02/2014-15) to GV.

CONFLICT OF INTEREST

There are no potential conflicts of interest to report.

REFERENCES

1. Gelder MG. Biological psychiatry in perspective. Brit Med Bull. 1996;52:401-7.
2. Walter H. The third wave of biological psychiatry. Front Psychol. 2013;4:582.
3. Rapoport JL, Addington AM, Frangou S, Psych MR. The neurodevelopmental model of schizophrenia: update 2005. Mol Psychiatry. 2005;10:434-49.
4. Venkatasubramanian G. Schizophrenia is a disorder of aberrant neurodevelopment: a synthesis of evidence from clinical and structural, functional and neurochemical brain imaging studies. Indian J Psychiatry. 2007;49:244-9.
5. Nicodemus KK, Marenco S, Batten AJ, Vakkalanka R, Egan MF, Straub RE, et al. Serious obstetric complications interact with hypoxia-regulated/vascular-expression genes to influence schizophrenia risk. Mol Psychiatry. 2008;13:873-7.
6. Schlotz W, Phillips DI. Fetal origins of mental health: evidence and mechanisms. Brain Behav Immun. 2009;23:905-16.
7. Bale TL, Baram TZ, Brown AS, Goldstein JM, Insel TR, Mccarthy MM, et al. Early life programming

8. Cannon M, Jones PB, Murray RM. Obstetric complications and schizophrenia: historical and meta-analytic review. Am J Psychiatry. 2002;159:1080-92.
9. Van Os J, Kenis G, Rutten BP. The environment and schizophrenia. Nature. 2010;468:203-12.
10. Schmidt-Kastner R, Van Os J, Esquivel G, Steinbusch HW, Rutten BP. An environmental analysis of genes associated with schizophrenia: hypoxia and vascular factors as interacting elements in the neurodevelopmental model. Mol Psychiatry. 2012;17:1194-205.
11. Brown AS, Derkits EJ. Prenatal infection and schizophrenia: a review of epidemiologic and translational studies. Am J Psychiatry. 2010;167:261-80.
12. Tochigi M, Okazaki Y, Kato N, Sasaki T. What causes seasonality of birth in schizophrenia? Neurosci Res. 2004;48:1-11.
13. Brown AS. Prenatal infection as a risk factor for schizophrenia. Schizophr Bull. 2006;32:200-2.
14. Patterson PH. Neuroscience. Maternal effects on schizophrenia risk. Science. 2007;318:576-7.
15. Smith SE, Li J, Garbett K, Mirnics K, Patterson PH. Maternal immune activation alters fetal brain development through interleukin-6. J Neurosci. 2007;27:10695-702.
16. Meyer U, Schwendener S, Feldon J, Yee BK. Prenatal and postnatal maternal contributions in the infection model of schizophrenia. Exp Brain Res. 2006;173:243-57.
17. Meyer U, Feldon J, Yee BK. A review of the fetal brain cytokine imbalance hypothesis of schizophrenia. Schizophr Bull. 2009;35:959-72.
18. Potvin S, Stip E, Sepehry AA, Gendron A, Bah R, Kouassi E. Inflammatory cytokine alterations in schizophrenia: a systematic quantitative review. Biol Psychiatry. 2008;63:801-8.
19. Paul-Samojedny M, Kowalczyk M, Suchanek R, Owczarek A, Fila-Danilow A, Szczygiel A, et al. Functional polymorphism in the interleukin-6 and interleukin-10 genes in patients with paranoid schizophrenia—a case-control study. J Mol Neurosci. 2010;42(1):112-9.
20. Marsland AL, Gianaros PJ, Abramowitch SM, Manuck SB, Hariri AR. Interleukin-6 covaries inversely with hippocampal grey matter volume in middle-aged adults. Biol Psychiatry. 2008;64:484-90.
21. Behrens MM, Ali SS, Dugan LL. Interleukin-6 mediates the increase in NADPH-oxidase in the ketamine model of schizophrenia. J Neurosci. 2008;28:13957-66.
22. Debnath M, Cannon DM, Venkatasubramanian G. Variation in the major histocompatibility complex [MHC] gene family in schizophrenia: associations and functional implications. Prog Neuropsychopharmacol Biol Psychiatry. 2013;42:49-62.
23. Sekar A, Bialas AR, De Rivera H, Davis A, Hammond TR, Kamitaki N, et al. Schizophrenia risk from complex variation of complement component 4. Nature. 2016;530:177-83.
24. Chhabra H, Shivakumar V, Agarwal SM, Bose A, Venugopal D, Rajasekaran A, et al. Transcranial direct current stimulation and neuroplasticity genes: implications for psychiatric disorders. Acta Neuropsychiatr. 2016;28:1-10.
25. Kandel ER, Pittenger C. The past, the future and the biology of memory storage. Philos Trans R Soc Lond B Biol Sci. 1999;354:2027-52.
26. Kandel ER. The molecular biology of memory storage: a dialog between genes and synapses. Biosci Rep. 2004;24:475-522.
27. Balu DT, Coyle JT. Neuroplasticity signaling pathways linked to the pathophysiology of schizophrenia. Neurosci Biobehav Rev. 2011;35:848-70.
28. Voineskos D, Rogasch NC, Rajji TK, Fitzgerald PB, Daskalakis ZJ. A review of evidence linking disrupted neural plasticity to schizophrenia. Can J Psychiatry. 2013;58:86-92.
29. Nakata K, Lipska BK, Hyde TM, Ye T, Newburn EN, Morita Y, et al. DISC1 splice variants are upregulated in schizophrenia and associated with risk polymorphisms. Proc Natl Acad Sci USA. 2009;106:15873-8.
30. Bailey CH, Bartsch D, Kandel ER. Toward a molecular definition of long-term memory storage. Proc Natl Acad Sci USA. 1996;93:13445-52.
31. Guo AY, Sun J, Riley BP, Thiselton DL, Kendler KS, Zhao Z. The dystrobrevin-binding protein 1 gene: features and networks. Mol Psychiatry. 2009;14:18-29.
32. Alizadeh F, Tabatabaiefar MA, Ghadiri M, Yekaninejad MS, Jalilian N, Noori-Daloii MR. Association of P1635 and P1655 polymorphisms in dysbindin (DTNBP1) gene with schizophrenia. Acta Neuropsychiatr. 2012;24:155-9.
33. Desbonnet L, Waddington JL, O'tuathaigh CM. Mutant models for genes associated with schizophrenia. Biochem Soc Trans. 2009;37:308-12.

34. Jonsson EG, Edman-Ahlbom B, Sillen A, Gunnar A, Kulle B, Frigessi A, et al. Brain-derived neurotrophic factor gene (BDNF) variants and schizophrenia: an association study. Prog Neuropsychopharmacol Biol Psychiatry. 2006; 30:924-33.
35. Allen NC, Bagade S, Mcqueen MB, Ioannidis JP, Kavvoura FK, Khoury MJ, et al. Systematic meta-analyses and field synopsis of genetic association studies in schizophrenia: the SzGene database. Nat Genet. 2008;40:827-34.
36. Venkatasubramanian G, Rao NP, Behere RV. Neuroanatomical, neurochemical, and neurodevelopmental basis of obsessive-compulsive symptoms in schizophrenia. Indian J Psychol Med. 2009;31:3-10.
37. Busatto GF, Kerwin RW. Perspectives on the role of serotonergic mechanisms in the pharmacology of schizophrenia. J Psychopharmacol. 1997;11:3-12.
38. Agid O, Kapur S, Remington G. Emerging drugs for schizophrenia. Expert Opin Emerg Drugs. 2008;13:479-95.
39. Murphy DL, Zohar J, Benkelfat C, Pato MT, Pigott TA, Insel TR. Obsessive-compulsive disorder as a 5-HT subsystem-related behavioural disorder. Br J Psychiatry Suppl. 1989;(8):15-24.
40. Bengel D, Greenberg BD, Cora-Locatelli G, Altemus M, Heils A, Li Q, et al. Association of the serotonin transporter promoter regulatory region polymorphism and obsessive-compulsive disorder. Mol Psychiatry. 1999;4:463-6.
41. Mundo E, Richter MA, Zai G, Sam F, Mcbride J, Macciardi F, et al. 5HT1Dbeta receptor gene implicated in the pathogenesis of obsessive-compulsive disorder: further evidence from a family-based association study. Mol Psychiatry. 2002;7:805-9.
42. Sodhi M, Wood KH, Meador-Woodruff J. Role of glutamate in schizophrenia: integrating excitatory avenues of research. Expert Rev Neurother. 2008;8:1389-406.
43. Tascedda F, Blom JM, Brunello N, Zolin K, Gennarelli M, Colzi A, et al. Modulation of glutamate receptors in response to the novel antipsychotic olanzapine in rats. Biol Psychiatry. 2001;50:117-22.
44. Bhattacharyya S, Chakraborty K. Glutamatergic dysfunction—newer targets for anti-obsessional drugs. Recent Pat CNS Drug Discov. 2007;2:47-55.
45. Rosenberg DR, Macmaster FP, Keshavan MS, Fitzgerald KD, Stewart CM, Moore GJ. Decrease in caudate glutamatergic concentrations in pediatric obsessive-compulsive disorder patients taking paroxetine. J Am Acad Child Adolesc Psychiatry. 2000;39:1096-103.
46. Macmaster FP, O'neill J, Rosenberg DR. Brain imaging in pediatric obsessive-compulsive disorder. J Am Acad Child Adolesc Psychiatry. 2008;47:1262-72.
47. Dickel DE, Veenstra-Vanderweele J, Cox NJ, Wu X, Fischer DJ, Van Etten-Lee M, et al. Association testing of the positional and functional candidate gene SLC1A1/EAAC1 in early-onset obsessive-compulsive disorder. Arch Gen Psychiatry. 2006;63:778-85.
48. Chakrabarty K, Bhattacharyya S, Christopher R, Khanna S. Glutamatergic dysfunction in OCD. Neuropsychopharmacology. 2005;30:1735-40.
49. Coric V, Taskiran S, Pittenger C, Wasylink S, Mathalon DH, Valentine G, et al. Riluzole augmentation in treatment-resistant obsessive-compulsive disorder: an open-label trial. Biol Psychiatry. 2005;58:424-8.
50. Keshavan MS, Tandon R, Boutros NN, Nasrallah HA. Schizophrenia, "just the facts": what we know in 2008 Part 3: neurobiology. Schizophr Res. 2008;106:89-107.
51. Duncan GE, Sheitman BB, Lieberman JA. An integrated view of pathophysiological models of schizophrenia. Brain Res Brain Res Rev. 1999;29:250-64.
52. Marazziti D, Hollander E, Lensi P, Ravagli S, Cassano GB. Peripheral markers of serotonin and dopamine function in obsessive-compulsive disorder. Psychiatry Res. 1992;42:41-51.
53. Goodman WK, Mcdougle CJ, Price LH, Riddle MA, Pauls DL, Leckman JF. Beyond the serotonin hypothesis: a role for dopamine in some forms of obsessive-compulsive disorder? J Clin Psychiatry. 1990;51 Suppl:36-43; discussion 55-8.
54. Bloch MH, Landeros-Weisenberger A, Kelmendi B, Coric V, Bracken MB, Leckman JF. A systematic review: antipsychotic augmentation with treatment refractory obsessive-compulsive disorder. Mol Psychiatry. 2006;11:622-32.
55. Jiang Z, Cowell RM, Nakazawa K. Convergence of genetic and environmental factors on parvalbumin-positive interneurons in schizophrenia. Front Behav Neurosci. 2013;7:116.
56. Shivakumar V, Kalmady SV, Venkatasubramanian G, Ravi V, Gangadhar BN. Do schizophrenia patients age early? Asian J Psychiatr. 2014;10:3-9.
57. Prabakaran S, Swatton JE, Ryan MM, Huffaker SJ, Huang JT, Griffin JL, et al. Mitochondrial dysfunction in schizophrenia: evidence for compromised brain metabolism and oxidative stress. Mol Psychiatry. 2004;9:684-97, 643.

58. Gysin R, Kraftsik R, Sandell J, Bovet P, Chappuis C, Conus P, et al. Impaired glutathione synthesis in schizophrenia: convergent genetic and functional evidence. Proc Natl Acad Sci USA. 2007;104:16621-6.
59. Chittiprol S, Venkatasubramanian G, Neelakantachar N, Babu SV, Reddy NA, Shetty KT, et al. Oxidative stress and neopterin abnormalities in schizophrenia: a longitudinal study. J Psychiatr Res. 2010;44:310-3.
60. Murr C, Widner B, Wirleitner B, Fuchs D. Neopterin as a marker for immune system activation. Curr Drug Metab. 2002;3:175-87.
61. Gangadhar BN, Jayakumar PN, Subbakrishna DK, Janakiramaiah N, Keshavan MS. Basal ganglia high-energy phosphate metabolism in neuroleptic-naive patients with schizophrenia: a 31-phosphorus magnetic resonance spectroscopic study. Am J Psychiatry. 2004;161:1304-6.
62. Berk M, Copolov D, Dean O, Lu K, Jeavons S, Schapkaitz I, et al. N-acetyl cysteine as a glutathione precursor for schizophrenia—a double-blind, randomized, placebo-controlled trial. Biol Psychiatry. 2008;64:361-8.
63. Venkatasubramanian G. The 'boon and bane' of antipsychotic-induced metabolic syndrome. Acta Psychiatr Scand. 2009;120:500-1; author reply 501.
64. Venkatasubramanian G. The 'Holy Grail' and 'Poisoned Chalice' effects of antipsychotics on oxidative stress in schizophrenia: can 'hormesis' explain this paradox? Indian J Psychol Med. 2012;34:97-8.
65. Polimeni J, Reiss JP. Evolutionary perspectives on schizophrenia. Can J Psychiatry. 2003;48:34-9.
66. Brune M. Schizophrenia—an evolutionary enigma? Neurosci Biobehav Rev. 2004;28:41-53.
67. Waddell C. Creativity and mental illness: is there a link? Can J Psychiatry. 1998;43:166-72.
68. Jeste DV, Harless KA, Palmer BW. Chronic late-onset schizophrenia-like psychosis that remitted: revisiting Newton's psychosis? Am J Psychiatry. 2000;157:444-9.
69. Karlsson JL. Inheritance of schizophrenia. Acta Psychiatr Scand Suppl. 1974;247:1-116.
70. Karlsson JL. Mental abilities of male relatives of psychotic patients. Acta Psychiatr Scand. 2001;104:466-8.
71. Friston KJ, Stephan KE, Montague R, Dolan RJ. Computational psychiatry: the brain as a phantastic organ. Lancet Psychiatry. 2014;1:148-58.
72. Montague PR, Dolan RJ, Friston KJ, Dayan P. Computational psychiatry. Trends Cogn Sci. 2012;16:72-80.
73. Dauvermann MR, Whalley HC, Schmidt A, Lee GL, Romaniuk L, Roberts N, et al. Computational neuropsychiatry—schizophrenia as a cognitive brain network disorder. Front Psychiatry. 2014;5:30.
74. Maia TV, Frank MJ. From reinforcement learning models to psychiatric and neurological disorders. Nat Neurosci. 2011;14:154-62.
75. Huys QJ, Maia TV, Frank MJ. Computational psychiatry as a bridge from neuroscience to clinical applications. Nat Neurosci. 2016;19:404-13.
76. Venkatasubramanian G, Keshavan MS. Biomarkers in psychiatry—a critique. Ann Neurosci. 2016;23:3-5.
77. Turner JA. The rise of large-scale imaging studies in psychiatry. Gigascience. 2014;3:29.
78. Deco G, Kringelbach ML. Great expectations: using whole-brain computational connectomics for understanding neuropsychiatric disorders. Neuron. 2014;84:892-905.
79. Wright R, Rethelyi JM, Gage FH. Enhancing induced pluripotent stem cell models of schizophrenia. JAMA psychiatry. 2014;71:334-5.

CHAPTER 3

Interface with Neurology

Adarsh Tripathi, Erika Pahuja, Sujita Kumar Kar

ABSTRACT

Neuropsychiatry as a branch comprised both neurology and psychiatry till around 20th century after which brain/mind dichotomy arose and neurology and psychiatry parted their ways. Recent advances in neuroscience make it almost impossible at this time to precisely draw the line between neurological and psychiatric disorders. Because of the vast increase in knowledge in recent years, most of the psychiatric disorders have been found to have neuropathological basis. This chapter focuses on the areas of cross fertilization between the two branches. Clearly, keeping in view the inseparability of these branches, it is also imperative to liaison between the branches.

INTRODUCTION

Ramsay in 1979 rightly quoted "Neurology and psychiatry are a pair of Siamese twins who cannot be separated".[1] Till 20th century, Neurology and Psychiatry were considered a single branch of medicine, "Neuropsychiatry". Brain and mind were considered one entity.[2]

The founding father of neuropsychiatry, Wilhelm Griesinger (1817–1868), professor of neurology and psychiatry stated, "Psychische Krankheiten sind Erkrankungen des Gehirns," or "Mental illnesses are diseases of the brain".[3] In his revolutionary textbook of psychiatry, Pathologie und Therapie der Psychischen Krankheiten (1845), Griesinger emphasized on a change of attitude toward the psychiatric patient from that of sinner who should be punished and isolated, to sufferer of a biological disease who requires curing.[3] Charcot, Freud, Jackson, Bleuler, Meynert, Liepmann, Pick, Oppenheim, Korsakoff, von Monakow, Babinski, Janet, Kraepelin, Bonhoeffer, and Alzheimer thought in terms of unified study of brain and mind. They were considered Neuropsychiatrists and worked in both the specialties.[4] These neuropsychiatrists were influenced by Griesinger's work and hoped to discover organic causes of mental illnesses.[3]

During 20th century, with the development of psychodynamics, brain/mind dichotomy arose and neurology and psychiatry parted their ways.[4] Neurology laid claim to those disorders of the nervous system with cognitive and behavioral abnormalities with elicitable physical signs, established etiologies and demonstrable anatomic pathology. Psychiatry claimed those disorders of mentation, mood and thought for which there was no or minor elicitable physical signs and no visible pathology, i.e., idiopathic functional illnesses.[4] Hence psychiatry remained more dependent on symptoms whereas neurology became dependent on signs and laboratory tests/imaging. This led to the emergence of "organic versus functional" dichotomy.[4]

After World War II, the division between neurology and psychiatry became explicit with the separation of the journal "The Archives of Neurology and Psychiatry" into two journals,[5] foundation of The American Academy of Neurology in 1948 to deal with "pure" neurological issues, and establishment of separate neurology departments throughout the United States, deletion of compulsory psychiatry training for neurologists by the Residency Review Committee for Psychiatry and Neurology in 1965.[4]

But even till date there are certain disorders, gray zones, which pose a difficulty drawing a line between neurology and psychiatry. This is because however, far these specialties drift away, they have "the common roots: Brain".

NEUROPSYCHIATRY

Neuropsychiatry has been defined in a variety of ways. International Neuropsychiatric Association defines the flavor of Neuropsychiatry in the most plausible way as "a field of scientific medicine that concerns itself with the complex relationship between human behavior and brain function, and endeavors to understand abnormal behavior and behavioral disorders on the basis of an interaction of neurobiological and psychological—social factors".[6] As stated by Arzy et al. in their work The Science of Neuropsychiatry: Past, Present, and Future (2014), the suggested definitions of "Neuropsychiatry" may be divided into two main categories—minimal and maximal. The minimal approach puts neuropsychiatry in the borderland between neurology and psychiatry, and sees its subject matter as "disorders that cross the boundary between the two disciplines", as well as neurological aspects of psychiatric disorders and psychiatric aspects of neurological disorders. The maximal approach includes the full range of central nervous system (CNS) diseases (occurring "above the foramen magnum"), as well as most of the psychiatric disorders, within the scope of neuropsychiatry.[3]

Describing the disorders in maximal approach is beyond the scope of this chapter. The disorders in minimal approach are described herewith.

DISORDERS THAT CROSS THE BOUNDARY BETWEEN TWO DISCIPLINES

Delirium

Delirium in the Diagnostic and Statistical Manual of Mental Disorders, Fifth Edition (DSM-5) is defined as acute decline in both the level of awareness and cognition with particular impairment in attention.[7] Delirium often involves perceptual disturbances, abnormal psychomotor activity, and sleep cycle impairment and can be life-threatening. Term delirium is derived from a Latin word *Delirio* which means *to be crazy*. It is actually decompensation of cerebral functions. The core features include altered consciousness, global disturbance of cognition, perceptual disturbance in the background of a physical abnormality with a rapid onset and fluctuating course.[8] Delirium tremens (DT) is alcohol withdrawal delirium characterized by core features of delirium and tremors, usually has an onset 3-4 days after the last drink. A number of short-term and long-term negative consequences follow delirium. Short-term consequences include stress to the patient and family members, prolonged hospital stay, delay in postoperative mobilization and rehabilitation and increased mortality. Long-term consequences include functional and cognitive decline which may progress to dementia.[9]

Epidemiology

Data suggest an incidence rate of delirium is 3–42% in hospitalized patients and prevalence to vary from 5 to 44% among the hospitalized patients. Indian studies reveal that prevalence of delirium in intensive care units (ICUs) varies from 26.2 to 68.2% and the incidence rates vary from 9.27 to 59.6%.[9]

Clinical Features

Delirium is characterized by acute onset of symptoms, fluctuating course, and resolution between days to weeks.[10] Prolonged delirium lasting >6 months has been observed in studies by Levkoff et al.[10,11] and Mori and Yamadori.[12] Delirium is of three types: (1) hyperactive, (2) hypoactive, and (3) mixed (fluctuating between hyperactive and hypoactive). Hyperactive is a more common subtype and hypoactive is associated with prolonged hospital stay and higher mortality rates.[10,13]

Clinical features of delirium have been categorized in a number of ways. They are categorized as cognitive, noncognitive, and motoric symptoms.[9] Taylor and Lewis divided delirium symptoms into six subheadings: (1) impairment of consciousness, (2) thinking, (3) memory, (4) psychomotor disturbances, (5) perceptual, and (6) emotional disturbances.[10,14] Impaired attention, fluctuating orientation, reduced or excessive awareness to environmental stimuli, hallucinations predominantly visual, fluctuating delusions, altered sleep wake cycle, sundowning (worsening symptoms after sunset) are characteristic features of delirium.[8,10]

Risk Factors[8,10]

Risk factors for delirium are described in **Table 1**.

Pathophysiology[8]

Multiple theories have been proposed to understand pathophysiology of delirium:[8]

TABLE 1: Risk factors for delirium.

Predisposing factors	Precipitating factors
Elderly	Severe acute illness
Male sex	Poor nutritional status/anemia
Sensory deficits	*Metabolic abnormalities:* Hyponatremia, hypokalemia
Dementia	Hypoxemia
Past history of delirium	Shock
Depression	Bladder catheter use and urinary tract infections
Immobility	Infections
History of falls	Intensive care unit admissions
Underlying physical illness: DM, renal, hepatic, endocrine disease, CAD, etc.	Dehydration
Substance use: Alcohol, BZPs	Fever/hypothermia
Compromised brain	Use of physical restraints
Dehydration and malnutrition	Pain
Use of psychotropics (particularly medications with anticholinergic properties)	• Cardiac and noncardiac surgeries • Orthopedics surgery • *Neurological disorders:* Stroke, meningitis • *Use of drugs:* BZPs and alcohol withdrawal, polypharmacy, anticholinergic drugs

(BZPs: benzodiazepines; CAD: coronary artery disease; DM: diabetes mellitus)

- Disturbance in brain oxygen supply versus demand
- Generalized disruption in higher cortical function
- Neurochemical disturbances affecting cholinergic, dopaminergic, glutamatergic, and gamma-aminobutyric acid (GABA) neurotransmission
- Inflammation

Differential Diagnosis

Differential diagnosis of delirium includes dementia, depression, and psychosis **(Table 2)**. Catatonia is a differential diagnosis for hypoactive delirium.[8,9]

Assessment[9]

Screening instruments: Delirium Observation Scale, Clinical Assessment of Confusion—A and B, Confusion Assessment Method (CAM).

Diagnostic instrument: CAM-ICU (Confusion Assessment Method for ICU)[9]

Management

Following key points need to considered during management:[9]
- Evaluate for the underlying cause, predisposing, precipitating, maintaining factors, and correct the cause
- Stop unnecessary medications
- Maintain hydration and correct biochemical abnormalities
- Monitor vitals, input/output, symptoms regularly
- Maintain liaison with the primary treating team (treating the underlying cause)
- Prevent secondary complications

Pharmacological management includes use of low-dose antipsychotics (haloperidol, olanzapine, risperidone, quetiapine). The dictum "start low and go slow" needs to be followed. Cholinesterase inhibitors also show improvement in some patients. DT requires adequate benzodiazepine replacement.[9]

Nonpharmacological methods include repeated reorientation and support, unambiguous environment, ensure proper sleep, correct sensory impairments by providing vision glasses, hearing aids, encourage mobilization.[9]

Psychoeducation of the family members about the course and prognosis.

TABLE 2: Differential diagnosis of delirium.

	Delirium	Dementia
Onset	Acute	Insidious
Consciousness	Altered	Intact
Course	Fluctuating/reversible	Progressive/downhill
	Delirium	Depression
Mood	Mood lability	Persistent sadness
Diurnal variation	Sundowning/evening worsening of symptoms	Morning worsening of symptoms
	Delirium	Psychosis
Onset	Sudden	Acute to insidious
Course	Fluctuating, sundowning	Stable
Consciousness	Reduced	Clear
Attention	Impaired	May be impaired
Cognition	Globally impaired	Selectively impaired
Orientation	Fluctuating/impaired	Usually intact
Delusions	Fleeting/poorly formed	Well formed
Hallucinations	Usually visual	Usually auditory
Cause	Organic	Organicity usually absent

Dementia

Dementia is defined as a disease process marked by progressive cognitive impairment in clear consciousness. It is cognitive impairment in one or more of the domains of complex attention, executive functions, learning and memory, language, perceptual motor ability, and social cognition.[8]

According to the World Health Organization (WHO), around 50 million people have dementia worldwide and every year around 10 million new cases are diagnosed.[15]

Describing dementia and its types in detail is beyond the scope of the chapter, hence only a brief introduction is given.

Dementia has multiple etiologies and each type differs in some features from each other. Some are reversible causes such as endocrine and nutritional causes whereas others are irreversible such as neurodegenerative, vascular, and neurological causes.[8] Dementia may be subcortical or cortical. Alzheimer's disease is the most common dementia globally **(Table 3)**.[8]

Scales for Assessment[8]

- Mini-Mental State Examination (MMSE): Screening tool. MMSE score <23 points toward dementia. Most commonly used tool for screening.
- Mini Cog
- Addenbrooke's Cognitive Assessment-revised
- Montreal Cognitive Assessment (MoCA)

Neuroimaging is advised to rule out neurological causes that can cause or contribute to dementia severity.

Treatment

Both pharmacological and nonpharmacological treatment have equal importance.[8]

TABLE 3: Etiology of dementia.

Neurodegenerative	• Alzheimer's disease • Dementia with Lewy body • Frontotemporal dementia • Parkinson's disease • Huntington's disease • Corticobasal syndrome • Progressive supranuclear palsy • Prion-related: Creutzfeldt–Jakob disease, variant Creutzfeldt–Jakob disease, Gerstmann–Straussler–Scheinker disease, fatal familial insomnia
Vascular	• Infarction • Binswanger's disease • Hemodynamic insufficiency • Small vessel disease • Watershed area hypoperfusion
Neurological	• Multiple sclerosis • Normal pressure hydrocephalus • Brain tumor • Nonconvulsive status epilepticus • Acute intermittent porphyria
Endocrine	• Hypothyroidism • Hypoparathyroidism • Hyperparathyroidism • Cushing's syndrome • Adrenal insufficiency • Hypoglycemia
Nutritional	• Vitamin B_{12} deficiency • Thiamine deficiency • Niacin deficiency • Folate deficiency
Infectious	• Human immunodeficiency virus (HIV) • Neurosyphilis • *Cryptococcus* • Whipple's disease

Contd...

Contd...	
	• Progressive multifocal leukoencephalopathy
• Tuberculosis
• Sarcoidosis
Metabolic	• Hepatic insufficiency
• Renal insufficiency
• Wilson's disease
• Metachromatic leukodystrophy
• Neuroacanthosis
Brain injuries	• Subdural hematoma
• Dementia pugilistica
• Post anoxic
• Post encephalitic
Exposure	• Alcohol
• Wernicke–Korsakoff syndrome
• Marchiafava–Bignami disease
• Heavy metals
• Irradiation
• Anticholinergic medications
• Carbon monoxide
• Industrial/environmental toxins (fertilizers, pesticides)
Vasculitides	• Lupus erythematosus
• Sjögren's syndrome

Pharmacological treatment involves use of cholinesterase inhibitors, N-methyl-D-aspartic acid (NMDA) receptor antagonist.[8]

Nonpharmacological interventions include psychoeducation of patient and family members, cognitive retraining, stimulation-oriented therapies, safety awareness and management, and caregiver support.[8]

Behavioral and Psychological Symptoms of Dementia

Behavioral and psychological symptoms of dementia (BPSD) include mood changes (depression—most common), anxiety, personality changes, psychosis, sleep disturbances, agitation, impulsivity, disinhibition, wandering, and suspiciousness. These symptoms are treated accordingly.[8]

NEUROLOGICAL DISORDERS WITH PSYCHIATRIC MANIFESTATIONS

Multiple Sclerosis

Multiple sclerosis (MS) is the most common chronic disabling CNS disease in young adults.[16] It affects 1 in 1,000 people in Western countries.[16] It is an autoimmune, demyelinating disorder with symptoms of muscle weakness, vision loss, spasticity, sexual dysfunction, bladder dysfunction, and fatigue. It is characterized by immune system attacking the myelin sheath, oligodendrocytes, and nerve itself. MS is diagnosed by McDonald criteria (revised in 2017).[17]

Neuropsychiatric manifestations of MS: Neuropsychiatric symptoms (NPSs) are found in up to 60% of patients of MS. These symptoms contribute to morbidity and mortality associated with MS and have significant impact on quality of life of people with MS.[18,19] Generally, neurological symptoms precede NPS, but in around 2–3% concomitant neurological and psychiatric symptoms; and in around 0.2–2% psychiatric manifestations precede the neurological symptoms.[20,21] Most common psychiatric disorders observed with MS are described in **Table 4**.

Major Depressive Disorder

Major depressive disorder (MDD) is the most common psychiatric disorder seen in patients of MS.[22] Fatigue, poor concentration, anorexia, memory deficits, and sleep issues are shared symptoms between MS and MDD and pose a difficulty in diagnosis of comorbid MDD in MS.

The 7-item Beck Fast Screen for medically ill patients, the Hospital Anxiety and Depression

TABLE 4: Most common psychiatric disorders in multiple sclerosis.

Psychiatric disorder	Prevalence
MDD	• 15% annual prevalence[22] • 50% of MS patients experience it in lifetime[23,24]
BPAD	• 0.3–2.4%[18] • Twice as that of general population[25]
Psychosis	• 2–4% • Thrice as that of general population[26]
Anxiety disorders	• 36% • GAD—19%; panic disorder—10%; OCD—9%; social anxiety disorder—8%[27]
Alcohol—harmful use/dependence	13.6%[19,28]
Pseudobulbar affect	10%[19]

(BPAD: bipolar affective disorder; GAD: generalized anxiety disorder; MDD: major depressive disorder; MS: multiple sclerosis; OCD: obsessive-compulsive disorder)

Scale, and the Beck Depression Inventory have been used in MS patients with MDD but should be interpreted cautiously due to common symptoms between the two disorders. Beck Fast Screen for medically ill patients excludes the physical symptoms that would normally confound other screening tools.[19]

One of the important causes of mortality in patients with MS is suicide with rates as high as 3% (completed suicide).[19,29] This is approximately 7.5 times of the general population.[19]

Etiological factors implicated in development of MDD in patients of MS include dysfunctional hypothalamic pituitary adrenal axis; psychosocial factors such as lower socioeconomic status, inadequate coping, unpredictable disease course, limited social support, loss of recreational activities, severe physical disability, perceived physical incapacity, hopelessness together with uncertainty about prognosis.[19,30] Treatment with disease-modifying agents interferon beta-1a and 1b has been linked with development of depression in MS patients though no conclusive evidences are available till date.[19,31]

Neuroimaging studies show that around 40% of patients with comorbid MDD and MS have lesions in medial inferior prefrontal cortex and the anterior temporal lobe.[32] Abnormalities in white matter connectivity and regional integration in frontal lobes and limbic regions; including the hippocampus and amygdala and subcortical regions have been observed.[19] These findings are suggestive of a biological correlation between demyelination of nerve fibers and psychiatric signs and symptoms.

There is a crunch in randomized controlled trials (RCTs) evaluating treatment options for MDD in MS. Available options include use of antidepressants such as selective serotonin reuptake inhibitor (SSRI)—sertraline, paroxetine; tricyclic antidepressant (TCA) like desipramine; cognitive behavioral therapy (CBT).[19] SSRIs can potentially reduce demyelination by reducing inflammation, reducing axonal degeneration by induction of glycogenolysis.[33] Studies on animal models show that lithium abolishes experimental autoimmune encephalomyelitis (EAE) and reduces demyelination. So, lithium may be used with caution in cases of treatment-resistant MDD.[34] Electroconvulsive therapy (ECT) has also been seen effective in treatment-resistant cases.

Bipolar Affective Disorder

Incidence of mania is almost twice as compared to general population, and develops later in the course of illness.[25] Etiological factors contributing are use of steroids,[19,35] antidepressant-induced manic switch, other agents including baclofen, dantrolene, tizanidine.[19,36] Genetic contributions with reports of familial clustering of both disorders and genetic loci 6q21-22 in close approximation with HLA are being studies.[37]

Treatment options include use of mood stabilizers such as valproate, lithium (additional disease-modifying benefits; used with caution due to risk of polyuria), atypical antipsychotics such as olanzapine.[19]

Psychosis

Affective as well as nonaffective psychosis with reports showing predominance of positive symptoms have been observed in patients with MS. Etiological factors include inflammatory process, psychosocial circumstances, medicinal use of cannabis, and use of steroids.[16]

Magnetic resonance imaging (MRI) findings show demyelination in periventricular white matter, temporal, and frontotemporal regions.[26]

Treatment options include use of low doses of second-generation antipsychotics with fewer propensities for extrapyramidal symptoms (EPS). Risperidone[38] and quetiapine[39] have demonstrated disease-modifying benefits in EAE mice models.

Anxiety Disorder

There is a dearth of research in relation anxiety disorders in MS. Risk factors for anxiety disorders include newly diagnosed MS, increased MS disease activity, experiencing pain, fatigue or sleep disturbance, female gender, social isolation, a past history of suicide and MDD, and comorbid alcohol or psychoactive substance misuse.[16] Development of self-injectable disease-modifying treatments (DMTs) has led to "self-injection anxiety" in around 50% of the patients.[40]

Treatment includes use of SSRI (first line), venlafaxine, buspirone, pregabalin, gabapentin, and beta-blockers. Psychotherapy may be considered.[19]

Psychoactive substance use: High rates of use of cannabis and alcohol have been observed in MS. Cannabis use alleviates certain neurological symptoms such as spasticity, tremors, pain, insomnia, and bladder dysfunction. Certain synthetic cannabinoid compounds are licensed for treatment of spasticity and neuropathic pain in MS in some European countries.[19,41]

Pseudobulbar Affect and Euphoria

Pseudobulbar affect (PBA), also known as pathological laughing and crying, emotional incontinence, involuntary emotional expression disorder, occurs in chronic sufferers and in progressive stages; with uncontrollable crying more common than laughing.

PBA is possibly due to lesions in cerebropontocerebellar pathways.[42] Monoaminergic system involvement has also been implicated.[19]

Treatment options include use of combination of dextromethorphan and quinidine, SSRI, norepinephrine reuptake inhibitor (SNRI), mirtazapine, levodopa, and amantadine.[19,43,44]

Epilepsy

According to the International League Against Epilepsy, 2014; a person is considered to have epilepsy if they meet any of the following conditions:[45]

- At least two unprovoked (or reflex) seizures occurring >24 hours apart
- One unprovoked (or reflex) seizure and a probability of further seizures similar to the general recurrence risk (at least 60%) after two unprovoked seizures, occurring over the next 10 years
- Diagnosis of an epilepsy syndrome

Epilepsy is considered to be resolved for individuals who had an age-dependent epilepsy syndrome but are now past the applicable age or those who have remained seizure-free for the last 10 years, with no seizure medicines for the last 5 years.[45]

According to WHO, approximately 50 million people currently have epilepsy worldwide. The current prevalence of active epilepsy (i.e., continuing seizures or with the need for treatment) at a given time is between 4 and 10 per 1,000 people. However, some studies suggest a higher prevalence between 7 and 14 per 1,000 people in the low- and middle-income countries (LMICs). Around 70% of people with epilepsy respond to antiepileptics and can live apparently normal lives. Measured in disability-adjusted life years (DALYs), epilepsy forms 0.5% of the global burden of disease, with 80% of that burden corresponding to the developing countries.[46] Epilepsy is associated with a number of neuropsychiatric manifestations; which also reflect the severity of the illness. There are a number of associations between epilepsy and psychiatric disorders:
- Associated social limitations, discrimination and stigmatization
- Neurobiological involvement
- Seizures increase the vulnerability for psychiatric disorder and vice versa as both are caused by abnormality of brain.
- Psychotropics (clozapine, clomipramine, bupropion) decrease seizure threshold. Antiepileptics such as levetiracetam are associated with behavioral problems.

Prevalence of various psychiatric disorders in epilepsy are described in **Table 5**.

Psychiatric disorders are also commonly found comorbid with pediatric epilepsy. Studies have found that attention-deficit hyperactivity disorder (ADHD) and autism spectrum disorder (ASD) are frequently associated with pediatric epilepsy.[51] Other commonly associated disorders include anxiety disorders, depression, conduct disorder, and developmental delay (National Survey of Children's Health).[51,52]

TABLE 5: Prevalence of various psychiatric disorders in epilepsy.

Psychiatric disorder	Prevalence
Any mental health disorder	35.5%[47]
Mood disorder	24.4%[47]
Anxiety disorder	22.8%[47]
Suicidal ideations	25%[47]
Psychosis	7–8%[48,49]
Personality disorder	18%[50]

Psychiatric problems associated with epilepsy are divided between ictal, peri-ictal, and interictal.[48]

Ictal Features
Epileptic aura may be characterized by mood changes, anxiety, depersonalization, derealization, hallucinations (visual, auditory, gustatory, olfactory), forced thinking, and pleasurable auras.

Peri-ictal
Prodromal symptoms occurring before a seizure episode are irritability, depression, headache, and confusion. Postictal symptoms include postictal psychosis (PIP) (60% of all psychotic experiences associated with epilepsy).[47] PIPs usually occur in patients with temporal lobe epilepsy (TLE), and extratemporal structural lesions.[47,53] PIP is characterized by lucid interval of 24–72 hours,[48] florid psychomotor excitation, mystic delusions, mood swings, paranoia. It lasts for days to week,[47] shows increased slowing in electroencephalogram (EEG), usually resolve spontaneously but may require low dose of antipsychotics in some patients to reduce mortality and morbidity.

Interictal

Mood disorder: Depression is the most common psychiatric comorbidity in epilepsy.[48] Most common mood state is dysthymia or interictal dysphoric disorder of epilepsy.[48,54] Involvement of the mesiotemporal structures (hippocampus and amygdala) and the modulation of major neurotransmitter pathways (serotonin) by the epilepsy accounts for comorbid mood disorders.[47] Treatment involves use of antidepressants with low potential to reduce seizure threshold.

Psychosis: It occurs in chronic/treatment refractory TLE.[47,48] A fraction of patients have psychotic symptoms with worsening seizure frequency or antiepileptic withdrawal and other fraction exhibits Landolt's phenomenon/forced normalization/paradoxical normalization/alternating psychosis, i.e., improving seizure frequency and EEG normalization with worsening psychosis.[47,48,55,56] Patients with early onset of seizures, long interval of poorly controlled partial complex seizure with secondary generalization, left temporal focus, mediobasal temporal lesions, recently diminished seizure frequency are predisposing factors for development of interictal psychosis (IIP).[48] Treatment involves adequate control of seizures with antiepileptics. Antipsychotics may be required in some patients.

Personality disorder: Most common personality disorder associated with epilepsy is borderline personality disorder (BPD). Gastaut–Geschwind syndrome occurs in a subset of patients with TLE. It is characterized by intensified mental life, viscosity of speech, hypergraphia, hyper-religiosity, hyposexuality.[48]

Anxiety: Anxiety may occur as an ictal, peri-ictal phenomenon, associated with depression or an isolated anxiety disorder. It is more common in focal epilepsy (TLE) as compared to generalized epilepsy.[48]

Suicide: Risk of completed suicide is four to five times higher as compared to general population. Patients with TLE, BPD, and PIP are predisposed to attempt suicide.[48]

Psychotropic Drugs and Epilepsy[57]

The effects of psychotropic drugs on seizure threshold are described in **Table 6**.

Pseudoseizures

Psychogenic nonepileptic seizures (PNESs)/pseudoseizures are episodic seizure-like behavioral events that occur in the absence of abnormal electrical discharge in the brain. An underlying psychological stress phenomenon or psychological conflict is usually present. Around 30–50% of patients who have PNESs have epilepsy,[56,58] and 20–60% of patients who have epilepsy have PNESs.[56,59] Differences between true and pseudoseizures are described in **Table 7**.

TABLE 6: Effects of psychotropic drugs on seizure threshold.

Fluoxetine, fluvoxamine	Lowers seizure threshold
Clomipramine, amitriptyline, dosulepin	Epileptogenic, particularly at high doses
Bupropion	Epileptogenic, should be avoided
Lithium	Low proconvulsive effect at therapeutic dose; epileptogenic in overdose
Risperidone, olanzapine, quetiapine	Caution required. May lower seizure threshold
Clozapine	Highly epileptogenic. Avoid if possible
Chlorpromazine	Most epileptogenic in first-generation antipsychotics

TABLE 7: Differentiating features between true and pseudoseizures.[56,60]

Clinical features	True seizures	Pseudoseizures
Ictal features		
Stereotyped nature	Yes	No
Episodes during sleep	Yes	No
Duration	Brief (1–2 min)	Usually long
Onset	Abrupt	Usually gradual
Precipitant	Usually absent	Usually present
Consciousness	Lost	Preserved
Aura	Usually present	Absent
Synchronous movements	Yes	No
Jactitation	No	Yes
Pelvic thrusting	No, though occurs only in around 24% of frontal lobe epilepsy and 2–4% of TLE[61]	Yes
Prolonged body flaccidity	No	Yes
Eye closure in tonic phase	No	Yes
Jaw clenching in tonic phase	No	Yes
Tongue bites	Yes, lateral	Usually absent. Rarely tip of tongue bite may be present
Pupillary reflex	May be normal	Normal
Plantar	Extensor	Flexor
Ictal moaning and crying	Absent	Present
Emotive speech	Absent	Present
Ictal stuttering	Absent	Present
Postictal features		
Stertorous breathing	Yes	No
Postictal nose rubbing	Yes	No
Postictal headache	Yes	No
Recall of items during ictus	No	Yes
Postictal confusion	Yes	No
Investigations		
EEG ictal changes and postictal slowing	Yes	No
pH after attack	May change	Same
Prolactin after attack	Rises	Normal

Pseudoseizures are diagnosed clinically by eliciting detailed history and examination. EEG and brain scanning may be done in confusing cases.

Treatment involves establishing rapport and therapeutic alliance, treat the underlying psychiatric comorbidity, development of insight into the symptoms, psychosocial explanation of symptoms, solving the psychosocial problems, cut secondary gains.

Parkinson's Disease

An essay on the shaking palsy by James Parkinson reported 6 cases of *paralysis agitans* in 1817 and described predominant motor symptoms of Parkinson's disease (PD).[62] Today we know that PD has a variety of motor and nonmotor symptoms. Motor symptoms include tremors, rigidity, bradykinesia and nonmotor symptoms include the cognitive and behavioral abnormalities.[63]

TABLE 8: Various psychiatric disorders associated with Parkinson's disease (PD).

Psychiatric disorder	Prevalence
Depression	20–40%[64,65]
Anxiety	40%[65,66]
Psychosis	• 10% of untreated PD • 15–40% of treated PD[65,67]
Dementia	• 30% • 80% with course >10 years[65,68]
Impulse control disorders	15%[65]
Sleep disorders	40–90%[65]
Apathy	40%[69]

Various psychiatric disorders associated with PD are enlisted in **Table 8**.

Depression

Depression and PD follow a vicious cycle increasing the risk of each other. PD is 3.24 times more likely to occur in patients with depression.[63,70] Patients on antiparkinsonian medications have higher rates of depression as compared to drug naïve patients (75.5% vs. 59.2%).[63,71] Features of depression in PD differ from idiopathic depression. Patients with PD have higher rates of anxiety, dysphoria, irritability, pessimism, suicidal ideation without suicidal behavior, and less rates of self-guilt and reproach.[65,72] Depressive symptoms usually fluctuate with motor symptoms and may be present only in the off phase. Risk factors include female gender, right-sided motor symptoms, akinetic rigid subtype, severe cognitive decline, advanced disease, longer duration of illness, associated anxiety or psychotic symptoms, younger age, motor disability, higher daily doses of levodopa.[63,65]

Dysfunction of the striatothalamic frontal and basotemporal limbic circuits, disruption in serotonergic and dopaminergic pathways have been implicated in development of depression in PD.[65]

Treatment involves assessing the relationship between depression and the antiparkinsonian drugs being given and adjust their dose accordingly.[63]

- *Mild depression:* Supportive therapy, CBT
- *Moderate depression:*
  - Antidepressants or CBT
  - Tricyclics have more evidences as compared to other antidepressants.
  - TCAs with least sedative and anticholinergic effects such as desipramine and nortriptyline are recommended.
- *Severe depression:*
  - ECT may be considered along with antidepressants.
  - Deep brain stimulation (DBS) and repetitive transcranial magnetic stimulation (rTMS) have also been found effective.[63]

Anxiety

The most common anxiety disorders associated with PD are panic disorder, generalized anxiety disorder (GAD), and social phobia.[73] Risk factors include female gender, younger age, young age at onset, severity of illness, comorbid depressive symptoms, sleep disturbances, motor fluctuations, dystonia, and dyskinesias.[63] Noradrenergic dysfunction has a role in pathophysiology of anxiety in PD.[74] These symptoms may occur as a part of off periods where adjustment of antiparkinsonian drugs is required. SSRIs are considered first-line treatment. Benzodiazepines may be used with caution for acute control of symptoms. TCAs, DBS, rTMS, and CBT also have some evidences.[63]

Psychosis

The most common presentation of psychosis in PD is visual hallucinations; benign hallucinosis in the initial state and complex, formed, moving hallucinations in later stage with severe cognitive decline.[65] The most common delusion experiences are of infidelity and phantom boarders. Risk factors for psychosis are old age, severe illness, severe cognitive decline, long duration of illness, exposure to antiparkinsonian drugs and polypharmacy, visual impairment, comorbid depression, anxiety, and sleep disturbances.[63,67]

Treatment includes ruling out delirium. Reduce the dose to lowest effective dose or discontinue antiparkinsonian drugs in the order of least efficacy: anticholinergics, selegiline, amantadine, dopamine receptor agonists, catechol-O-methyltransferase inhibitors, and lastly levodopa. If this does not resolve psychotic symptoms, antipsychotics may be used in low dose.[65] 5-HT2A inverse agonist pimavanserin is the first US Food and Drug Administration (FDA)-approved drug (May 2016) for treatment of psychosis in PD.[75] Clozapine[76] and quetiapine[77] are also considered safe in PD.

Dementia

Onset of dementia at least after 12 months of onset of PD favors PD dementia and helps to distinguish it from Lewy body dementia. This is known as "12-month rule".[65] PD-mild cognitive impairment (PD-MCI) and dementia are commonly seen in patients with PD.[63] The mean time estimated from onset of PD to dementia is around 10 years.[78] Risk factors include old age, severity of motor symptoms, postural and gait disturbances, PD-MCI, visual hallucinations, and nontremor predominant type.[63,65]

Dementia in PD is subcortical dementia with impaired attention, executive and visuospatial dysfunction and relative sparing of memory and language functions. Neuropathological changes show both *alpha-synuclein* (Lewy bodies) and Alzheimer's disease like changes (senile plaques and neurofibrillary tangles).[79]

Treatment includes ruling out other reversible causes of dementia. FDA has approved rivastigmine for mild-to-moderate Parkinson's disease dementia (PDD). Memantine can also be used.[65]

Impulse Control Disorders

Impulse control disorders (ICDs) arise due to excessive dopamine receptor stimulation.[63] ICDs include pathological gambling, compulsive sexual behavior, compulsive buying, binge eating, punding, hoarding and aimless wandering.[80,81] These disorders may occur at both low and high doses of dopamine agonists whereas occur at very high doses of levodopa (>1,000 mg/day) and are more common in individuals receiving dopamine agonists as compared to levodopa.[82] Treatment involves lowering or stopping the culprit drug.

Dopamine Dysregulation Syndrome

Some authors consider it a part of ICD. It is characterized by addiction to dopaminergic drugs particularly levodopa with behavioral symptoms and dysfunction in social functioning.[63]

Sleep Disorders

Sleep disorders impair quality of life of people with PD. The various sleep disorders in PD [according to the International Classification of Sleep Disorders, 2nd Edition (ICSD-2)][65] are elucidated in **Table 9**.

Most common sleep problem reported by PD patients is "sleep fragmentation" which commonly occurs in stage 1 and 2 of sleep.[83]

Management of sleep disturbances includes correct diagnosis by obtaining history from both patient and bed partner. Sleep fragmentation may be corrected by

TABLE 9: Various sleep disorders in Parkinson's disease.

Category	Specific disorders
Insomnias	Insomnia due to medical conditions
Sleep-related breathing disorders	Obstructive sleep apnea
Hypersomnia	• Hypersomnia due to medical condition • Hypersomnia due to drugs
Parasomnias	• Rapid eye movement (REM) sleep behavior disorder • Nightmare • Night terrors • Nocturnal vocalizations
Sleep-related movement disorders	• Restless legs syndrome • Periodic limb movement sleep disorder

optimizing antiparkinsonian drugs,[83] periodic leg movements respond to dopaminergic drugs.[84] Clonazepam is the drug of choice for rapid eye movement (REM) sleep behavior disorder.[85] Modafinil may be given for excessive daytime somnolence and sleep attacks.[86]

Apathy

Apathy in PD is classified as emotional affective apathy, cognitive apathy, and autoactivation apathy. There are some evidences of improvement of apathy with rivastigmine, methylphenidate and some antidepressants.[65]

Cerebrovascular Disorders

According to WHO, every year around 15 million people are diagnosed with stroke.[87] Incidence of stroke increases as age advances. Stoke is the second leading cause of death globally.[88] Stroke is of two types: (1) ischemic and (2) hemorrhagic. Stokes may have variety of neuropsychiatric implications. These implications affect the quality of life of patients as well as the caregivers. They increase the burden of care and negative care giving experiences and are an important reason of hospitalization of these patients.[89]

Depression

Poststroke depression (PSD) is of three types: (1) major depressive like episode, (2) depressive symptoms not fulfilling the criteria for MDD, and (3) mixed depressive and manic symptoms.[7,90] In a review by Hackett et al. published in 2014, the prevalence of PSD anytime between 1 and 5 years after stroke was estimated around 31%.[91] A similar prevalence rate of 29% was estimated in a review by Ayerbe et al. in 2013.[92] Suicide is an important cause of mortality in PSD. Predictors of PSD are past history of depression, anxiety and cognitive symptoms, severity of neurological deficit and physical disability, subcortical lesions interfering with the monoaminergic pathways, patient's personality and coping strategies, lifestyle, and social support.[92,93] In a meta-analysis by Narushima et al. (2003), patients with left frontal or left basal ganglia lesion were twice more likely to suffer from depression as compared to lesions on right side. Though conclusive evidences for these finding are not yet present.[94]

Management: Psychotherapy has some role in preventing PSD. No robust evidences are till date available for treatment of PSD by psychotherapy.

Pharmacotherapy is the treatment of choice for PSD. SSRIs have been found effective. Choice of SSRI differs from patient to patient considering the adverse effects, comorbidity, drug reactions, and past responses.

Neurostimulation is not generally used in PSD as these patients are prone for seizures.

Mania

Mania is a rare complication of stroke occurring in about 1–2% of poststroke patients. It is more common in patients with lesions of right cerebral hemispherical structures with connections to the limbic system.[95] Recurrence of manic episodes may occur. Treatment involves use of appropriate mood stabilizers such as lithium, valproate, carbamazepine. Choice of mood stabilizers varies from patient to patient.[89]

Anxiety Disorders

Generalized anxiety disorder (GAD) is the most common anxiety disorder observed in stroke survivors.[96] According to meta-analysis and systematic review conducted by Campbell et al. (2013), the prevalence of anxiety is between 20 and 24% within first 6 months after stroke.[97] Its prevalence remains elevated even years after stroke. Predictors for anxiety disorder are past history of depression, anxiety, alcohol abuse; young age, female sex, physical disability, lack of social support.[8,89] Treatment involves psychotherapy and pharmacotherapy with SSRIs. Benzodiazepines may be used cautiously for small periods of time for acute control of symptoms.

Psychosis

Poststroke psychosis is a rare and very less studied phenomenon. Available data suggests right hemispheric lesion, seizures, and subcortical atrophy as important factors in poststroke psychosis. Management involves use of anticonvulsants as poststroke psychosis is usually associated with seizures. If symptoms persist, low-dose atypical antipsychotics may be used with "start low, go slow" method.[8]

Pseudobulbar Affect

Frontopontocerebellar pathway has been implicated in development of PBA. Pathological Laughter and Crying Scale (PLACS) has been specifically designed to assess poststroke pathological emotions. Treatment involves use of FDA-approved combination of dextromethorphan and quinidine. Antidepressants such as SSRI, SNRI, and TCAs have also shown response in PBA.[8]

Personality Change

According to DSM-5, personality changes due to medical condition are of following types: labile, disinhibited, aggressive, apathetic, paranoid, other, combined type.[7] Predominant personality changes observed after a stroke are disinhibition and irritability. Irritability is characterized by impatience, flashes of anger, rapid mood changes, or quarrelling. Disinhibition is characterized by impulsivity, tactlessness or sexual disinhibition.[98] Assessment can be done using the "Neuropsychiatric Inventory".[89] No consistent results regarding association of a brain lesion with personality changes have been obtained.

Apathy

Apathy is defined by lack of motivation plus two of the three symptoms: (1) lack of emotions, (2) slowed motor activity, and (3) impaired cognitive activity present most of the time for at least a period of 4 weeks.[8] Apathy scale is used to rate severity of apathy. Dopaminergic drugs such as bromocriptine, amantadine; and adrenergic drugs such as methylphenidate, nortriptyline, reboxetine have been used with benefits. Nefiracetam also shows promising results in apathy.[8,89]

Traumatic Brain Injury

The Centers for Disease Control and Prevention (CDC) defines a traumatic brain injury (TBI) as a disruption in the normal function of the brain that can be caused by a bump, blow, or jolt to the head, or penetrating head injury.[99] Each year around 69 million (95% CI 64–74 million) individuals suffer TBI from all causes. Southeast Asian and Western Pacific regions experiencing the greatest overall burden of disease. The prevalence of TBI is nearly three times in LMICs as compared to high-income countries (HICs). The peak incidence is observed in age group 15-24 and >64 years. Males are affected twice as compared to females. According to CDC, falls are the most frequent cause of TBI.[99,100]

Traumatic brain injury affects not only the affected person but has an impact on the entire family. Psychiatric complications are an important cause of long-term morbidity associated with TBI. TBI may lead to psychiatric complications due to cerebral edema, diffuse axonal injury, cerebral hypoxia/anoxia, neuronal death, changes in biogenic amine pathways.[100,101] Psychiatric complications in patients of TBI are more common in patients with past history of psychiatric illness, poor social support, premorbid personality, marital discords, problems at work, financial instability.[101,102] Psychiatric complications associated with TBI are explained below.

Depression

Sadness is the most prevalent reaction after TBI.[101] Kreutzer et al. found that the most frequent symptoms of depression were fatigue (46%), frustration (41%), and poor concentration (38%).[103] Increased risk of suicide has been reported in many studies and should be evaluated. Alcoholism and interpersonal difficulties contribute to the increased risk of suicide and an association with lesions in frontal and temporal lobes has been reported.[104] Depression occurs more frequently with left dorsolateral frontal and left basal ganglia lesions.[105] Depression is responsive to treatment by antidepressants.

Mania

Mania after TBI is less common as compared to depression.[101] Irritable mania is more common than euphoric mania after TBI.[106,107] Basal region of right temporal lobe[108] and right orbitofrontal cortex (OFC) damage[109] along with genetic loading of bipolar disorder causes mania in patients with TBI. Management includes use of mood stabilizers preferably sodium valproate as it acts as an antiepileptic as well as a mood stabilizer.[100]

Cognitive Sequelae

Attention and memory followed by executive functions are the most common domains affected after TBI.[101] Post-traumatic amnesia >24 hours increases chances of post-TBI cognitive impairment.[100]

Psychosis

Damage to temporal and less commonly frontal lobes lead to psychotic symptoms after TBI.[110-112] Paranoid delusions are the most common cause followed by auditory hallucinations.[112,113] Latency time for onset of psychotic symptoms may vary from few days to 20 years with a mean of 4-5 years.[104]

Anxiety Disorders

Anxiety disorders include GAD, post-traumatic stress disorder (PTSD), panic disorder, phobias, and obsessive-compulsive disorder (OCD). They are more commonly associated with right hemispheric lesion.[104] Mayou et al. in 1993 found that PTSD is associated with horrific memories of the accident.[114] Imaging studies have shown small hippocampal volumes in patients with PTSD.[101] Treatment involves psychotherapy and use of serotonergic drugs. Benzodiazepines may be used for acute symptom control.

Others

Other psychiatric complications with TBI include aggression, apathy, personality changes, hypersexuality, sleep disturbances, dissociative disorders, emotional instability,

TABLE 10: Other disorders in traumatic brain injury.

Klüver–Bucy syndrome	• Damage to anterior temporal lobes • Characterized by inappropriate sexual behaviors, mouthing of objects, loss of normal fear and anger responses, memory loss, distractibility and seizures[115,116]
Kleine–Levin syndrome	• Hypothalamus pathology • Characterized by intermittent hypersomnolence, behavioral and cognitive disturbances, hyperphagia, and in some cases hypersexuality in teenage boys[117,118]
Autoimmune encephalitis	Characterized by acute confusional mania, catatonia, perceptual disturbances
Wernicke's encephalopathy	• Characterized by global confusion, ataxia, ophthalmoplegia • Seen in chronic alcoholics with thiamine deficiency • MRI changes are altered signal intensity in medial thalami, mammillary bodies, tegmentum, periaqueductal region, and tectal plate[119]

TABLE 11: Neurological soft signs.[120,124]

Category	Localization	Sign
Sensory integration	Parietal lobe	• Audiovisual integration • Bilateral extinction • Stereognosis • Graphesthesia • Right/left confusion
Motor coordination	Frontal lobe and cerebellum	• Tandem walk • Dysdiado-chokinesia • Finger-thumb opposition • Finger-nose test • Intentional tremors • Hopping • Gait
Motor sequencing	Prefrontal cortex	• Fist-edge-palm test • Fist-ring test • Ozeretski test • Go-no-go test • Rhythm tapping
Primitive reflexes	Frontal lobe	• Glabellar tap • Jaw jerk • Palmomental reflex • Pout/snout reflex • Sucking reflex • Grasp reflex
Others		• Romberg test • Adventitious overflow • Tremor • Mirror movements • Convergence

fatigue, post-TBI headache, postconcussion syndrome (constellation of cognitive, emotional/behavioral and physical symptoms).[100,101,104]

Other disorders in TBI are depicted in **Table 10**.

NEUROLOGICAL ASPECTS OF PSYCHIATRIC DISORDERS

Neurological Soft Signs (Table 11)

Neurological signs are of two types: (1) hard and (2) soft. Hard neurological signs are focal localizing signs and are impairments in basic motor, sensory, and reflex behaviors. Soft signs are nonlocalizing neurological abnormalities that cannot be related to impairment of a specific brain region or are not believed to be part of a well-defined neurological syndrome.[120] A *neurological soft sign* (NSS) is a non-normative performance on a *motor or sensory test* in the neurological examination.[121] The word "soft" indicates that there is no association between the observed abnormalities and fixed or transient neurological lesion or disorder and they lack specificity, validity, and localizing value.[122,123] Scales for assessment of NSS include:[123]

- Neurological Evaluation Scale—most commonly used
- The Cambridge Neurological Inventory
- The Heidelberg Scale
- The Brief Motor Scale.

Schizophrenia

Schizophrenia is considered a neurodevelopmental disorder with dysfunction in corticothalamo-cerebellar cortical circuit causing a "cognitive dysmetria".[123] More and more research is pointing toward an organic cause of schizophrenia. NSS in patients of schizophrenia is evidence pointing toward primary neurological dysfunction.

Prevalence studies of NSS have reported a prevalence rate of 50–73% in patients of schizophrenia. Early studies showed low prevalence (50–65%) and chronicity of illness and prior use of neuroleptics were confounding variables. Later studies reported prevalence rates up to 73%.[123] NSSs are found in patients > nonpsychotic relatives of schizophrenia > healthy controls; pointing toward genetic component in NSS.[123,125] According to systematic review conducted by Dazzan et al. in 2002, patients with first-episode psychosis have more positive NSSs particularly in the areas of motor coordination and sequencing, sensory integration and in developmental reflexes.

NSS have been associated with psychopathology.[126] According to a meta-analysis conducted by Bachmann et al. in 2014, NSS scores decrease with remission of psychopathological symptoms in schizophrenia. NSS has been strongly correlated with neurophysiologic deficits and negative symptoms of schizophrenia.[127]

NSS have been considered as the candidate neurological and cognitive endophenotypes for schizophrenia. NSS have been associated with the genetic risk for schizophrenia and afford greater predictive validity when used as a composite endophenotype in genetic association studies.[123]

Bipolar Disorder

There is an extensive research on NSS and schizophrenia. Data on association of NSS and bipolar disorder is limited but sufficient to demonstrate an association between the two.

According to a study by Negash et al. in 2004, neurological dysfunction, particularly in the area of sequencing of complex motor acts, is more common in bipolar I disorder patients as compared to healthy controls. As per the study, the presence of stable neurological abnormalities in the form of NSS in bipolar I disorder which can be identified from the onset of the illness represents the fact that it is a stable disease process that has been existing long before the onset of the symptoms.[128]

Meta-analysis by Bora et al. in 2018 demonstrated that increased NSS is a common feature of both schizophrenia and bipolar disorder. Increase in NSS in bipolar affective disorder (BPAD) is only moderately less severe than schizophrenia.[129]

In a study by Sagheer et al. in 2017, patients with bipolar disorder showed significantly more total NSS signs, motor coordination signs, and sensory-integration signs as compared to healthy controls. Patients with bipolar disorder showed significantly more sensory integration signs and a trend of difference in the sequencing of complex motor acts and other subscales as compared to patients with unipolar disorder.[124]

Obsessive-Compulsive Disorder

Evidences suggest that OCD is also a neurodevelopmental disorder such as schizophrenia. Which led to the hypothesis of possibility of NSS in OCD. Evidences of NSS in OCD are inconsistent. Study by Jaafari et al. in 2011 did not find any association between NSS and OCD.[130] Whereas association has been established in other studies. Meta-analysis of 15 studies by Jaafari et al. in 2013 reported that patients of OCD scored significantly higher on NSS scales (motor coordination, sensory integration, and primitive reflexes) as compared to controls.[131] A study by Malhotra et al. in 2016 reported higher NSS in OCD patients and their first-degree relatives as compared to healthy controls.[132]

Attention-Deficit Hyperactivity Disorder

Multiple studies have demonstrated an association between NSS and ADHD. Strong association between inattention and movement difficulties was established in a study by Pitcher et al. in 2003.[133] Persistence of overflow movements has been observed in children of ADHD134 pointing toward developmental origin of brain abnormalities in ADHD.[135]

Autism Spectrum Disorder

Motor deficits are among the earliest and most prominent symptoms in children with ASD.[136] There is dearth in this area though few studies point toward an association between ASD and NSS and favor the neurodevelopment origin of autism. Significant differences were found between ASD children and healthy controls in motor and sensory integration functions in a study by Halayem et al. in 2010.[137]

NEUROBIOLOGY OF PSYCHIATRIC DISORDERS

Over last 30 years, there has been enormous development in neurobiology of psychiatric disorders. With the advent of neuroimaging, genetics, molecular, and cellular biology, neurobiology has become one of the extensively researched areas over last three decades. This understanding is now pointing toward organic/neurological/impaired brain functions as cause of various psychiatric disorders which were once considered functional. Brain/mind dichotomy has now become a questionable idea. There are evidences that all mental illnesses have underlying dysfunctional neuronal circuits or abnormalities in neurotransmission. Dopaminergic and glutamatergic theory of schizophrenia, serotonergic dysfunction in mood disorders, cortico-striato-thalamo-cortical (CSTC) circuit involvement in OCD and ICDs, reward pathway (mesolimbic) involvement in addiction disorders, adrenergic dysfunction in ADHD; all point toward underlying organic causes of mental illnesses.

CONCLUSION

The advances in neurobiology of psychiatric disorders and the areas of cross-fertilization between neurology and psychiatry discussed above point toward the importance of collaboration of the two specialties. These advances have proved the well said statement that neurology and psychiatry are Siamese twins and favor what great neuropsychiatrists, such as Griesinger, Freud, Charcot, Jackson, Oppenheim, etc., believed. There is a huge burden of psychiatric and neurological illnesses globally. This burden and the treatment of cost may be reduced by interdisciplinary collaboration. There are certain countries where psychiatric training is mandatory for a neurologist and vice versa. Current status in India mandates neurology training for a psychiatrist. It is the need of the hour to encourage psychiatric training for a neurologist and potentiate the neurology training of a psychiatrist; so that both the facilities can work hand in hand, supplement each other in areas of cross-fertilization and lead to a successful future alliance of both the branches. As said by Alice Weaver Flaherty, "Neurology and psychiatry should be treating the same organ".

REFERENCES

1. Ramsay RA. Neurology and psychiatry: interface and integration. Psychosomatics. 1979;20(4):269-77.
2. Baird G, Santosh P. Interface between neurology and psychiatry in childhood. J Neurol Neurosurg Psychiatry. 2003;74(Suppl 1):i17-22.
3. Arzy S, Danziger S. The science of neuropsychiatry: past, present, and future. J Neuropsychiatry Clin Neurosci. 2014;26(4):392-5.
4. Price BH, Adams RD, Coyle JT. Neurology and psychiatry: closing the great divide. Neurology. 2000;54(1):8-14.
5. Boller F, Dalla Barba G. The evolution of psychiatry and neurology. In: Jeste DV, Friedman JH (Eds). Psychiatry for Neurologists. New York: Springer; 2006. pp. 11-5.
6. Sachdev PS, Mohan A. Neuropsychiatry: where are we and where do we go from here? Mens Sana Monogr. 2013;11(1):4-15.
7. American Psychiatric Association. Diagnostic and Statistical Manual of Mental Disorders, Fifth Edition. Washington, DC: American Psychiatric Association Publishing; 2013.
8. Sadock BJ, Sadock VA, Ruiz P. Kaplan and Sadock's Comprehensive Textbook of Psychiatry. Philadelphia: Wolters Kluwer Health; 2017.
9. Grover S, Avasthi A. Clinical practice guidelines for management of delirium in elderly. Indian J Psychiatry. 2018;60(7):329-40.
10. Burns A, Gallagley A, Byrne J. Delirium. J Neurol Neurosurg Psychiatry. 2004;75(3):362-7.
11. Levkoff SE, Evans DA, Liptzin B, Cleary PD, Lipsitz LA, Wetle TT, et al. Delirium: the occurrence and persistence of symptoms among elderly hospitalized patients. Arch Intern Med. 1992;152(2):334-40.
12. Mori E, Yamadori A. Acute confusional state and acute agitated delirium. Occurrence after infarction in the right middle cerebral artery territory. Arch Neurol. 1987;44:1139-43.
13. Lipowski Z. Delirium (acute confusional states). JAMA. 1987;258(13):1789-92.
14. Taylor D, Lewis S. Delirium. J Neurol Neurosurg Psychiatry. 1993;56(7):742-51.
15. World Health Organization (2017). Dementia. [online] Available from: https://www.who.int/news-room/fact-sheets/detail/dementia [Last accessed June, 2021].
16. Chwastiak LA, Ehde DM. Psychiatric issues in multiple sclerosis. Psychiatr Clin North Am. 2007;30(4):803-17.
17. Thompson AJ, Banwell BL, Barkhof F, Carroll WM, Coetzee T, Comi G, et al. Diagnosis of multiple sclerosis: 2017 revisions of the McDonald criteria. Lancet Neurol. 2018;17(2):162-73.
18. Marrie R, Horwitz R, Cutter G, Tyry T, Campagnolo D, Vollmer T. The burden of mental comorbidity in multiple sclerosis: frequent, underdiagnosed, and undertreated. Mult Scler. 2009;15(3):385-92.
19. Murphy R, O'Donoghue S, Counihan T, McDonald C, Calabresi PA, Ahmed MA, et al. Neuropsychiatric syndromes of multiple sclerosis. J Neurol Neurosurg Psychiatry. 2017;88(8):697-708.
20. Asghar-Ali AA, Taber KH, Hurley RA, Hayman LA. Pure neuropsychiatric presentation of multiple sclerosis. Am J Psychiatry. 2004;161(2):226-31.
21. Lo Fermo S, Barone R, Patti F, Laisa P, Cavallaro TL, Nicoletti A, et al. Outcome of psychiatric symptoms presenting at onset of multiple sclerosis: a retrospective study. Mult Scler. 2010;16(6):742-8.
22. Patten SB, Beck CA, Williams JV, Barbui C, Metz L. Major depression in multiple sclerosis: a population-based perspective. Neurology. 2003;61(11):1524-7.
23. Feinstein A. The neuropsychiatry of multiple sclerosis. Can J Psychiatry. 2004;49(3):157-63.
24. Minden SL, Schiffer RB. Affective disorders in multiple sclerosis review and recommendations for clinical research. Arch Neurol. 1990;47(1):98-104.
25. Schiffer RB, Wineman NM, Weitkamp LR. Association between bipolar affective disorder and multiple sclerosis. Am J Psychiatry. 1986;143(1):94-5.
26. Patten SB, Svenson LW, Metz LM. Psychotic disorders in MS: population-based evidence of an association. Neurology. 2005;65(7):1123-5.

27. Korostil M, Feinstein A. Anxiety disorders and their clinical correlates in multiple sclerosis patients. Mult Scler. 2007;13(1):67-72.
28. Quesnel S, Feinstein A. Multiple sclerosis and alcohol: a study of problem drinking. Mult Scler. 2004;10(2):197-201.
29. Sadovnick A, Remick R, Allen J, Swartz E, Yee I, Eisen K, et al. Depression and multiple sclerosis. Neurology. 1996;46(3):628-32.
30. Ghaffar O, Feinstein A. The neuropsychiatry of multiple sclerosis: a review of recent developments. Curr Opin Psychiatry. 2007;20(3):278-85.
31. Neilley LK, Goodin DS, Goodkin DE, Hauser SL. Side effect profile of interferon beta-lb in MS: results of an open label trial. Neurology. 1996;46(2):552-3.
32. Feinstein A, Roy P, Lobaugh N, Feinstein K, O'connor P, Black S. Structural brain abnormalities in multiple sclerosis patients with major depression. Neurology. 2004;62(4):586-90.
33. Sijens PE, Mostert JP, Irwan R, Potze JH, Oudkerk M, De Keyser J. Impact of fluoxetine on the human brain in multiple sclerosis as quantified by proton magnetic resonance spectroscopy and diffusion tensor imaging. Psychiatry Res. 2008;164(3):274-82.
34. Chiu CT, Chuang DM. Molecular actions and therapeutic potential of lithium in preclinical and clinical studies of CNS disorders. Pharmacol Ther. 2010;128(2):281-304.
35. Bhangle SD, Kramer N, Rosenstein ED. Corticosteroid-induced neuropsychiatric disorders: review and contrast with neuropsychiatric lupus. Rheumatol Int. 2013;33(8):1923-32.
36. Baldessarini RJ, Faedda GL, Offidani E, Vazquez GH, Marangoni C, Serra G, et al. Antidepressant-associated mood-switching and transition from unipolar major depression to bipolar disorder: a review. J Affect Disord. 2013;148(1):129-35.
37. Nurnberger J Jr, Foroud T, Eckstein G, Ekelund J, Faraone S, Goldman D, et al. Chromosome 6 workshop report. Am J Med Genet. 1999;88(3):233-8.
38. O'Sullivan D, Green L, Stone S, Zareie P, Kharkrang M, Fong D, et al. Treatment with the antipsychotic agent, risperidone, reduces disease severity in experimental autoimmune encephalomyelitis. PLoS One. 2014;9(8):e104430.
39. Zhornitsky S, Wee Yong V, Koch MW, Mackie A, Potvin S, Patten SB, et al. Quetiapine fumarate for the treatment of multiple sclerosis: focus on myelin repair. CNS Neurosci Ther. 2013;19(10):737-44.
40. Mohr DC, Cox D, Merluzzi N. Self-injection anxiety training: a treatment for patients unable to self-inject injectable medications. Mult Scler. 2005;11(2):182-5.
41. Chong M, Wolff K, Wise K, Tanton C, Winstock A, Silber E. Cannabis use in patients with multiple sclerosis. Mult Scler. 2006;12(5):646-51.
42. Parvizi J, Anderson SW, Martin CO, Damasio H, Damasio AR. Pathological laughter and crying: a link to the cerebellum. Brain. 2001;124(9):1708-19.
43. Pioro EP. Review of dextromethorphan 20 mg/quinidine 10 mg (NUEDEXTA®) for pseudobulbar affect. Neurol Ther. 2014;3(1):15-28.
44. Stahl SM. Dextromethorphan-quinidine-responsive pseudobulbar affect (PBA): psychopharmacological model for wide-ranging disorders of emotional expression? CNS Spectr. 2016;21(6):419-23.
45. Fisher RS, Acevedo C, Arzimanoglou A, Bogacz A, Cross JH, Elger CE, et al. ILAE official report: a practical clinical definition of epilepsy. Epilepsia. 2014;55(4):475-82.
46. World Health Organization (2019). Epilepsy. [online] Available from https://www.who.int/news-room/fact-sheets/detail/epilepsy [Last accessed June, 2021].
47. Mula M. Neuropsychiatric Symptoms of Epilepsy. Switzerland: Springer; 2016.
48. Mohapatra S, Rath N. Psychiatric aspects of epilepsy: a review. Eastern J Psychiatry. 2016;17(2).
49. Torta R, Keller R. Behavioral, psychotic, and anxiety disorders in epilepsy: etiology, clinical features, and therapeutic implications. Epilepsia. 1999;40:s2-20.
50. Swinkels W, Duijsens I, Spinhoven P. Personality disorder traits in patients with epilepsy. Seizure. 2003;12(8):587-94.
51. Kar SK. Psychiatric aspects of pediatric epilepsy: focus on anxiety disorder. Med J DY Patil Univ. 2015;8(4):425-30.
52. Russ SA, Larson K, Halfon N. A national profile of childhood epilepsy and seizure disorder. Pediatrics. 2012;129(2):256-64.
53. Kanemoto K, Kawasaki J, Kawai I. Postictal psychosis: a comparison with acute interictal and chronic psychoses. Epilepsia. 1996;37(6):551-6.
54. Blumer D. Antidepressant and double antidepressant treatment for the affective disorder of epilepsy. J Clin Psychiatry. 1997;58(1):3-11.
55. Krishnamoorthy E, Trimble M. Forced normalization: clinical and therapeutic relevance. Epilepsia. 1999;40:s57-64.
56. Marcangelo MJ, Ovsiew F. Psychiatric aspects of epilepsy. Psychiatr Clin North Am. 2007;30(4):781-802.

57. Taylor DM, Paton C, Kapur S. The Maudsley Prescribing Guidelines in Psychiatry, 12th Edition. Oxford: Wiley-Blackwell; 2015.
58. Reuber M, Fernandez G, Helmstaedter C, Qurishi A, Elger C. Evidence of brain abnormality in patients with psychogenic nonepileptic seizures. Epilepsy Behav. 2002;3(3):249-54.
59. D'Alessio L, Giagante B, Oddo S, Silva W, Solís P, Consalvo D, et al. Psychiatric disorders in patients with psychogenic non-epileptic seizures, with and without comorbid epilepsy. Seizure. 2006;15(5):333-9.
60. Devinsky O, Gazzola D, LaFrance WC Jr. Differentiating between nonepileptic and epileptic seizures. Nat Rev Neurol. 2011;7(4):210-20.
61. Geyer JD, Payne TA, Drury I. The value of pelvic thrusting in the diagnosis of seizures and pseudoseizures. Neurology. 2000;54(1):227-9.
62. Parkinson J. An essay on the shaking palsy. J Neuropsychiatry Clin Neurosci. 2002;14(2):223-36.
63. Grover S, Somaiya M, Kumar S, Avasthi A. Psychiatric aspects of Parkinson's disease. J Neurosci Rural Pract. 2015;6(1):65-76.
64. Cummings JL. Depression and Parkinson's disease: a review. Am J Psychiatry. 1992;149(4):443-54.
65. Kharbanda P, Sharma S, Mehta S. Neuropsychiatric aspects of Parkinson's disease. Astrocyte. 2015;2(1):25-30.
66. Dissanayaka NN, Sellbach A, Matheson S, O'Sullivan JD, Silburn PA, Byrne GJ, et al. Anxiety disorders in Parkinson's disease: prevalence and risk factors. Mov Disord. 2010;25(7):838-45.
67. Fénelon G, Mahieux F, Huon R, Ziégler M. Hallucinations in Parkinson's disease: prevalence, phenomenology and risk factors. Brain. 2000;123(4):733-45.
68. Aarsland D, Andersen K, Larsen J, Lolk A, Nielsen H, Kragh-Sørensen P. Risk of dementia in Parkinson's disease: a community-based, prospective study. Neurology. 2001;56(6):730-6.
69. Pagonabarraga J, Kulisevsky J, Strafella AP, Krack P. Apathy in Parkinson's disease: clinical features, neural substrates, diagnosis, and treatment. Lancet Neurol. 2015;14(5):518-31.
70. Shen CC, Tsai SJ, Perng CL, Kuo BI, Yang AC. Risk of Parkinson disease after depression: a nationwide population-based study. Neurology. 2013;81(17):1538-44.
71. Ossowska K, Lorenc-Koci E. Depression in Parkinson's disease. Pharmacol Rep. 2013;65(6):1545-57.
72. Brown R, MacCarthy B, Gotham AM, Der G, Marsden C. Depression and disability in Parkinson's disease: a follow-up of 132 cases. Psychol Med. 1988;18(1):49-55.
73. Nuti A, Ceravolo R, Piccinni A, Dell'Agnello G, Bellini G, Gambaccini G, et al. Psychiatric comorbidity in a population of Parkinson's disease patients. Eur J Neurol. 2004;11(5):315-20.
74. Péron J, Dondaine T, Le Jeune F, Grandjean D, Vérin M. Emotional processing in Parkinson's disease: a systematic review. Mov Disord. 2012;27(2):186-99.
75. US Food and Drug Administration (2019). FDA approves first drug to treat hallucinations and delusions associated with parkinson's disease. [online] Available from: https://www.fda.gov/newsevents/newsroom/pressannouncements/ucm498442.htm [Last accessed June, 2021].
76. Seppi K, Weintraub D, Coelho M, Perez-Lloret S, Fox SH, Katzenschlager R, et al. The Movement Disorder Society evidence-based medicine review update: treatments for the non-motor symptoms of Parkinson's disease. Mov Disord. 2011;26(S3):S42-80.
77. Juncos JL, Roberts VJ, Evatt ML, Jewart RD, Wood CD, Potter LS, et al. Quetiapine improves psychotic symptoms and cognition in Parkinson's disease. Mov Disord. 2004;19(1):29-35.
78. Aarsland D, Kurz MW. The epidemiology of dementia associated with Parkinson disease. J Neurol Sci. 2010;289(1-2):18-22.
79. Caballol N, Martí MJ, Tolosa E. Cognitive dysfunction and dementia in Parkinson disease. Mov Disord. 2007;22(S17):S358-66.
80. Hassan A, Bower JH, Kumar N, Matsumoto J, Fealey R, Josephs KA, et al. Dopamine agonist-triggered pathological behaviors: surveillance in the PD clinic reveals high frequencies. Parkinsonism Relat Disord. 2011;17(4):260-4.
81. Weintraub D, Koester J, Potenza MN, Siderowf AD, Stacy M, Voon V, et al. Impulse control disorders in Parkinson disease: a cross-sectional study of 3090 patients. Arch Neurol. 2010;67(5):589-95.
82. Ondo WG, Lai D. Predictors of impulsivity and reward seeking behavior with dopamine agonists. Parkinsonism Relat Disord. 2008;14(1):28-32.
83. Kales A, Ansel RD, Markham CH, Scharf MB, Tan TL. Sleep in patients with Parkinson's disease and normal subjects prior to and following levodopa administration. Clin Pharmacol Ther. 1971;12(2):397-406.
84. Partinen M, Hirvonen K, Jama L, Alakuijala A, Hublin C, Tamminen I, et al. Efficacy and safety of pramipexole in idiopathic restless legs syndrome: a polysomnographic dose-finding study—the PRELUDE study. Sleep Med. 2006;7(5):407-17.
85. Olson EJ, Boeve BF, Silber MH. Rapid eye movement sleep behaviour disorder:

demographic, clinical and laboratory findings in 93 cases. Brain. 2000;123(2):331-9.
86. Ondo W, Fayle R, Atassi F, Jankovic J. Modafinil for daytime somnolence in Parkinson's disease: double blind, placebo controlled parallel trial. J Neurol Neurosurg Psychiatry. 2005;76(12):1636-9.
87. World Health Organization. The world health report 2002: reducing risks, promoting healthy life. World Health Organization; 2002.
88. Johnson W, Onuma O, Owolabi M, Sachdev S. Stroke: a global response is needed. Bull World Health Organ. 2016;94(9):634.
89. Ferro JM, Caeiro L, Figueira ML. Neuropsychiatric sequelae of stroke. Nature Rev Neurol. 2016;12(5):269-80.
90. Robinson RG, Jorge RE. Post-stroke depression: a review. Am J Psychiatry. 2015;173(3):221-31.
91. Hackett ML, Pickles K. Part I: frequency of depression after stroke: an updated systematic review and meta-analysis of observational studies. Int J Stroke. 2014;9(8):1017-25.
92. Ayerbe L, Ayis S, Wolfe CD, Rudd AG. Natural history, predictors and outcomes of depression after stroke: systematic review and meta-analysis. Br J Psychiatry. 2013;202(1):14-21.
93. Kutlubaev MA, Hackett ML. Part II: predictors of depression after stroke and impact of depression on stroke outcome: an updated systematic review of observational studies. Int J Stroke. 2014;9(8):1026-36.
94. Narushima K, Kosier J, Robinson RG. A reappraisal of poststroke depression, intra- and inter-hemispheric lesion location using meta-analysis. J Neuropsychiatry Clin Neurosci. 2003;15(4):422-30.
95. Santos CO, Caeiro L, Ferro JM, Figueira ML. Mania and stroke: a systematic review. Cerebrovasc Dis. 2011;32(1):11-21.
96. Ferro JM. Neuropsychiatric Symptoms of Cerebrovascular Diseases. London: Springer; 2013.
97. Burton CA, Murray J, Holmes J, Astin F, Greenwood D, Knapp P. Frequency of anxiety after stroke: a systematic review and meta-analysis of observational studies. Int J Stroke. 2013;8(7):545-59.
98. Hackett ML, Köhler S, T O'Brien J, Mead GE. Neuropsychiatric outcomes of stroke. Lancet Neurol. 2014;13(5):525-34.
99. Centers for Disease Control and Prevention. (2021). Traumatic brain injury and concussion. [online] Available from: https://www.cdc.gov/traumaticbraininjury/index.html [Last accessed June, 2021].
100. Ghosh S, Nayek S. Neuropsychiatric aspects of head injury—an overview. Eastern J Psychiatry. 2017;19(1).
101. Ahmed S, Venigalla H, Mekala HM, Dar S, Hassan M, Ayub S. Traumatic brain injury and neuropsychiatric complications. Indian J Psychol Med. 2017;39(2):114-21.
102. Rao V, Lyketsos CG. Psychiatric aspects of traumatic brain injury. Psychiatr Clin North Am. 2002;25(1):43-69.
103. Kreutzer JS, Seel RT, Gourley E. The prevalence and symptom rates of depression after traumatic brain injury: a comprehensive examination. Brain Inj. 2001;15(7):563-76.
104. Chaudhury S, Biswas P, Kumar S. Psychiatric sequelae of traumatic brain injury. Med J DY Patil Univ. 2013;6(3):222-8.
105. Van Reekum R, Bolago I, Finlayson M, Garner S, Links P. Psychiatric disorders after traumatic brain injury. Brain Inj. 1996;10(5):319-27.
106. Schwarzbold M, Diaz A, Martins ET, Rufino A, Amante LN, Thais ME, et al. Psychiatric disorders and traumatic brain injury. Neuropsychiatr Dis Treat. 2008;4(4):797-816.
107. Shukla S, Cook BL, Mukherjee S, Godwin C, Miller MG. Mania following head trauma. Am J Psychiatry. 1987;144(1):93-6.
108. Starkstein SE, Mayberg HS, Berthier ML, Fedoroff P, Price TR, Dannals RF, et al. Mania after brain injury: neuroradiological and metabolic findings. Ann Neurol. 1990;27(6):652-9.
109. Starkstein SE, Boston JD, Robinson RG. Mechanisms of mania after brain injury: 12 case reports and review of the literature. J Nerv Ment Dis. 1988;176(2):87-100.
110. Achté K, Jarho L, Kyykkä T, Vesterinen E. Paranoid disorders following war brain damage. Psychopathology. 1991;24(5):309-15.
111. Davison K. Schizophrenia-like psychoses associated with organic disorders of the central nervous system: review of literature. Br J Psychiatry. 1969;4:113-84.
112. Fujii D, Ahmed I. Psychotic disorder following traumatic brain injury: a conceptual framework. Cogn Neuropsychiatry. 2002;7(1):41-62.
113. Sachdev P, Smith J, Cathcart S. Schizophrenia-like psychosis following traumatic brain injury: a chart-based descriptive and case-control study. Psychol Med. 2001;31(2):231-9.
114. Mayou R, Bryant B, Duthie R. Psychiatric consequences of road traffic accidents. BMJ. 1993;307(6905):647-51.
115. Lanska DJ. The Klüver-Bucy syndrome. Front Neurol Neurosci. 2018;41:77-89.
116. National Organization of Rare Disorders (2017). Klüver-Bucy syndrome. [online] Available from:

https://rarediseases.org/rare-diseases/kluver-bucy-syndrome/ [Last accessed June, 2021].
117. National Center for Advancing Translational Sciences (2019). Kleine Levin syndrome. [online] Available from: https://rarediseases.info.nih.gov/diseases/3117/kleine-levin-syndrome [Last accessed June, 2021].
118. Kleine-Levin Syndrome Foundation. Kleine-Levin syndrome. 2019.
119. Cerase A, Rubenni E, Rufa A, Vallone I, Galluzzi P, Coratti G, et al. CT and MRI of Wernicke's encephalopathy. Radiol Med. 2011;116(2):319-33.
120. Bombin I, Arango C, Buchanan RW. Significance and meaning of neurological signs in schizophrenia: two decades later. Schizophr Bull. 2005;31(4):962-77.
121. Fountoulakis KN, Panagiotidis P, Kimiskidis V, Nimatoudis I, Gonda X. Prevalence and correlates of neurological soft signs in healthy controls without family history of any mental disorder: a neurodevelopmental variation rather than a specific risk factor? Int J Dev Neurosci. 2018;68:59-65.
122. Sanders RD, Keshavan MS. The neurologic examination in adult psychiatry: from soft signs to hard science. J Neuropsychiatry Clin Neurosci. 1998;10(4):395-404.
123. Varambally S, Venkatasubramanian G, Gangadhar BN. Neurological soft signs in schizophrenia—the past, the present and the future. Indian J Psychiatry. 2012;54(1):73-80.
124. Sagheer TA, Assaad S, Haddad G, Hachem D, Haddad C, Hallit S. Neurological soft signs in bipolar and unipolar disorder: a case-control study. Psychiatry Res. 2018;261:253-8.
125. Kinney DK, Woods BT, Yurgelun-Todd D. Neurologic abnormalities in schizophrenic patients and their families. II. Neurologic and psychiatric findings in relatives. Arch Gen Psychiatry. 1986;43(7):665-8.
126. Dazzan P, Murray RM. Neurological soft signs in first-episode psychosis: a systematic review. Br J Psychiatry Suppl. 2002;43:s50-7.
127. Bachmann S, Degen C, Geider FJ, Schroder J. Neurological soft signs in the clinical course of schizophrenia: results of a meta-analysis. Front Psychiatry. 2014;5:185.
128. Negash A, Kebede D, Alem A, Melaku Z, Deyessa N, Shibire T, et al. Neurological soft signs in bipolar I disorder patients. J Affect Disord. 2004;80(2-3):221-30.
129. Bora E, Akgul O, Ceylan D, Ozerdem A. Neurological soft signs in bipolar disorder in comparison to healthy controls and schizophrenia: a meta-analysis. Eur Neuropsychopharmacol. 2018;28(11):1185-93.
130. Jaafari N, Baup N, Bourdel MC, Olie JP, Rotge JY, Wassouf I, et al. Neurological soft signs in OCD patients with early age at onst, versus patients with schizophrenia and healthy subjects. J Neuropsychiatry Clin Neurosci. 2011;23(4):409-16.
131. Jaafari N, Fernandez de la Cruz L, Grau M, Knowles E, Radua J, Wooderson S, et al. Neurological soft signs in obsessive-compulsive disorder: two empirical studies and meta-analysis. Psychol Med. 2013;43(5):1069-79.
132. Malhotra DS, Borade DP, Sharma DP, Satija DY, Dr G. A qualititative study of neurological soft signs in obsessive compulsive disorder and effect of comorbid psychotic spectrum disorders and familiality on its expression in Indian population. Asian J Psychiatr. 2017;25: 6-12.
133. Pitcher TM, Piek JP, Hay DA. Fine and gross motor ability in males with ADHD. Dev Med Child Neurol. 2003;45(8):525-35.
134. Mostofsky SH, Newschaffer CJ, Denckla MB. Overflow movements predict impaired response inhibition in children with ADHD. Percept Mot Skills. 2003;97(3 Pt 2):1315-31.
135. D'Agati E, Casarelli L, Pitzianti MB, Pasini A. Overflow movements and white matter abnormalities in ADHD. Prog Neuropsychopharmacol Biol Psychiatry. 2010;34(3):441-5.
136. Green D, Charman T, Pickles A, Chandler S, Loucas T, Simonoff E, et al. Impairment in movement skills of children with autistic spectrum disorders. Dev Med Child Neurol. 2009;51(4):311-6.
137. Halayem S, Hammami M, Fakhfakh R, Gaddour N, Tabbane K, Amado I, et al. Adaptation and validation of the neurological soft sign's scale of Krebs et al. to children. Encephale. 2017;43(2):128-34.

CHAPTER 4

Interface with Obstetrics and Gynecology

Debadatta Mohapatra, Biswa Ranjan Mishra, Sweta Singh

INTRODUCTION

Psychiatric disorders are equally prevalent in both male and female. However, there exists some gender-specific differences in onset, clinical course, prognosis, treatment resistance. Also, some disorders are specific to females. Women experience various stages of life starting from menarche, menstrual cycle, pregnancy, postpartum period, and menopause, which are greatly influenced by hormonal changes and impact the psychological vulnerability and, in turn, leading to the predisposition of women to certain psychiatric illnesses. While a woman passes through these times along with the transitional stages, she has to go through tremendous hormonal and psychological challenges and biological alterations, which have potential consequences in women's mood, behavior, and thought processes. Hormones such as estrogens, thyroid hormones, progesterone, and hormonal drugs in contraceptives and postmenopausal hormone replacement therapy influence many psychiatric conditions. Furthermore, in countries like India, where unplanned pregnancy is around 50–60%, it is even more challenging to assess the mental health condition.

Laterally, there are numerous biological differences among males and females, influencing a drug's pharmacokinetics and pharmacodynamics. Women have more body fat that may increase distribution volumes for lipophilic drugs like benzodiazepines. Drug absorption rates are slightly lower in women, whereas bioavailability is higher in women. Renal processes of glomerular filtration, tubular secretion, and reabsorption are slower in females leading to dose adjustments of drugs with renal excretion. Slower gastrointestinal motility, delayed gastric emptying, less intestinal enzymatic activity, and slower gastric emptying significantly affect the pharmacokinetics in females. Phase I metabolism such as oxidation, reduction, and hydrolysis usually catalyzed by cytochrome P isoenzymes.

Pregnancy can lead to alterations in pharmacokinetics in terms of increased renal plasma flow and glomerular filtration due to expansion of total body water. Oral contraceptives, which are the most widely prescribed, are microsomal enzyme inducers leading to strong drug interactions.

INTRODUCTION/PREAMBLE

Reproductive medicine is an inclusive term that includes holistic concepts of obstetrics, gynecology, adolescent gynecology, infertility, gynecologic oncology, contraception, menopause, reproductive biology, etc., implying women' health. Reproductive events have both physiological and psychological concomitants; likewise, psychological states affect reproductive physiology, thereby establishing a strong bidirectional interrelationship between reproductive biology and psychiatric conditions.

Gender refers to a person's self-image and sex-role identity, which is determined by the exposure and responsiveness of a person to sex steroids and the learning in early childhood, societal models, and cultural expectations. Carol Gilligan conceptualized that preadolescent girls have a sense of self-confidence and belief in their efficacy. In contrast, after adolescence, they express less confidence, accompanied by a sense of intimidation and passiveness. Women in the adolescent and adult age group focus on the intimacy of the relationship and try to build an affiliative style in social relationships. In comparison, men tend to focus on individualization and assertiveness in social relationships, along with a sense of achievement in work, activities, and sports. By the age of 15 years, girls experience lifetime depressive episodes twice more than boys. Negative life stress, psychosocial stressors, differential interpersonal goals, personal self-views also contribute to the predisposition of girls to depression. The need for dominance in a relationship is precipitated by a testosterone surge in males, whereas estrogen produces aggression in girls. Hypothalamic neurohormone oxytocin facilitates some behaviors like caregiving and adult pair-bond formation. Shelley Taylor proposed the existence of a uniquely female *response* to stress called a *tend-and-befriend* response. The biological mechanism of this response is females bear a more significant role in caregiving and protection of young offsprings mediated by oxytocin that reduces sympathetic hypothalamic pituitary adrenal responses to stress and increase affiliative responses.

The following discussion will be based on the reproductive cycle, which can be classified as:
- Menarche and menstrual cycle
- Perinatal
- Postmenopausal

PREMENSTRUAL DYSPHORIC DISORDER

Premenstrual symptoms are pretty common in women. Almost 80% of women experience physical, behavioral, or psychological symptoms without affecting socio-occupational function. Premenstrual symptoms, characterized by recurrent physical and psychological symptoms during the menstrual cycle's luteal phase, are prevalent in around 20–32% of women. The severe one, premenstrual dysphoric disorder (PMDD), affects 3–8% of premenopausal women **(Box 1)**.[1]

Women with PMDD present with various physical symptoms (bloating, breast tenderness, cramping, and headache) and emotional symptoms (depression, anxiety, irritability, and insomnia). While a woman presents with symptoms of PMDD, gynecological conditions such as endometriosis, fibrocystic diseases, and migraine headaches should be ruled out. Family history of PMDD should be included in the assessment as it runs a familial course. In order to rate the symptoms, several scales.

Management

The management of PMDD includes non-pharmacological and pharmacological management.[2]

Nonpharmacological Management
- Use of caffeine, alcohol, red meat, salt, and nicotine should be avoided.
- Consumption of fruits, legumes, adequate water, whole grains, smaller and more frequent meals can be helpful.

> **BOX 1:** Diagnostic criteria for premenstrual dysphoric disorder according to the Diagnostic and Statistical Manual of Mental Disorders, 5th Edition (DSM-5).
>
> A. In majority of menstrual cycles, at least five symptoms must be present in the final week before the onset of menses, start to *improve* within a few days and after the onset of menses, and become *minimal* or absent in the week postmenses
> B. One (or more) of the following symptoms must be present:
>   1. Marked affective lability (e.g., mood swings; feeling suddenly sad or tearful, or increased sensitivity to rejection)
>   2. Marked irritability or anger or increased interpersonal conflicts
>   3. Marked depressed mood, feelings of hopelessness, or self-deprecating thoughts
>   4. Marked anxiety, tension, and/or feelings of being keyed up or on edge
> C. One (or more) of the following symptoms must additionally be present, to reach a total of *five* symptoms when combined with symptoms from criterion B above:
>   1. Decreased interest in usual activities (e.g., work, school, friends, hobbies)
>   2. Subjective difficulty in concentration
>   3. Lethargy, easy fatigability, or marked lack of energy
>   4. Marked change in appetite; overeating; or specific food cravings
>   5. Hypersomnia or insomnia
>   6. A sense of being overwhelmed or out of control
>   7. Physical symptoms such as breast tenderness or swelling, joint or muscle pain, a sensation of bloating, or weight gain
>
>   *Note:* The symptoms in criteria A-C must have been met for most menstrual cycles that occurred in the preceding year.
> D. The symptoms are associated with clinically significant distress or interference with work, school, usual activities, or relationships with others (e.g., avoidance of social activities; decreased productivity and efficiency at work, school or home)
> E. The disturbance is not merely an exacerbation of the symptoms of another disorder, such as major depressive disorder, panic disorder, persistent depressive disorder (dysthymia), or a personality disorder (although it may co-occur with any of these disorders)
> F. Criterion A should be confirmed by prospective daily ratings during at least two symptomatic cycles. (*Note:* The diagnosis may be made provisionally prior to this confirmation)
> G. The symptoms are not attributable to the physiological effects of a substance (e.g., a drug of abuse, a medication, other treatment) or another medical condition (e.g., hyperthyroidism)

- Proper sleep hygiene, exercise, relaxation therapy, and cognitive-behavioral therapy (CBT) are among some nonpharmacological management that can benefit patients with mild PMDD.

Pharmacological Management

Among pharmacological management, none of the existing literature supports a single or few agents for PMDD treatment. However, few studies found that:
- A high intake of calcium and vitamin D may lessen moderate-to-severe premenstrual symptoms.
- Seventy percent of women with PMDD respond adequately to selective serotonin reuptake inhibitors (SSRIs). Among SSRIs, fluoxetine, paroxetine, sertraline, and citalopram are significantly beneficial and can be used during the luteal phase (2 weeks) until menses start.
- Continuous use of SSRI can be recommended for those with comorbid depression or anxiety disorder.
- Intermittent use of SSRI is best for those having PMDD restricted to the premenstrual phase.

- There are also some roles of buspirone and alprazolam as anxiolytics.

PERINATAL PSYCHIATRIC ILLNESS

The perinatal period is eventful in a woman's life associated with various biological and psychological alterations and physical changes. The changes eventually might lead to psychiatric conditions like anxiety, depression, affective, and nonaffective psychosis. The manifestations are not only limited to immediate illnesses but also some long-term consequences. Perinatal mental illnesses are a significant complication occurring during pregnancy and postpartum period having variable clinical manifestation and contributing to substantial morbidity and mortality. The history of the conception of perinatal mental illness can be dated back to the Hippocrates era.

The perinatal psychiatric illness primarily includes postpartum blues, postpartum depression, and postpartum psychosis. The first 6 months following delivery is a critical period, creating much emotional instability in a woman. Maternal sleep deprivation is pervasive and an essential factor for the evolution of postpartum psychiatric illness.

Postpartum Blues

Postpartum blues, otherwise called baby blues, is usually a benign condition prevalent in 90% of women after delivery. It is a transient condition characterized by the onset of symptoms 2–4 days after delivery of a patient when the mother is discharged from the hospital with a peak of symptoms by 5–7 days. The symptoms usually resolve by 10 days postpartum. Characteristic symptoms of postpartum blues are tearfulness, rapid mood shifts, irritability, loss of appetite, lack of energy and anxiety, and overwhelmed feelings mainly related to the baby's caregiving. About 75% of women experiencing postpartum blues face resolution of symptoms by 10 days to 2 weeks, whereas 20–25% of them continue to have a severe form of this called postpartum depression.[3] The management includes careful assessment of the patient and observation for progression of symptoms, psychoeducation, reassurance, support, and validation of mother's account.

Postpartum Depression

Postpartum depression is a common and severe psychiatric disorder that has a tremendous effect on the mother's physical and mental health and has negative consequences on the child. The initial 6 months following delivery has the highest risk for developing depression, with a 13–19% prevalence. Despite being a significant health concern, it usually remains undiagnosed.

The Diagnostic and Statistical Manual of Mental Disorders, 5th Edition (DSM-5) recognizes this type of illness using a specifier "peripartum onset" with depressive disorder. "Peripartum onset" is used as a specifier when the symptoms meet full criteria of depressive episode and the onset is either during pregnancy or within 4 weeks of the postpartum period.

More than 50% of postpartum depression has onset during pregnancy. Women with peripartum depression usually present with panic attacks and severe anxiety. Prepartum depressive disorder can present with or without psychotic symptoms. Severe depression with psychotic symptoms can present with infanticide in response to command hallucination or as an acting out behavior of delusion. Longitudinal studies have found that postpartum depression with psychotic symptoms is increased in women with prior history of mood disorder or family history of bipolar disorder. The chances of recurrence of postpartum depression in subsequent deliveries are increased up to 30–50% after a woman experiences severe depression with psychotic symptoms.

The risk factors that strongly predict the occurrence of postpartum depression are:
- Previous history of depression in woman
- Poor social support in the female
- Stressful life events
- Depression and anxiety in the woman during pregnancy

Risk factors that are moderate predictors of the occurrence of postpartum depression are:
- Stress-related to child care
- Low self-esteem in women
- The difficult temperament of the infant
- Maternal neuroticism

The risk factors that are small predictors of the occurrence of postpartum depression are:
- Pregnancy-related complications
- Single parent
- The negative cognitive style of attribution
- Low-socioeconomic status
- Low income
- Poor relationship with the partner

However, some risk factors that do not have any relationship with postpartum depression are the mother's age, race and ethnicity, gender of the child, level of education, and parity.[4]

Effects of Postpartum Depression on the Mother-Infant Relationship

Recent studies have found that there are various negative consequences of postpartum depression on the infant. Some studies have also found long-term complications that affect the child's emotional and social life. Young children of a mother with postpartum depression suffer from cognitive, emotional, and interpersonal problems compared to nondepressed mothers. With regard to the child's growth and development, studies also support the same finding.[5]

Management of Postpartum Depression

Detailed and comprehensive history taking is a must to diagnose postpartum depression and excludes other differential diagnoses. A thorough investigation, including a thyroid function test, is required to look for thyroid dysfunction as the postpartum period is a time for increased risk for thyroid dysfunction. The management needs to be comprehensive, including psychoeducation, individual psychotherapy and group psychotherapy, supportive psychotherapy, and pharmacological management.[6]

While considering pharmacotherapy, few important things need to be taken into consideration:
- If a woman is newly diagnosed with postpartum depression, then the decision regarding which antidepressant should be chosen for treatment depends on the breastfeeding status of the patient. It is vital to consider drugs that are safe during lactation.
- If a woman has a previous history of postpartum depression or major depression, then antidepressant needs to be started 24–48 hours after delivery. However, all women with a history of postpartum depression need to be carefully monitored for relapse or signs of the severity of depression. The choice of antidepressant will also depend on past history of response to medication.

Postpartum Psychosis

Postpartum psychosis is the most severe and life-threatening condition for both the mother and the infant, with a prevalence of 1–2 every 1,000 births. According to DSM-5, it is diagnosed as a "brief psychotic disorder" with postpartum onset as a specifier if the onset is during pregnancy or within 4 weeks of delivery. Mood lability, delusion, hallucination, extreme impulsivity leading to suicide and infanticide, agitation, disturbed sleep and thought disorganization feature the condition. The course is usually mercurial changing rapidly during the day and the postpartum period. The usual onset of illness is within 2 weeks of postpartum, but sometimes onset may be after 3-5 months.[7]

Women with postpartum depression are at higher risk of developing bipolar disorder. In females with a history of bipolar disorder, there is a 25-35% chance of developing postpartum depression. If a woman has both history of bipolar disorder and prior history of postpartum mood disorder **(Table 1)** is having a 50% chance of having postpartum depression in the subsequent delivery. Family history of bipolarity also increases the risk of postpartum depression. These findings suggest that postpartum depression is associated with bipolar disorder.

Management of Postpartum Psychosis

There is an increased chance of suicide, infanticide, and child neglect in postpartum depression, which warrants hospitalization. Detailed history taking and medical evaluation is essential to rule out medical conditions like postpartum thyroiditis, Sheehan's syndrome, pregnancy-related autoimmune disorders, human immunodeficiency virus (HIV) related infection, etc. Acute management includes antipsychotics and benzodiazepines for agitation and sedation. Long-term management includes continuation of antipsychotics for 1 year because of the chance of recurrence.[8] Prognosis of postpartum psychosis is usually considered as favorable whenever early treatment is done. However, it may lead to chronic and refractory to treatment if treatment is delayed.[9]

Postpartum Bipolar Disorder

Females with a past history of bipolar disorder are at higher risk for developing postpartum bipolar disorder. Compared to postpartum depression, in women with postpartum bipolar disorder, the chances of hospitalization are more.[10]

Etiological factors for postpartum bipolar disorder are:
- Abrupt changes in estrogen and progesterone
- Erratic sleep pattern due to infant care
- Increased psychosocial stress associated with young motherhood and child care

TABLE 1: Postpartum mood disorder.

Disorder	Incidence	Presentation	Treatment
Postpartum blues	Common 80%	Mood lability, emotional sensitivity, crying spells	• Support, reassurance • Usually, resolve within 10–12 days • If severe beyond 12 days, consider another diagnosis
Postpartum depression	13–18%	Meet full criteria of major depression	Individual psychotherapy, psychoeducation, antidepressant, hospitalization if required, electroconvulsive therapy (ECT)
Postpartum psychosis	0.1%	• Early-onset, usually by 2–3 days, often presents with mixed/rapid cycling features • Risk of infanticide	• Hospitalization, education, reassurance, and supportive care. • Antipsychotics, mood stabilizers if required, ECT

- Hypothalamic-pituitary-thyroid axis dysfunction

Pharmacotherapy is usually the mainstay of therapy in this condition. Women should be maintained on mood stabilizers within 24 hours of delivery in severe cases to prevent the risk of relapse.

POSTMENOPAUSAL

Menopause refers to the cessation of ovulation which usually occurs by the age of 45–55 years. Perimenopause is referred to as the period around menopause when ovarian function declines.

The underlying hormonal changes that occur in postmenopausal women are ovarian decline in estrogen that subsequently leads to an increase in luteinizing hormone (LH) and follicular-stimulating hormone (FSH) levels (40 mIU/mL) and low levels of estradiol (<25 pg/mL). Increased FSH level just after a cycle is an indicator of perimenopausal age. The decline in ovarian function leads to vasomotor symptoms, cardiovascular diseases, sexual dysfunction, the decline in cognitive function, and reduced bone density.

Factors associated with an earlier transition to menopause are:
- Cigarette smoking
- Lower educational level
- Separated, widowed, or divorced
- Unemployment
- History of cardiac disease

About 80% of women experience perimenopausal hot flushes and cold sweats due to a reduction in ovarian estrogen. Hot flushes are usually mistaken as panic attacks, and panic attacks might be confused as hot flushes also. Night sweats may be associated with sleep deprivation, ultimately leading to worsening of fatigue, reduced concentration, irritability and subsequently predisposing to depression.

Perimenopausal Depression

Women in the perimenopausal age group might experience first-onset depression. The faster the rise in FSH levels, the shorter the transition to menopause and the less likely she is to experience depression.

Risk Factors

The risk factors for developing depression in the postmenopausal age group are:
- Being divorced, separated, or widow
- Empty nest
- Having significant caregiving responsibilities
- Being in a socially disadvantaged position
- Chronic illness
- History of depression
- Sleep-related problems
- Prominent vasomotor symptoms

Management

- Hormone replacement therapy is being used for vasomotor symptoms.[11]
- Antidepressants like SSRI have some role in relieving postmenopausal depression.
- Psychotherapy also has some roles.

PSYCHOLOGICAL ASPECTS OF OTHER CONDITIONS

Infertility

Around 15–20% of couples cannot conceive and suffer from the problem of infertility. The etiology of infertility can be attributed to male factors in approximately 40–60%, and female factors also contribute equally. Among the common female causes of infertility, ovulatory, uterine, and tubal causes are most common. Some psychiatric conditions such as anorexia nervosa and stress-induced amenorrhea result in hypothalamic hypopituitary syndrome associated with infertility. Current or past history of depression is also associated with a decline in ovarian function, leading to infertility. Infertile couples feel isolated and struggle with lowered self-esteem and depression, which causes a vicious cycle of depression leading to infertility and infertility depression. The cost of workup and treatment of infertility is time-consuming and needs lots of money. The long-term treatment of infertility also determines the working hours and their vacation.[12]

Psychological Effects of Infertility

The challenging and demanding aspects of infertility and its treatment imposes various psychological consequences in women.

- The need for sexual relationships in the time, as advised by the treating doctor, harms intimacy and affects spontaneity.
- The daily monitoring of reproductive-related functions may be cumbersome.
- Success rates are uncertain, and high cost produces stress in the couple.
- Women who postponed pregnancy face guilt and self-blame.
- The drugs used in treating infertility like clomiphene and gonadotropin-releasing hormone (GnRH) produce changes in mood, anxiety, and insomnia in women.

Management

Mild psychiatric symptoms may be treated with psychotherapy, but moderate to severe symptoms need psychotropics like antidepressants and antianxiety drugs.

Induced Abortion

Induced abortion may be because of some medical reasons or unwanted pregnancy.

If abortion is because of detected congenital malformations, the women might be at a stage of ambivalence or feeling guilty. Impending fetal demise and mourning for the loss are also quite prevalent, where preabortion counseling and sensitive education about the malformation is very much needed.[13]

If abortion is performed due to unwanted pregnancy caused by rape or other mishaps, counseling becomes an integral part of the treatment.

If abortion is due to unwanted pregnancy, counseling for effective contraception is also essential.

When a woman with chronic mental illness induces abortion, there is a chance of exacerbating preexisting mental disorder. Here, the role of a psychiatrist is critical, and psychotropics might be required.

Loss of Pregnancy

It is found that up to 50% of pregnancies are not sustained, although all are not documented. Loss of pregnancy leads to severe mental trauma, and the women feel isolated from their social life. If pregnancy loss is after 6 months, there is more chance of anxiety and depression in women. Some risk factors for major depression in women after miscarriage are previous history of depression, childlessness, or young mother. Stillbirth is the most traumatic event. However, normal bereavement needs to be differentiated from depression here. A psychiatric referral should be considered for women who have a late-trimester fetal loss and previous history of depression.

Contraception and its Effects on Mood

Contraceptives are available in oral, implants, or transdermal patches containing various combinations of estrogen, progesterone, or progesterone-only. Studies found that there is not much difference in women using oral contraceptives compared to untreated in terms of mood instability.[14,15] However, oral contraceptive pills may precipitate depression in some women with following risk factors like:

- Women with a history of dysmenorrhea, depression, premenstrual mood symptoms, or pregnancy-related mood symptoms.
- Women in the postpartum period
- Family history of oral contraceptive-associated negative mood states
- Triphasic oral contraceptive agents are more likely to precipitate depressive symptoms.

PSYCHOTROPICS DURING PREGNANCY

There exists lots of controversial clinical issue for the use of psychotropics during pregnancy and breastfeeding. There has been misperception that pregnancy exerts protective effect against mental illness, with alongside genuine concerns that women during pregnancy should avoid extraneous exposure to the minimum, eventually undermining the seriousness of emergence or exacerbation of psychiatric illness during pregnancy or the postpartum period. The perinatal period is a high-risk time period for the occurrence of maternal severe mental illnesses such as major depressive disorder (MDD), bipolar disorder, psychosis, and high suicidal rates. Again, maternal mental illness during pregnancy has been associated with adverse perinatal outcomes, including fetal distress, intrauterine growth retardation, neonatal hypoglycemia, and adverse neurodevelopmental effects.

The safety of psychotropics during pregnancy has been debatable because robust, prospective trials are unethical, with limited future data from teratology shreds of evidence. Individual decisions on psychotropic use in pregnancy are majorly influenced by published case reports which are known to be biased toward selective reporting of adverse outcomes. Again, there is an increased risk of relapse in late pregnancy and early postpartum, irrespective of medication use. Hence, the psychiatrist's decision largely depends upon the risk-benefit analysis of psychotropics from the patient's perspective.

Changes in Metabolism and Drug Clearance during Pregnancy

Major adaptive physiologic changes happen during pregnancy, which can significantly affect the pharmacokinetics and pharmacodynamics of the psychotropics. The changes might begin early and continue during the 3rd trimester, resulting in about a 50% increase in plasma volume and increased drug distribution volume. Changes in liver enzyme activation occur (for example, CYP1A2 activity decreases; CYP2D6 activity and CYP3A activity increase), and glomerular filtration rate can increase, influencing the clearance of psychotropics from our body. In view of the high inter-individual pharmacodynamic variability during pregnancy and the postpartum period, therapeutic monitoring of serum levels of psychotropics becomes important.

Psychotropics and Risks to Offspring

All the psychotropics in the maternal circulatory system can cross the placental barrier and eventually leading to risk of fetal exposure to some degree. The description in the literature regarding psychotropic-induced fetal exposure has revolved mainly around the 1st trimester involving the phase of organogenesis; however, the intrauterine exposure during the 2nd and 3rd trimester can also lead to postnatal fetal complications. The risks can be divided into teratogenicity, perinatal syndromes, obstetrical complications, and long-term postnatal behavioral sequelae.

To guide physicians about the reproductive safety of various psychotropics, the US Food and Drug Administration (FDA) has classified medications into five risk categories (A, B, C, D, and X) based on human and animal data. Category A medications are designated as safe during pregnancy (no psychotropics are included), while category X drugs are contraindicated as they have demonstrable fetal risks that outweigh benefits to the patient. Most psychotropic drugs are classified as category C agents for which adequate human studies are lacking. Evidence of fetal effects seen in animal studies may be insufficient (except for lithium, which is classified under category D).

Treatment with Psychotropics during Pregnancy

Antipsychotics

First-generation or typical antipsychotics (FGAs) are usually considered to have minimal risk of teratogenicity. Even though, few case studies have reported an association between typical antipsychotic, haloperidol and limb defects, the actual risk is extremely low. Low-potency antipsychotics such as chlorpromazine are usually avoided because of side effects, such as hypotension. Neonatal jaundice has been reported with phenothiazines, and there are case studies related to neonatal dyskinesia with the use of FGAs. However, the wide use over several decades of FGAs suggests that any risk is small, and they are safe during pregnancy.[16]

Atypical antipsychotics or second-generation antipsychotics (SGAs) are less safe to use in pregnancy than FGAs, with evidence of increased risk of maternal weight gain, increased risk of gestational diabetes, and increased infant birth weight. Several case series and population-based observational studies have reported the development of gestational diabetes with the use of olanzapine and clozapine. Several studies advocate that the use of SGAs in pregnancy is linked with an increased risk of hypoglycemia. Therefore, radiological monitoring of fetal size in late pregnancy and appropriate glucose monitoring may be beneficial in women on atypical antipsychotics.

Clozapine being the only antipsychotic belonging to category B of FDA classification has no definitive association found between maternal exposure and congenital anomalies in either animals or humans. However, there are reports of clozapine use during pregnancy being associated with floppy baby syndrome, neonatal seizures, and worsening of gestational diabetes with shoulder dystocia. It is also recommended that infants with exposure to clozapine in utero should be monitored for agranulocytosis weekly for the first 6 months of life.

Antidepressants

Tricyclic antidepressants (TCAs) use in pregnancy are usually safe, with less risk of congenital fetal malformation. However, their use during the delivery period may occasionally result in transient neonatal withdrawal symptoms anticholinergic side effects. Among TCAs, nortriptyline and desipramine are preferably used in view of their less chances of anticholinergic and hypotensive side effects.

Selective serotonin reuptake inhibitors are generally considered to be safe during pregnancy, with the majority of the prospective or retrospective studies not finding any association with miscarriage or congenital malformation. According to studies, there is no consistent association between SSRI use during pregnancy and cardiovascular malformations. However, the use of antidepressants in early pregnancy has been reported with a modestly increased risk of spontaneous abortion. The rate of preterm birth is higher among mothers who take SSRIs, with anecdotal reports of their association with low birth weight. In persistent pulmonary hypertension of the newborn

(PPHN), the resistance of the pulmonary vasculature fails to decrease at birth, resulting in breathing difficulties and leading to hypoxia of the newborn. Studies evaluating the link between SSRIs and PPHN in the newborn have found the odds ratio not to be significant. Babies exposed to antidepressants in the uterus may present with "withdrawal symptoms" known as poor neonatal adaptation syndrome (PNAS). But, this entity is poorly defined, with limited evidence to recommend tapering antidepressants in the 3rd trimester of pregnancy.

Mood Stabilizers and Antiepileptics

Lithium is labeled as a category D drug during pregnancy. There is an excess of cardiovascular malformations, particularly Ebstein's anomaly with the use of lithium as per the reports from an early International Register of Lithium Babies. The estimated risk of Ebstein's anomaly in lithium exposed infants is 10–20 times higher than that of general population. The absolute risk is small (0.05–0.1%), and lithium has been concluded to be a safe mood stabilizer during pregnancy. Although there are case-based descriptions of lithium-associated congenital abnormalities, including large for gestational age infants, anencephaly, and oromandibular-limb hypogenesis. During delivery, exposure to lithium has been rarely associated with muscular hypotonia, with impaired breathing known as "floppy baby syndrome". Isolated cases of lithium-induced neonatal hypothyroidism, polyhydramnios, and diabetes insipidus have also been described. In view of the blood volume changes during the 3rd trimester and postdelivery, frequent monitoring of serum lithium levels and dose titration is recommended to maintain lithium's "therapeutic window".

Antiepileptic mood stabilizers pose higher teratogenic potential compared to lithium. Factors increasing the risk for teratogenesis are high maternal serum anticonvulsant levels and exposure to more than one anticonvulsant. Carbamazepine exposure in the 1st trimester is associated with about a 1.0% risk of neural tube defects, increased risk for craniofacial abnormalities, growth retardation, microcephaly, fingernail hypoplasia, cardiac abnormalities, and developmental delay. Fetal exposure to carbamazepine has also been associated with transient hepatic toxicity. Carbamazepine may also increase the risk of neonatal hemorrhage, as it is a competitive inhibitor of prothrombin precursors.

Exposure to valproic acid during 1st trimester has been associated with higher rates of neural tube defects in the range of 1.0–5.0%. The neural tube defect found in exposed infants is more likely to be lumbosacral rather than anencephalic, suggesting the effect of the drug on neural crest closure. Prenatal exposure to valproate has also been associated with some other characteristic craniofacial abnormalities, limb defects, cardiovascular malformations, genital anomalies, and intrauterine growth retardation. Valproate use during delivery is associated with other neonatal complications like heart rate deceleration, hypoglycemia, hepatotoxicity, and reductions in neonatal fibrinogen levels. Lamotrigine monotherapy does not increase the risk of congenital defects. Animal studies with the use of topiramate and gabapentin have demonstrated craniofacial and skeletal abnormalities. However, their possible teratogenic effects in humans are lacking.

It is recommended that the pregnant women on anticonvulsants should take high-dose folate (5 mg/day), which theoretically reduces the risk of neural tube defects. Therapeutic blood monitoring should be encouraged, and 2nd-trimester ultrasound to screen for major congenital anomalies.

Benzodiazepines

Benzodiazepine use during pregnancy has produced contradictory and controversial results. All benzodiazepines diffuse readily across the placenta to the fetus. When the fetus is exposed between 2 and 8 weeks after conception the risk of malformation is highest. If the drugs are administered at or near term, they may cause fetal dependence and eventual withdrawal symptoms. Benzodiazepine use during pregnancy has been associated with perinatal toxicity, including temperature dysregulation, hypotonia, and poor feeding according to some anecdotal case reports. In addition, early studies identified an increased risk of oral cleft palate defects. However, more recent prospective and retrospective studies have shown no increased risk of cleft lip or palate with benzodiazepine use in pregnancy. When considering the risks and benefits of benzodiazepines, it is needed to consider the risks of untreated insomnia and anxiety in pregnancy, which may lead to physiological effects, worsening of mood, and impaired functioning.

General Recommendations

- Patients with a history of psychosis and are maintained on antipsychotic medication should be advised to discuss a planned pregnancy as early as possible.
- In women with depression planning for pregnancy, SSRIs can be safely considered, or antidepressants with a past response may be initiated. Women who are at a high risk of relapse are best maintained on the same antidepressant during and after pregnancy.
- Valproate should be stopped if a woman becomes pregnant. Other anticonvulsants should be avoided unless the risks and consequences of relapse outweigh the known risk of teratogenesis. The patient can be maintained on mood-stabilizing antipsychotic. Therapeutic drug level monitoring and 2nd-trimester ultrasound to screen for major congenital anomalies should be encouraged.
- When initiating an antipsychotic in a woman planning pregnancy, the previous response must be considered. FGAs are relatively safe in pregnancy, and with the use of SGAs, glycemic indices should be periodically monitored.
- Benzodiazepines, zopiclone, and zolpidem are probably not teratogenic but should be cautiously used when anxiety and insomnia are functionally disabling.
- Theoretically, high-dose folate supplementation should be encouraged throughout pregnancy for their protective effects against neural tube defects.

BREASTFEEDING AND PSYCHOTROPICS MEDICATION

Breastfeeding is usually advisable for 6 months postdelivery, but breastfeeding is influenced by the safety of drugs taken by the mother. All psychotropics are excreted in breast milk to some extent. Infant plasma levels are the most direct measure of infant exposure, which is rarely available. Another step that is commonly used to measure infant exposure is breast milk drug concentrations. The infant weight-adjusted dose expressed as a maternal weight-adjusted dose is called relative infant dose (RID). Drugs with RID <10% or infant plasma level <10% of maternal plasma level is considered safe in breastfeeding.

General Consideration of Prescribing Psychotropics in Breastfeeding

- The safety of a drug in breastfeeding should always be taken into consideration while prescribing psychotropics in breastfeeding.

- Discussion about safety of drugs should be done before conception or early in pregnancy.
- While a mother is taking a drug during pregnancy, continuation of the drug is usually considered.
- The benefits of breastfeeding to the mother and infant should always be weighed against the risk of infant exposure.
- Neonates and infants do not have the same capacity for drug clearance. Hence, caution should be there while prescribing drugs in premature infants and infants with renal, hepatic or neurological impairment.
- Monitoring the infant for specific adverse effects and feeding patterns and growth and development is essential.
- Infant plasma levels should be monitored whenever toxicity is suspected.
- The lowest effective dose should be used.
- Polypharmacy should be avoided.
- The regimen prescribed during pregnancy should be continued during breastfeeding.
- It is crucial to consider the previous response to treatment and half-lives of the drugs.

Specific Considerations

- *Antidepressants:* While initiating an antidepressant during the postpartum period, *sertraline* or *mirtazapine* should be considered.
- *Antipsychotics:* It is usually advisable to continue the same drug that is continued during pregnancy, except *clozapine*. Women taking clozapine should be advised against breastfeeding, and clozapine should be continued. While initiating an antipsychotic postpartum, *olanzapine* or *quetiapine* should be considered.
- *Mood stabilizers:* It is usually advisable to continue the same drug that is continued during pregnancy, except lithium. Women taking lithium should be advised against breastfeeding, and lithium should be continued. While initiating a mood stabilizer postpartum, mood-stabilizing antipsychotics, *olanzapine*, or *quetiapine* should be considered.
- *Sedatives:* Usually to be avoided. If required, a drug with a short half-life should be used. *Lorazepam* should be considered.

TREATMENT OF PSYCHIATRIC DISORDERS DURING PREGNANCY

The mental health of the expectant mother is an important determinant of health of the fetus and neonate. Psychiatric disorders compromising the cognitive function of mothers increase the risk of poor obstetrics outcomes, thereby leading to the compromised physical health of neonates. Hence, it is the responsibility of both the gynecologist and psychiatrist to liaise with each other and work for the betterment of the newborn and the parents.

Schizophrenia

Previously, it was thought that there is no gender difference in schizophrenia, but recent studies indicate male preponderance. The protecting factors in females may be:

- Antidopaminergic effects of estrogen
- Good premorbid history
- Later age of onset
- Less structural brain abnormality
- Better language function in females
- Less substance abuse
- More likely to have a family history
- More affective symptoms
- More positive symptoms
- Better social functioning

Gender Issues on the Treatment of Schizophrenia

Females have a better prognosis as compared to males. Treatment response is better in females, and they require lower doses of antipsychotics.

Antipsychotic-induced hyperprolactinemia is more in women. Women with schizophrenia are at increased risk of pregnancy because of chances of sexual assault and ineffective contraception. There is an increased risk of preterm delivery, low birth weight babies, low Apgar score, abruptio placentae, congenital abnormalities, sudden infant death, etc.[17]

Special attention should be given to regular antenatal checkups, adequate psychosocial support, proper nutrition, and compliance with antipsychotics and prenatal instructions.

Depression

Women tend to develop depression usually in response to their interpersonal difficulties, whereas men are due to occupational and financial stress. Studies found that the heritability of depression is also more in women, probably because of hormonal changes during the menstrual cycle, pregnancy and postpartum period leading to genetic alterations. Seasonal affective episodes are more in women. Depression during pregnancy increases the risk of postpartum depression. Depression is 1.7-2 times more prevalent in women as compared to men. Women with a history of perinatal mood disorder, PMDD, perimenopausal depression, and oral contraceptive-induced depression are at more risk for developing other reproductive-related depressive episodes.[18]

Management of Depression in Pregnancy and Lactation

- While considering the treatment of women with depression, the risk of treatment should be weighed against the dangers of untreated psychiatric illness.
- Risk-benefit decisions should be based on case-to-case basis along with parents and doctors.
- Mild-to-moderate depression should be treated with nonpharmacological methods such as psychotherapy, bright light therapy, supportive psychotherapy.
- Severe depression psychotropics can be considered the specific risk of each drug.
- If a patient is already on antidepressants and becomes pregnant, medication should be withheld if possible (mild depression, first episode or previous episodes also improved without medication).
- If already on antidepressants, with severe depression or chronic depression, history of relapse after withdrawing medication, then antidepressants should be considered. However, in these cases, regular antenatal monitoring and scan for risk of congenital malformations should be considered.
- Women with a history of depression are at increased risk for postpartum depression; consideration should be given to prophylactic initiation of antidepressants immediately after delivery.

Bipolar Disorder

Bipolar disorder is equally prevalent in both men and women, but mixed features and rapid cycling are approximately twice as common in women. History of bipolar disorder in women increases the risk for postpartum recurrence. Women having bipolar disorder are at higher risk for comorbid substance use disorder. It is essential to ensure that all bipolar women of childbearing age need to be managed carefully using the safest possible medications, maximizing clinical stability.[19]

Anxiety Disorder

Women are at increased risk to experience anxiety disorder than men. Women are twice as likely to suffer from post-traumatic stress disorder than men, with two to three times more chances of developing panic disorder with agoraphobia. Prevalence of obsessive-compulsive disorder (OCD) is roughly equal in both sexes, with earlier onset in women.[20]

Nonpharmacological interventions like CBT, elimination of caffeine and nicotine, reduction of psychosocial stressors, couples' therapy should be considered in case of mild to moderate anxiety disorder. For severe anxiety, antianxiety drugs can be considered.

Substance Use Disorder

Prevalence of alcohol use disorder is much more common in males compared to males. However, this is rising in females. While women take alcohol, it reaches higher blood alcohol levels because of more body fat and less body water. Hence, they become more intoxicated than men with an equal amount of alcohol. In women, the complications of alcohol use like anemia, peptic ulcer, liver disease, and cerebral atrophy develop more quickly. Risk factors for drug abuse in women are family history of abuse, antisocial personality disorder, and depression.

Alcohol use in pregnancy might lead to preterm labor, abruptio placentae, stillbirth, teratogenic complications associated with alcohol and its metabolite acetaldehyde. A lifelong disabling condition, fetal alcohol syndrome occurring in around 1.5/1,000 live birth due to in utero exposure to alcohol. The features are mental retardation, microcephaly, abnormal facial features, conduct disorder, and attention-deficit/hyperactivity disorder (ADHD) in childhood. There is no established safe quantity of alcohol use in the prenatal period. Fetal exposure to any substance is determined by the teratogenic effects of the drug and other high-risk behaviors of the mother.[21]

In utero, cocaine use also leads to preterm labor, abruptio placentae, and other obstetric complications due to the vasoconstriction property of cocaine. Heroin use also leads to irritability and withdrawal symptoms in the child, also sudden infant death. Neonatal use in tobacco may lead to intrauterine growth retardation, low birth weight, spontaneous abortion, and preterm delivery. Smoking more than 10 cigarettes can be associated with chromosomal instability. Intrauterine caffeine use might increase the risk of early spontaneous abortion.

Eating Disorder

Anorexia nervosa and bulimia nervosa are a few conditions that need to be considered as they are more prevalent in women, around 0.3–1%. They have excessive concern about their body image, and to compensate for their food intake, they can fast, do exercise, self-induced vomiting, etc. Various medical complications can be associated with eating disorders like metabolic abnormalities, hypokalemia, hypotension, esophageal perforation, atrial and ventricular abnormalities, metabolic acidosis, dental erosion, osteoporosis—some gynecological conditions like amenorrhea.[22] The treatment includes multidisciplinary management. Psychological management includes serotonergic drugs, antipsychotics use, psychoeducation, individual psychotherapy, CBT, etc.[23]

Sleep Disorder

Insomnia is more evident in females than men, probably due to various reasons during different phases of life of a woman like the perimenstrual period and sleep-related difficulties in the reproductive cycle starting from pregnancy, postpartum, and postmenopausal time. Other common causes include depression, anxiety disorder, substance use, and medical comorbidities. The prevalence of insomnia is more in women with breast cancer.[24]

The management of insomnia includes an initial evaluation of the causes of insomnia, and if there are psychiatric disorders, they should be treated. Proper sleep hygiene should be advised, and sedative medication should be prescribed if required. Use of sedating antidepressants is also advocated if needed.

Polycystic Ovarian Syndrome

Women and adolescents with polycystic ovarian syndrome (PCOS) have higher rates of moderate to severe anxiety, depression, and perceived stress.[25-27] The exact etiology for the increased risk in PCOS is still unclear. It is hypothesized that obesity, insulin resistance, stress, hirsutism, elevated androgens, and infertility may contribute to the association of PCOS with depression. Healthcare professionals should be aware that women with PCOS have a higher prevalence of weight gain and obesity, presenting significant concerns for women, impacting on health and emotional well-being.[3] When assessing weight, related stigma, negative body image and/or low self-esteem need to be considered and assessment needs to be respectful and considerate. Treatment of PCOS-related symptoms with lifestyle modification and/or oral contraceptive pills may benefit the above associated conditions. If treatment is warranted, psychological therapy and/or pharmacological treatment should be offered.[27] However, caution is needed to avoid inappropriate treatment with antidepressants or anxiolytics.

The PCOS is a common disorder affecting around 15% of women. It is associated with an increased risk of depression, anxiety disorder, bipolar disorder, and OCD. Along with these, it is also associated with worsening of depression, somatoform disorder, and OCD.[28] Psychotropics used in women, like mood stabilizers, especially sodium valproate, can have some issues related to the menstrual cycle like amenorrhea, oligomenorrhea, and delayed menstrual cycle.[29,30] Menstrual irregularities are also quite common with carbamazepine which is around 30%.[30]

Where mental health disorders are clearly documented and persistent, or if suicidal symptoms are present, treatment of depression or anxiety needs to be informed by clinical regional practice guidelines.[30] Use of agents that exacerbate PCOS symptoms, including weight gain, need careful consideration. Screening for anxiety and depression, along with increased focus on emotional well-being and quality of life is recommended in women and adolescents with PCOS at the time of diagnosis.[29,30]

GYNECOLOGICAL ONCOLOGY

Anxiety, depression, and poorer quality of life are experienced by women after gynecological cancer diagnosis and during gynecologic cancer treatment.[31,32] It is recommended that healthcare professionals strengthen the early assessment of anxiety, depression, and social support in women with gynecologic cancers.[4] In addition, sensitivity toward their emotional status should be increased. Helping women diagnosed with gynecological cancers identify benefits from their cancer experience, also known as benefit-finding, may reduce depression by paving the way for them to accept their emotional reactions, accept life changes associated with cancer and facilitate supportive reactions from friends and family.[5] Psychological and social support and related interventions should be provided based on patient needs in order to maintain quality of life.[32]

COVID, PREGNANCY AND MENTAL ILLNESS

The novel coronavirus has a profound impact on the mental health of all human beings. The most common psychological impact being anxiety, probably because of overloaded and inadequate information. Pregnant women also have a major concern for transmission of infection to their child and its consequences on the baby if they will be infected during pregnancy. The other matters affecting the parents are the inability to do regular antenatal checkups because of the infection and imposed lockdown, and unavailability of facilities.

Studies have shown that there is approximately a 35% chance of increased anxiety, 18% depression, and 11% for stress.[33,34]

TAKE-HOME POINTS

1. Women and men are at equal risk of developing a psychiatric disorder, but there are some gender-specific differences in prevalence, clinical presentation, course, and treatment of the illness.
2. Prevalence of mood disorder is particularly more in women at times of reproductive transition.
3. Premenstrual dysphoric disorder responds to SSRIs.
4. The mental health of a woman is essential for the health and well-being of a child.
5. Decisions regarding psychotropic use should be based on assessment and balancing of risk and benefit.
6. Up to 60% of women with bipolar disorder need mood stabilizers as there is relapse when discontinued.
7. Comprehensive and careful assessment of psychological, genetic, reproductive, medical and psychosocial risks is essential for treating psychiatric disorders in women.

REFERENCES

1. Sadock BJ, Sadock VA. Kaplan and Sadock's Comprehensive Textbook of Psychiatry. Philadelphia: Lippincott Williams and Wilkins; 2000.
2. Carlini SV, Deligiannidis KM. Evidence-based treatment of premenstrual dysphoric disorder: a concise review. J Clin Psychiatry. 2020;81(2):19ac13071.
3. Šebela A, Hanka J, Mohr P. Diagnostics and modern trends in therapy of postpartum depression. Ceska Gynekol. 2019;84(1):68-72.
4. Pariente G, Broder OW, Sheiner E, Battat TL, Mazor E, Salem SY, et al. Risk for probable post-partum depression among women during the COVID-19 pandemic. Arch Womens Ment Health. 2020;23(6):767-73.
5. Takács L, Kandrnal V, Kaňková Š, Bartoš F, Mudrák J. The effects of pre-and post-partum depression on child behavior and psychological development from birth to pre-school age: a protocol for a systematic review and meta-analysis. Syst Rev. 2020;9(1):146.
6. Guille C, Newman R, Fryml LD, Lifton CK, Epperson CN. Management of postpartum depression. J Midwifery Womens Health. 2013;58(6):643-53.
7. Gilden J, Kamperman AM, Munk-Olsen T, Hoogendijk WJ, Kushner SA, Bergink V. Long-term outcomes of postpartum psychosis: a systematic review and meta-analysis. J Clin Psychiatry. 2020;81(2):19r12906.
8. Teodorescu A, Dima L, Popa MA, Moga MA, Bîgiu NF, Ifteni P. Antipsychotics in postpartum psychosis. Am J Ther; 2020.
9. Kapfhammer HP, Reininghaus EZ, Fitz W, Lange P. Clinical course of illness in women with early onset puerperal psychosis: a 12-year follow-up study. J Clin Psychiatry. 2014;75(10):1096-104.
10. Khan SJ, Fersh ME, Ernst C, Klipstein K, Albertini ES, Lusskin SI. Bipolar disorder in pregnancy and postpartum: principles of management. Curr Psychiatry Rep. 2016;18(2):13.
11. Maki PM, Kornstein SG, Joffe H, Bromberger JT, Freeman EW, Athappilly G, et al. Guidelines for the evaluation and treatment of perimenopausal depression: summary and recommendations. J Womens Health (Larchmt). 2019;28(2):117-34.
12. Yazdi HZ, Sharbaf HA, Kareshki H, Amirian M. Infertility and psychological and social health of Iranian infertile women: a systematic review. Iran J Psychiatry. 2020;15(1):67-79.
13. Horvath S, Schreiber CA. Unintended pregnancy, induced abortion, and mental health. Curr Psychiatry Rep. 2017;19(11):77.
14. Schaffir J, Worly BL, Gur TL. Combined hormonal contraception and its effects on mood: a critical review. Eur J Contracept Reprod Health Care. 2016;21(5):347-55.
15. Taylor DM, Barnes TR, Young AH. The Maudsley Prescribing Guidelines in Psychiatry, 13th edition. John Wiley and Sons; 2018.
16. Breadon C, Kulkarni J. An update on medication management of women with schizophrenia in pregnancy. Expert Opin Pharmacother. 2019;20(11):1365-76.

17. Abel KM, Drake R, Goldstein JM. Sex differences in schizophrenia. Int Rev Psychiatry. 2010;22(5):417-28.
18. Sramek JJ, Murphy MF, Cutler NR. Sex differences in the psychopharmacological treatment of depression. Dialogues Clin Neurosci. 2016;18(4):447-57.
19. Clark CT, Wisner KL. Treatment of peripartum bipolar disorder. Obstet Gynecol Clin North Am. 2018;45(3):403-17.
20. Gdańska P, Drozdowicz-Jastrzębska E, Grzechocińska B, Radziwon-Zaleska M, Węgrzyn P, Wielgoś M. Anxiety and depression in women undergoing infertility treatment. Ginekol Pol. 2017;88(2):109-12.
21. Frazer Z, McConnell K, Jansson LM. Treatment for substance use disorders in pregnant women: motivators and barriers. Drug Alcohol Depend. 2019;205:107652.
22. Arnold C, Johnson H, Mahon C, Agius M. The effects of eating disorders in pregnancy on mother and baby: a review. Psychiatr Danub. 2019;31(Suppl 3):615-8.
23. Treasure J, Duarte TA, Schmidt U. Eating disorders. Lancet. 2020;395(10227):899-911.
24. Kwak A, Jacobs J, Haggett D, Jimenez R, Peppercorn J. Evaluation and management of insomnia in women with breast cancer. Breast Cancer Res Treat. 2020;181(2):269-77.
25. Damone AL, Joham AE, Loxton D, Earnest A, Teede HJ, Moran LJ. Depression, anxiety and perceived stress in women with and without PCOS: a community-based study. Psychol Med. 2019;49(9):1510-20.
26. Cooney LG, Dokras A. Depression and anxiety in polycystic ovary syndrome: etiology and treatment. Curr Psychiatry Rep. 2017;19(11):83.
27. Teede HJ, Misso ML, Costello MF, Dokras A, Laven J, Moran L, et al. Recommendations from the international evidence-based guideline for the assessment and management of polycystic ovary syndrome. Fertil Steril. 2018;110(3):364-79.
28. Brutocao C, Zaiem F, Alsawas M, Morrow AS, Murad MH, Javed A. Psychiatric disorders in women with polycystic ovary syndrome: a systematic review and meta-analysis. Endocrine. 2018;62(2):318-25.
29. Rodriguez-Paris D, Remlinger-Molenda A, Kurzawa R, Głowińska A, Spaczyński R, Rybakowski F, et al. Psychiatric disorders in women with polycystic ovary syndrome. Psychiatr Pol. 2019;53(4):955-66.
30. Viswanathan LG, Satishchandra P, Bhimani BC, Reddy JY, Rama Murthy BS, Subbakrishna DK, et al. Polycystic ovary syndrome in patients on antiepileptic drugs. Ann Indian Acad Neurol. 2016;19(3):339-43.
31. Yeh YC, Huang SF, Lu CH. Correlation among anxiety, depression, and quality of life in women with gynecologic cancer. Hu Li Za Zhi. 2019;66(6):43-53.
32. Manne SL, Kashy DA, Virtue S, Criswell KR, Kissane DW, Ozga M, et al. Acceptance, social support, benefit-finding, and depression in women with gynecological cancer. Qual Life Res. 2018;27(11):2991-3002.
33. Rasgon N. The relationship between polycystic ovary syndrome and antiepileptic drugs: a review of the evidence. J Clin Psychopharmacol. 2004;24(3):322-34.
34. Ng QJ, Koh KM, Tagore S, Mathur M. Perception and feelings of antenatal women during COVID-19 pandemic: a cross-sectional survey. Ann Acad Med Singap. 2020;49(8):543-52.

CHAPTER 5

Interface with Rheumatology

Sandeep Grover, Anish Shouan

ABSTRACT

The rheumatoid arthritis (RA) was included as one of the seven psychosomatic disorders in the original description of "holy seven" by Alexander. Over the years with the improvement in the understanding of various rheumatological disorders, there is also an improvement in understanding about the prevalence of various psychiatric disorders in patients with rheumatic diseases, especially systemic lupus erythematosus (SLE) and RA. Available data suggest a wide range of psychiatric morbidity in patients with SLE and RA, with depression and anxiety disorders being the most commonly reported morbidities. SLE is also characterized by neuropsychiatric SLE. The medications, especially corticosteroids used for management for various rheumatological diseases are also associated with a wide range of psychiatric manifestations. Assessment of psychiatric disorders in patients with rheumatological diseases involves detailed evaluation for the type, severity, and cause of the disorder. Management of various psychiatric disorders needs to take into consideration the severity of physical illness, complications, ongoing medications, and comorbid illnesses. Psychotropics should be used judiciously with regular monitoring of the patients.

INTRODUCTION

Rheumatological diseases have been long recognized to have been associated with psychiatric disorders. The original description of "holy seven" psychosomatic disorders by Alexander included rheumatoid arthritis (RA) as one of the prototypes of psychosomatic diseases.[1] Over the years, the nomenclature of rheumatic diseases has broadened. Rheumatic diseases include autoimmune disorders involving the musculoskeletal system. Some of the commonly encountered rheumatic diseases in the clinical practice include RA, systemic lupus erythematosus (SLE), osteoarthritis (OA), psoriatic arthritis (PA), ankylosing spondylitis (AS), gouty arthritis, scleroderma, Sjögren's syndrome (SS), polymyositis, and dermatomyositis.

Compared to other medical diseases, evaluation of psychiatric issues in patients with rheumatic diseases is more challenging for the psychiatrist because of their multifaceted and variable clinical features.[2] Patients with various rheumatological diseases can present with a wide range of psychiatric disorders. The disease state influences the psychiatric presentations (acute illness vs. patients in clinical remission), and the type of the underlying rheumatic disease. Besides the underlying biological underpinnings explaining the psychiatric morbidity in patients with rheumatological diseases, social factors, personality features, the doctor-patient relationship between the rheumatologist and the patient, opportunistic infections, concurrent medical illnesses and treatments, complications of the primary rheumatological disease and the medications used for the treatment of various rheumatological diseases, also contribute to the development of various psychological morbidities.[2] This chapter attempts to evaluate the interface between psychiatry and rheumatology.

EPIDEMIOLOGY OF PSYCHIATRIC MORBIDITY IN PATIENTS WITH RHEUMATOLOGICAL DISEASES

The epidemiology of various psychiatric disorders in patients with various rheumatological diseases varies widely, depending on the assessment methods (use of screening or diagnostic instruments), disease severity, and the type of psychiatric morbidity assessed (single disorder or a whole range of disorders being evaluated).

A systematic review and meta-analysis, which included 72 studies and data of 13,189 patients, showed that researchers used 43 methods to define depression in patients with RA. The prevalence of depression ranged from 0.04 to 66.3%. The prevalence of major depression as per the Diagnostic and Statistical Manual of Mental Disorders (DSM) diagnostic criteria was estimated to be 16.8% (95% CI: 10–24%) and that of dysthymia was 18.7% (95% CI: -2–39%). However, when the authors considered the specific scales, the prevalence of depression was 38.8% when evaluated by using Patient Health Questionnaire-9 (PHQ-9). According to Hospital Anxiety and Depression Scale (HADS), the prevalence of depression was 34.2% when the cutoff of 8 was used, and this prevalence reduced to 14.8% when the cutoff of 11 was used.[3] Overall data suggested that lower age was associated with a higher prevalence of depression.[3] One large sample size study (n = 1,026) based on population-based administrative data from Canada reported that various psychiatric disorders' incidence was higher in patients with RA than controls. The incidence rate ratio (IRR) of depression over the study period was 1.46 (95% CI: 1.35–1.58), and the same for anxiety disorder was 1.24 (95% CI: 1.15–1.34), and bipolar disorder was 1.21 (95% CI: 1.00–1.47). However, the IRR (0.96; 95% CI: 0.61–1.50) for schizophrenia was comparable to the control group. There was a minimal decline in the incidence of psychiatric disorders over time.[4] The prevalence of anxiety disorders in patients with RA in different studies ranges from 13 to 70%.[5-7]

Neuropsychiatric manifestations are considered as part and parcel of diagnostic criteria of SLE, with neuropsychiatric manifestations seen in two-thirds of the patients with SLE.[8] In a large sample study (n = 384), authors reported prevalence of neuropsychiatric manifestations in 64.4% of patients with cognitive deficits (49.33%) being the most common neuropsychiatric manifestation, followed by lupus headache (23.11%, with more than half of the patients having tension-type), psychoses (12.00%), seizures (10.67%), and cerebrovascular events (9.78%).[9] Based on the prevalence of various clinical and laboratory parameters, authors suggested that the diagnosis of neuropsychiatric SLE (NPSLE) should be considered when the patient has at least one of the features from the first group of criteria (seizures, psychosis, cerebrovascular event, lesion of cranial nerves, motor disturbances, quantitative alterations of consciousness) and at least two indicators from the second group of criteria [cognitive dysfunction, headache due to lupus, peripheral neuropathy, magnetic resonance imaging changes, electroencephalogram changes, electroneuromyography changes, positive antireplication protein A (aRPA), positive anti-phospholipid (aPL) antibodies after ruling out other causes (except for SLE)].[9]

Besides, the NPSLE, available data also suggest a high prevalence of other psychiatric disorders in patients with SLE. Many systematic reviews have assessed the prevalence of depression and anxiety in patients with SLE.[10,11] A recent systematic review and meta-analysis included 59 studies, which included 10,928 adult patients with SLE. This review suggested that different studies have used 35 methods to assess depression, whereas the researchers used 13 methods to assess anxiety. The prevalence of depression in different studies varies from 2 to 91.7%. The prevalence of depression as per the DSM or International Classification of Diseases (ICD) criteria in patients with SLE is 24% (95% CI: 16–31%). Additionally, the prevalence of dysthymia is 12%, and adjustment disorder is 20%.[11] In terms of the prevalence of depression as per the various scales, the prevalence as per HADS was 30% (95% CI: 22–38%) when the cutoff of 8 was used, and the prevalence was 38% (95% CI: 32–44%) when the assessment of depression on Center for Epidemiologic Studies Depression Scale (CES-D) was considered. In terms of the Beck Depression Inventory, the prevalence of depression was 39% (95% CI: 29–49%).[11] The prevalence of anxiety in patients with SLE ranged from 4 to 85%, with the pooled prevalence in the meta-analysis being 37% as per DSM/ICD criteria, whereas it was 40% (95% CI: 30–49%) as per HADS with the cutoff of 8 (Zhang et al., 2017).[11] Further, the meta-analysis revealed that the prevalence of depression was higher in recent studies.[11] Another review suggested that the prevalence of mood disorders is higher among those with active disease than those with inactive disease.[10] Studies have also reported delirium in about one-sixth of patients during the acute phase of SLE.[12] Case reports have also documented the occurrence of catatonia in patients with SLE.[13]

Available data for other rheumatological disorders also suggest a high prevalence of depression and anxiety in patients with these diseases. One study estimated the prevalence of anxiety to be 48% and depression to be 32% in patients with primary SS.[14] Similarly, the prevalence of depression in patients with AS has been estimated to be 18%.[15]

Patients with various rheumatological diseases also experience significant sleep problems. A review, which included 9 studies, reported that 55–85% of patients with SLE experience one or more sleep disorders. Further, it is suggested that the sleep disorders in patients with SLE are related to the disease activity, pain, and fatigue.[16,17]

CLINICAL CONDITIONS AT THE INTERFACE OF RHEUMATOLOGY AND PSYCHIATRY

Other conditions that lie at the interface of rheumatology and psychiatry include fatigue and chronic fatigue syndrome (CFS). Available data also suggest that besides depression and anxiety, there is a high prevalence of fatigue in patients with various rheumatological disorders. It is suggested that a significant proportion of patients with fatigue have underlying psychiatric disorders.[18] The CFS is named differently, and it is characterized by significant debilitating fatigue and a combination of symptoms (impaired memory and concentration, postexertional malaise, unrefreshing sleep, muscle pain, pain in multiple joints without swelling or redness, headache, sore throat, and tender axillary or cervical lymph nodes) resulting in a substantial reduction in occupational, personal, social, and educational status.[19] CFS is said to be commonly misdiagnosed as depression.[19] Another issue that is important to understand in patients with the rheumatological disease is the role of psychological factors and psychiatric comorbidity in expression and perception of pain. It is well known that anxiety, depression, and sleep disturbances and other adverse psychosocial factors can influence the pain perception and the patients with rheumatological diseases can have noninflammatory pain.[17]

RHEUMATOLOGICAL CONDITIONS PRESENTING WITH PSYCHIATRIC DISORDERS

The clinicians should keep in mind that, at times, psychiatric manifestations may be the first set of symptoms in patients with rheumatological diseases. Due to this, the patients often visit the psychiatrist first rather than the rheumatologist. Consideration of underlying SLE is important in patients presenting with first-episode psychosis or catatonia.[20-23] The psychosis in patients with SLE can also mimic schizophrenia or schizoaffective disorder.[24,25] Hence, when a young patient, presents with first-episode psychosis/schizophrenia and catatonia, a thorough physical examination needs to be conducted to look for features of SLE, and if required, the clinician should order diagnostic tests.

The roles of autoimmune factors in the manifestation of obsessive-compulsive disorders are well known. Patients with pediatric autoimmune neuropsychiatric disorders associated with streptococcal infection (PANDAS) and pediatric acute-onset neuropsychiatric syndrome (PANS) can present to the psychiatrists with features of tics, obsessive-compulsive behavior, and other neuropsychiatric symptoms.[26,27] Other symptoms of PANS/PANDAS can include eating restrictions, anxiety (particularly separation anxiety), emotional lability or depression; irritability, aggression, and/or severely oppositional behaviors, attention-deficit/hyperactivity disorder (ADHD)-like behaviors, memory deficits, and cognitive changes leading to poor scholastic performance, sensory or motor abnormalities; sleep disturbances, enuresis, or urinary frequency.[28] Hence, in all children presenting with acute-onset neuropsychiatric symptoms, the clinician should consider a possibility of PANS/PANDAS and the clinician should order appropriate investigations.

PSYCHOSOCIAL OUTCOMES IN PATIENTS WITH RHEUMATOLOGICAL DISORDERS

Besides psychiatric disorders, various rheumatological disorders are also associated with adverse psychosocial outcomes because of the chronic nature of the illnesses, which are characterized by multiple relapses. Many patients report not being able to live a normal life,[29] experiencing body image disturbance,[30,31] stigma,[32,33] loneliness,[34] social isolation,[33] low self-esteem,[35] demoralization,[36] poor quality of life,[37] and sexual dysfunction.[38]

IMPACT OF STRESS AND PSYCHIATRIC DISORDERS ON THE COURSE OF RHEUMATOLOGICAL DISEASES

One of the major reasons for the relapse of SLE is considered to be poor adherence to medications. Besides poor medication adherence, other factors associated with the flare-up of the disease activity include psychological stress.[39] Available studies also suggest that the presence of psychiatric morbidity in patients with SLE and other rheumatological diseases are associated with poor medication adherence,[40] suggesting an indirect role of psychiatric disorders in the relapse of rheumatological diseases. Further, the data also shows the dose-response relationship with a higher level of nonadherence in patients with higher severity of depression.[41] On the other hand, poor medication adherence has also been shown to be associated with a higher number of outpatient, primary care, and emergency department visits.[40] Sleep disturbances, depression, and anxiety can influence the perception of the pain.[17]

CAUSAL ASSOCIATION OF PSYCHIATRIC DISORDERS IN PATIENTS WITH RHEUMATOLOGICAL DISEASES

As with other medical diseases, the psychiatric symptoms/disorders in patients with various rheumatological diseases could be due to the same etiology as the primary rheumatological disorder, could be due to the psychological reaction to the illness or burden due to illness could be due to complications of the primary illness, and could be due to the medications used for management of various rheumatological diseases. It is also possible for both psychiatric disorders and rheumatological diseases to coexist with no specific causal association **(Box 1)**.

There is a bidirectional relationship between various psychiatric disorders, psychosocial factors, and manifestations of rheumatological diseases. The role of inflammation is well known in various psychiatric disorders, which are considered to be at the core of all rheumatological diseases. It is suggested that in patients with rheumatological diseases, alteration in the inflammatory markers impacts the brain. Chronic inflammation leads to impairment in the normal physiological stress responses and results in psychiatric symptoms. The inflammatory changes also directly influence the brain and lead to the development of psychiatric manifestations.[16] Sleep disturbances can influence the perception of the pain, inflammatory response, and the levels of various cytokines.[17]

BOX 1: Reasons for psychiatric morbidity in patients with rheumatological diseases.

- *Psychiatric symptoms due to same etiological factors and integral part of rheumatological diseases:* The features of neuropsychiatric SLE are considered to be the outcome of the same underlying etiology as for other features of SLE
- *Psychiatric symptoms as a result of psychological reaction to the illness or burden due to illness:* Development of chronic disabling and disfiguring illness can lead to significant psychological reactions and, in the long run, can be burdensome for the patients
- *Psychiatric symptoms due to treatment agents of rheumatological diseases:* The various treatment modalities used for the management of rheumatological disorders can give rise to psychiatric manifestations, for example, steroids can give rise to a wide range of psychiatric manifestations
- *Psychiatric symptoms due to complications of rheumatological diseases:* The involvement of multiple organs in patients with SLE can lead to organ failure, and infections; these can lead to the development of delirium
- *No association of psychiatric disorders and rheumatological diseases:* Both the conditions coexist and run independent courses

PSYCHIATRIC EVALUATION IN PATIENTS WITH RHEUMATOLOGICAL DISEASES

Considering the high prevalence of psychiatric disorders in patients with various rheumatological diseases, it is essential to evaluate all the patients with various rheumatological diseases for psychiatric disorders, and adverse psychosocial outcomes. Hence, all patients with rheumatological disorders should be screened for psychiatric morbidity and adverse psychosocial outcomes throughout the course of illness. Besides the obvious psychiatric manifestations reported by the patients and their caregivers, which require psychiatric assessment, the patients presenting with frequent relapses of illnesses, especially due to poor medication adherence should also be assessed for psychiatric morbidity.

A mental health professional may be involved in the care of a patient with rheumatological disease, when the patient presents with acute symptoms of the primary illness, or when the patient is not responding adequately to the treatment (e.g., a patient with RA not responding adequately to the pain killers). As it is not possible to refer all the patients with various rheumatological diseases to the mental health professionals, the rheumatologists can screen their patients for common mental disorders such as depression, anxiety, sleep disorders, and delirium by using a simple screening questionnaire and those found to screen positive, can be referred to the mental health professionals. Further, considering the chronic nature of the illness, the mental health assessment should be an ongoing process rather than just a one-time assessment.

At every stage, the mental health professionals should carry out a thorough assessment **(Box 2)** to understand the type of psychiatric morbidity, the severity of psychiatric morbidity, the possible cause of psychiatric manifestations, the role of psychiatric/psychological factors in the manifestation of the primary rheumatological disease. The mental health professional should also focus on other psychological issues, which may be arising due to the primary rheumatological illness, and the relationship/therapeutic alliance of patient/family with the treating physician. A careful review of treatment history can provide important clues about the association of the psychiatric symptoms with the medication.

While considering a psychiatric disorder, the possibility of a medication-induced disorder should always be kept in mind, especially steroids. Steroids are known to be associated with a wide range of psychiatric disorders in the form of psychosis, mood disorders (hypomania, mania, mixed states, depression), suicidal behavior, anxiety and

> **BOX 2:** Psychiatric assessment of patients with rheumatological diseases.
> - Assess the premorbid personality and previous psychiatric history
> - Assess the type of symptoms, the severity of symptoms, level of dysfunction and disability, and suicidality
> - Assess the severity and extent of the primary rheumatological illness (e.g., a patient having an acute flare of systemic lupus erythematosus can have neuropsychiatric SLE)
> - Assess for the relationship of onset of psychiatric symptoms with the severity of physical illness, change in status of the illness, complications, and changes in medications
> - Evaluate for comorbid physical illnesses, as these can also contribute to the development of psychiatric disorders
> - *Understand other psychological issues, social issues, and outcomes:* Perceived loss by the patient and family due to the rheumatological illness, body image issues, stigma, isolation, sexual dysfunction, demoralization, selfesteem, quality of life, disability, coping mechanisms
> - Evaluate for comorbid substance dependence, medication adherence, medication abuse
> - Relationship/therapeutic alliance of patient/family with the treating physician
> - Mental status examination
> - Review the treatment chart and available investigations

panic disorder, delirium, agitation, aggression, catatonia, insomnia, depersonalization, isolated cognitive impairments (impaired attention, concentration, memory, and word-finding difficulties), and reversible dementia.[42-44] Additionally, the steroids may also lead to drug dependency and psychiatric manifestations during the withdrawal phase.[45,46] It is generally suggested that the incidence of psychiatric manifestations in patients receiving steroids is high with the use of higher doses, use of steroids for a longer duration[47] and during the initial phase of steroids (usually 1 day to 2 months).[42]

While establishing the association of psychiatric disorders with medications, the mental health professionals should take into account the temporal relationship between drug exposure and the development of psychiatric side effect, response to the withdrawal of drug, presence or absence of alternative explanations for symptoms (e.g., disease, other drugs) and the effect of rechallenge with the same drug.[48] If there is a temporal correlation between the use of medications, lack of other alternative explanations and withdrawal of medication leads to amelioration of symptoms, the possibility of medication-induced psychiatric disorders is high. If the clinicians are unsure about establishing the association of medication and psychiatric manifestation, they can rely on the Naranjo's Scale[49] or the World Health Organization and Uppsala Monitoring Centre Scale to establish the association.[50]

Besides steroids, other immunosuppressants and immunomodulators are also associated with psychiatric manifestations.

CONSIDER RHEUMATOLOGICAL DISEASES IN PATIENTS PRESENTING WITH PSYCHIATRIC MANIFESTATIONS

The usual clinical dictum to rule out underlying organic conditions applies to all psychiatric disorders. While evaluating underlying organic conditions, rheumatological diseases should always be considered. As discussed earlier, many patients with rheumatological and immunological diseases can also present with psychiatric manifestations as the first clinical feature. Hence, in all patients presenting with acute-onset neuropsychiatric syndromes for the first time in life, the possibility of underlying rheumatological diseases, especially SLE or other immunological diseases, must be considered. Appropriate investigations must be carried out in liaison with the rheumatologist to rule out the possible diseases.

MANAGEMENT OF PSYCHIATRIC DISORDERS IN PATIENTS WITH RHEUMATOLOGICAL DISEASES

Management of psychiatric disorders in patients with various rheumatological diseases requires a multidisciplinary approach. The management of psychiatric issues can be understood under the headings of general principles, pharmacological management, and nonpharmacological management.

General Principle

There is a need to establish a close liaison with the treating physician to understand the severity of the primary illness, need for the ongoing medications, and their further course of action. If the psychiatric manifestations are considered to be an outcome of the ongoing medications, a clear communication with the treating physician helps understand the possibility of reducing or changing the doses of medications. Additionally, a close liaison with the treating physician can also help the mental health professionals in understanding the severity of illness, possible outcome or prognosis, and their understanding of the patients' psychological reaction to the illness. The liaison can also facilitate in informing the clinician about the patients' psychological reaction to the illness, and conveying the expectations of the patients from the treatment and the clinician. This can, in the long run, improve the therapeutic alliance of the patient and the primary clinician.

In general, it is important to remember that the psychiatric morbidity should not be undertreated as it can have significant negative consequences for the underlying physical illness.

Further, mild symptoms should initially be managed with nonpharmacological interventions. Moderate to severe symptoms should be managed with pharmacological agents. However, if the psychiatric symptoms are severe and life-threatening, then the clinician should consider electroconvulsive therapy (ECT) (i.e., catatonia not responding to lorazepam, severe depression not responding to antidepressants, presence of risk of suicide, etc.).

Pharmacological Management of Psychiatric Disorders

The pharmacological management of various psychiatric disorders in patients with rheumatological diseases should follow the usual guidelines for the management of these disorders in terms of selection of medications.[51-53] However, while implementing the various pharmacological measures, additional principles of use of psychotropics in medically ill should be kept in mind.[54] Patients with SLE may have involvement of the central nervous system, renal system, eyes, skin, cardiopulmonary system, gastrointestinal system, joints, and blood cells. The involvement of some of these organs can influence the pharmacokinetics and pharmacodynamics of psychotropic medications.

Additionally, the risk of bleeding must be kept in mind, while using psychotropic in patients with SLE and those receiving non-steroidal anti-inflammatory drugs (NSAIDs). Similarly, the high risk of development of diabetes mellitus must be kept in mind while considering antipsychotics in patients who are already on steroids. Another important aspect to consider is the possibility of cumulative or similar side effects, while choosing psychotropics in patients with rheumatological diseases, such as QTc prolongation with concomitant use of hydroxychloroquine and antipsychotics.[55]

It is always advisable to carry out basic investigations in all medically ill patients before starting psychotropic medications. The investigation battery should include a complete hemogram (including bleeding and clotting time if felt so), renal function test, liver function test, fasting blood glucose levels, serum electrolytes, and electrocardiogram. Other investigations should be decided based on the underlying rheumatological illnesses and the specific psychotropic medications being considered. The factors to be considered before considering a psychotropic agent are listed in **Box 3**. The basic principles to be followed while using psychotropics are listed in **Box 4**.

While selecting various antidepressants, it is important to remember that certain class(es) of antidepressants have nociceptive properties and can have an additional advantage in the management of pain. However, it is to be remembered that the use of antidepressants only for the management of pain (in the absence of depression or anxiety) in patients with RA is not supported by the available evidence.[57]

BOX 3: Issues to be considered while choosing psychotropic medications in patients with rheumatological conditions.

- Severity of rheumatological illness
- *Organs involvement:* Type of organ involved, level of decompensation
- *Associated symptoms of the rheumatological disease:* Pain, seizures
- *Psychiatric syndrome:* Severity, type of symptoms
- *Possible cause of psychiatric syndrome:* Primary disease per se, ongoing medications, psychological distress
- *Ongoing medications:* Type, side effects
- *Comorbid diseases:* Hepatic, cardiac
- *Investigation findings:* QTc interval, serum sodium levels, platelet count, and risk of bleeding
- Substance use, including overuse of opioids
- Associated pain symptoms
- Possible drug interactions between psychotropics and ongoing medications
- Side effects profile of psychotropics

> **BOX 4:** Basic principles of psychopharmacology in patients with medical illnesses.[56]
> - Maintain close liaison with the physician and discuss the starting of medications, the expected side effects of medications and the safety issues
> - Start with a lower dose and increase the doses slowly, with close monitoring of psychopathology, investigations, and severity of the primary illness
> - Starting dose should be about half the normal starting dose in adults and one-fourth of the normal starting dose in elderly and children
> - Maintain a close follow-up
> - Repeat investigations before increasing the dose, e.g., serum electrolytes should be repeated before increasing the dose of selective serotonin reuptake inhibitors
> - Stop the medications whenever possible, e.g., if the delirium has resolved

Medication-associated psychiatric manifestations require special consideration. If it is felt that the psychiatric syndrome could be related to the ongoing medication, e.g., steroids, then the history should be more thoroughly reviewed to establish the same. However, it is important to remember that the diagnosis is always provisional initially, and it is confirmed by the resolution of symptoms with the stoppage of the offending agent. If a provisional diagnosis is considered that the same should be discussed with the primary team, and the possibility of stoppage (and switching to alternate agents) or reduction in the dose of medication needs to be considered. If any of this is not possible, then the use of psychotropics needs to be considered. If the psychotropics are considered for management of drug-induced psychiatric manifestations then the duration of use of psychotropics should take into account the duration of use, changes in the doses of the offending agent with time and the psychotropics must be stopped with the stoppage of the offending agent. Further, attempts also must be made to stop the psychotropics with the reduction in the doses of offending agents.

Another important aspect of pharmacological management is addressing the issues of NPSLE. If the neuropsychiatric manifestations are related to the underlying illness, it is important to remember that these symptoms will improve with treating underlying illness with steroids, cyclophosphamide, methotrexate, hydroxychloroquine, and rituximab.[58] However, if the NPSLE symptoms are severe, disruptive, and life-threatening, then the use of psychotropics must be considered.

Nonpharmacological Management of Psychiatric Disorders and Psychological Issues

Clinicians should preferably manage patients with mild symptoms with only nonpharmacological measures. Those with moderate-to-severe disorders should receive a combination of pharmacological and nonpharmacological treatments. Additionally, patients presenting with significant psychological issues not amounting to a psychiatric disorder should also be considered nonpharmacological treatments. These patients usually benefit from supportive psychotherapy and psychoeducation about the illness. All patients with diagnosed psychiatric disorders should also receive appropriate psychoeducation about their disorder.

The selection of the specific nonpharmacological measure is based on the type of psychiatric disorder, ease of the therapist in implementing the same and cooperation of the patient. Patients with mild to moderate depression can benefit from supportive psychotherapy, interpersonal therapy, or cognitive behavioral therapy. Cognitive behavioral therapy, guided imagery, diaphragmatic breathing, progressive muscle relaxation, and mindfulness-based stress reduction strategies can be used by clinicians to manage pain management strategies. Available evidence suggests that various psychosocial interventions in patients with SLE lead to a reduction in the level of anxiety, depression, stress, and disease activity.[59]

The evidence also suggests that when the evidence-based psychosocial interventions incorporate both social support and health education, these lead to a reduction in pain, improvement in functioning, and delaying of disability.[60]

Somatic Treatment for Psychiatric Disorders

As mentioned earlier, in patients with catatonia not responding to lorazepam, ECT may be considered. Case reports suggest the beneficial effect of ECT in patients with catatonia in the background of SLE.[13]

CONCLUSION

Psychiatric disorders are highly prevalent in patients with various rheumatological diseases. The psychiatric disorders in patients with rheumatological diseases could be due to the primary physical illness, use of medications for the management of the rheumatological diseases, complications arising due to the rheumatological diseases, and the adverse psychosocial impact of the illness on the sufferers. Hence, it is important that all patients with rheumatological diseases should undergo a frequent psychiatric evaluation to address the various psychiatric disorders and the emerging psychological issues, which adversely impact the outcome of the rheumatological disease. Management of psychiatric disorders should take into consideration the type of illness, associated complications, ongoing medications, and their side effects. When psychotropics are used, the patients should be closely monitored.

REFERENCES

1. Alexander F. Psychosomatic Medicine: Its Principles and Applications. New York: WW Norton and Company; 1950.
2. Moran MG. Psychiatric aspects of rheumatology. Psychiatr Clin North Am. 1996;19:575-87.
3. Matcham F, Rayner L, Steer S, Hotopf M. The prevalence of depression in rheumatoid arthritis: a systematic review and meta-analysis. Rheumatology (Oxford). 2013;52:2136-48.
4. Marrie RA, Hitchon CA, Walld R, Patten SB, Bolton JM, Sareen J, et al. Increased burden of psychiatric disorders in rheumatoid arthritis. Arthritis Care Res (Hoboken). 2018;70(7):970-8.
5. Isik A, Koca SS, Ozturk A, Mermi O. Anxiety and depression in patients with rheumatoid arthritis. Clin Rheumatol. 2007;26:872-8.
6. Lok EY, Mok CC, Cheng CW, Cheung EF. Prevalence and determinants of psychiatric disorders in patients with rheumatoid arthritis. Psychosomatics. 2010;51:338-e8.
7. VanDyke MM, Parker JC, Smarr KL, Hewett JE, Johnson GE, Slaughter JR, et al. Anxiety in rheumatoid arthritis. Arthritis Rheum. 2004;51:408-12.
8. Brey RL, Holliday SL, Saklad AR, Navarrete MG, Hermosillo-Romo D, Stallworth CL, et al. Neuropsychiatric syndromes in lupus: prevalence using standardized definitions. Neurology. 2002;58(8):1214-20.
9. Monov S, Monova D. Classification criteria for neuropsychiatric systemic lupus erythematosus: do they need a discussion? Hippokratia. 2008; 12:103-7.
10. Asano NM, Coriolano MD, Asano BJ, Lins OG. Psychiatric comorbidities in patients with systemic lupus erythematosus: a systematic review of the last 10 years. Rev Bras Reumatol. 2013;53(5):431-7.
11. Zhang L, Fu T, Yin R, Zhang Q, Shen B. Prevalence of depression and anxiety in systemic lupus erythematosus: a systematic review and meta-analysis. BMC Psychiatry. 2017;17(1):70.
12. Katsumata Y, Harigai M, Kawaguchi Y, Fukasawa C, Soejima M, Takagi K, et al. Diagnostic reliability of cerebral spinal fluid tests for acute confusional state (delirium) in patients with systemic lupus erythematosus: interleukin-6 (IL-6), IL-8, interferon-alpha, IgG index, and Q-albumin. J Rheumatol. 2007;34(10):2010-7.
13. Grover S, Parakh P, Sharma A, Rao P, Modi M, Kumar A. Catatonia in systemic lupus erythematosus: a case report and review of literature. Lupus. 2013;22(6):634-8.

14. Valtýsdóttir ST, Gudbjörnsson B, Lindqvist U, Hällgren R, Hetta J. Anxiety and depression in patients with primary Sjögren's syndrome. J Rheumatol. 2000;27(1):165-9.
15. Webers C, Vanhoof L, Leue C, Boonen A, Köhler S. Depression in ankylosing spondylitis and the role of disease-related and contextual factors: a cross-sectional study. Arthritis Res Ther. 2019; 21(1):215.
16. Lwin MN, Serhal L, Holroyd C, Edwards CJ. Rheumatoid arthritis: the impact of mental health on disease: a narrative review. Rheumatol Ther. 2020;7(3):457-71.
17. Palagini L, Tani C, Mauri M, Carli L, Vagnani S, Bombardieri S, et al. Sleep disorders and systemic lupus erythematosus. Lupus. 2014;23(2):115-23.
18. Sandıkçı SC, Özbalkan Z. Fatigue in rheumatic diseases. Eur J Rheumatol. 2015;2(3):109-13.
19. Griffith JP, Zarrouf FA. A systematic review of chronic fatigue syndrome: don't assume it's depression. Prim Care Companion J Clin Psychiatry. 2008;10(2):120-8.
20. Hanly JG, Li Q, Su L, Urowitz MB, Gordon C, Bae SC, et al. Psychosis in systemic lupus erythematosus: results from an International Inception Cohort Study. Arthritis Rheumatol. 2019;71(2):281-9.
21. Pai S, Kramer N, Rosenstein ED. Malignant catatonia as the presenting manifestation of systemic lupus erythematosus. Bull Hosp Jt Dis (2013). 2020;78(2):146-52.
22. Pustilnik S, Trutia A. Catatonia as the presenting symptom in systemic lupus erythematosus. J Psychiatr Pract. 2011;17(3):217-21.
23. Ali A, Taj A, Uz-Zehra M. Lupus catatonia in a young girl who presented with fever and altered sensorium. Pak J Med Sci. 2014;30(2):446-8.
24. Siu BW, Chow HM, Kwok SS, Li OL, Koo ML, Poon PW. Systemic lupus erythematosus as a cause of first-episode psychosis in the second trimester of pregnancy. East Asian Arch Psychiatry. 2010;20(3):145-50.
25. Mack A, Pfeiffer C, Schneider EM, Bechter K. Schizophrenia or atypical lupus erythematosus with predominant psychiatric manifestations over 25 years: case analysis and review. Front Psychiatry. 2017;8:131.
26. Kurlan R, Kaplan EL. The pediatric autoimmune neuropsychiatric disorders associated with streptococcal infection (PANDAS) etiology for tics and obsessive-compulsive symptoms: hypothesis or entity? Practical considerations for the clinician. Pediatrics. 2004;113(4):883-6.
27. Lepri G, Rigante D, Bellando Randone S, Meini A, Ferrari A, Tarantino G, et al. Clinical-serological characterization and treatment outcome of a large cohort of Italian children with pediatric autoimmune neuropsychiatric disorder associated with streptococcal infection and pediatric acute neuropsychiatric syndrome. J Child Adolesc Psychopharmacol. 2019;29(8):608-14.
28. Thienemann M, Murphy T, Leckman J, Shaw R, Williams K, Kapphahn C, et al. Clinical management of pediatric acute-onset neuropsychiatric syndrome: Part I-Psychiatric and Behavioral Interventions. J Child Adolesc Psychopharmacol. 2017;27(7):566-73.
29. Ahlmén M, Nordenskiöld U, Archenholtz B, Thyberg I, Rönnqvist R, Lindén L, et al. Rheumatology outcomes: the patient's perspective. A multicentre focus group interview study of Swedish rheumatoid arthritis patients. Rheumatology (Oxford). 2005;44(1):105-10.
30. Zhou C, Shen B, Gao Q, Shen Y, Cai D, Gu Z, et al. Impact of rheumatoid arthritis on body image disturbance. Arch Rheumatol. 2019;34(1):79-87.
31. Jolly M, Pickard AS, Mikolaitis RA, Cornejo J, Sequeira W, Cash TF, et al. Body image in patients with systemic lupus erythematosus. Int J Behav Med. 2012;19(2):157-64.
32. Sehlo MG, Bahlas SM. Perceived illness stigma is associated with depression in female patients with systemic lupus erythematosus. J Psychosom Res. 2013;74(3):248-51.
33. Drenkard C, Aspey L, Bao G, Dunlop-Thomas C, Lim SS. Role of stigma and social isolation on depression in patients with chronic cutaneous lupus erythematosus. Lupus Sci Med. 2019; 6(Suppl 1):A178.
34. Brennan KA, Creaven AM. Living with invisible illness: social support experiences of individuals with systemic lupus erythematosus. Qual Life Res. 2016;25(5):1227-35.
35. Zhao Q, Chen H, Yan H, He Y, Zhu L, Fu W, et al. The correlations of psychological status, quality of life, self-esteem, social support and body image disturbance in Chinese patients with systemic lupus erythematosus. Psychol Health Med. 2018;23(7):779-87.
36. Katz RC, Flasher L, Cacciapaglia H, Nelson S. The psychosocial impact of cancer and lupus: a cross validation study that extends the generality of "benefit finding" in patients with chronic disease. J Behav Med. 2001;24:561-71.
37. Pascual-Ramos V, Contreras-Yáñez I, Valencia-Quiñones KR, Romero-Díaz J. Rheumatoid

arthritis patients achieved better quality of life than systemic lupus erythematosus patients at sustained remission. Clin Exp Rheumatol. 2018;36(4):619-26.
38. Jin Z, Yang C, Xiao C, Wang Z, Zhang S, Ren J. Systemic lupus erythematosus and risk of sexual dysfunction: a systematic review and meta-analysis. Lupus. 2021;30(2):238-47.
39. Kakati S, Teronpi R, Barman B. Frequency, pattern and determinants of flare in systemic lupus erythematosus: a study from North East India. The Egyptian Rheumatologist. 2015; 37:S55-9.
40. Julian LJ, Yelin E, Yazdany J, Panopalis P, Trupin L, Criswell LA, et al. Depression, medication adherence, and service utilization in systemic lupus erythematosus. Arthritis Rheum. 2009; 61(2):240-6.
41. Alsowaida N, Alrasheed M, Mayet A, Alsuwaida A, Omair MA. Medication adherence, depression and disease activity among patients with systemic lupus erythematosus. Lupus. 2018;27(2): 327-32.
42. Kenna HA, Poon AW, de los Angeles CP, Koran LM. Psychiatric complications of treatment with corticosteroids: review with case report. Psychiatry Clin Neurosci. 2011;65:549-60.
43. Bhangle SD, Kramer N, Rosenstein ED. Corticosteroid-induced neuropsychiatric disorders: review and contrast with neuropsychiatric lupus. Rheumatol Int. 2013;33:1923-32.
44. Fardet L, Petersen I, Nazareth I. Suicidal behavior and severe neuropsychiatric disorders following glucocorticoid therapy in primary care. Am J Psychiatry. 2012;169(5):491-7.
45. Fardet L, Nazareth I, Whitaker HJ, Petersen I. Severe neuropsychiatric outcomes following discontinuation of long-term glucocorticoid therapy: a cohort study. J Clin Psychiatry. 2013; 74;e281-6.
46. Dixon R, Christy N. On the various forms of corticosteroid withdrawal syndrome. Am J Med. 1980;68:224-30.
47. Curtis JR, Westfall AO, Allison J, Bijlsma JW, Freeman A, George V, et al. Population-based assessment of adverse events associated with long-term glucocorticoid use. Arthritis Rheum. 2006;55:420-6.
48. Tango RC. Psychiatric side effects of medications prescribed in internal medicine. Dialogues Clin Neurosci. 2003;5:155-65.
49. Naranjo C, Busto U, Sellers E, Sandor P, Ruiz I, Roberts E, et al. A method for estimating the probability of adverse drug reactions. Clin Pharmacol Ther. 1981;30:239-45.
50. World Health Organization. The use of the WHO-UMC system for standardized case causality assessment. Uppsala: The Uppsala Monitoring Centre. 2005:2-7.
51. Grover S, Avasthi A. Clinical practice guidelines for management of delirium in elderly. Indian J Psychiatry. 2018;60(Suppl 3):S329-40.
52. Grover S, Chakrabarti S, Kulhara P, Avasthi A. Clinical practice guidelines for management of schizophrenia. Indian J Psychiatry. 2017;59 (Suppl 1):S19-33.
53. Gautam S, Jain A, Gautam M, Vahia VN, Grover S. Clinical practice guidelines for the management of depression. Indian J Psychiatry. 2017;59 (Suppl 1): S34-50.
54. Robinson MJ, Levenson JL. The use of psychotropics in the medically ill. Curr Psychiatry Rep. 2000;2(3):247-55.
55. Rani S, Grover S, Mehra A, Sahoo S. Psychiatric implications of the use of hydroxychloroquine in COVID-19 patients. Indian J Pharmacol. 2020;52(3):229-31.
56. Sarkar S, Kate N, Grover S. Consultation-liaison psychiatry: psychopharmacology dos and don'ts. J Mental Health Hum Behav. 2012;17:72-83.
57. Richards BL, Whittle SL, Buchbinder R. Antidepressants for pain management in rheumatoid arthritis. Cochrane Database Syst Rev. 2011;(11): CD008920.
58. Fanouriakis A, Kostopoulou M, Alunno A, Aringer M, Bajema I, Boletis JN, et al. 2019 update of the EULAR recommendations for the management of systemic lupus erythematosus. Ann Rheum Dis. 2019;78(6):736-45.
59. Zhang J, Wei W, Wang CM. Effects of psychological interventions for patients with systemic lupus erythematosus: a systematic review and meta-analysis. Lupus. 2012;21(10):1077-87.
60. Williams EM, Egede L, Faith T, Oates J. Effective self-management interventions for patients with lupus: potential impact of peer mentoring. Am J Med Sci. 2017;353(6):580-92.

CHAPTER 6

Interface with Gastroenterology

Samir Kumar Praharaj, Sonia Shenoy

INTRODUCTION

Functional gastrointestinal disorders (also known as FGIDs) are syndromes that include a set of gastrointestinal (GI) symptoms that cluster together, in the absence of any structural disease. These are also called *"disorders of gut-brain interaction"*.[1] It comprises of a group of disorders that have visceral hypersensitivity, altered motility, changes in the mucosal and immune function, alteration of the gut microbiome, and changes in the central nervous system (CNS) processing of gut signals.[2]

The *Rome IV criteria* for FGIDs are based on symptoms **(Box 1)**. The classification of the disorders into anatomic regions (i.e., esophageal, gastroduodenal, bowel, biliary, and anorectal) presumes unifying features underlying diagnosis and management that relate to these organ locations. There are 33 adult and 20 pediatric FGIDs in Rome IV.[3] In the International Classification of Diseases, 10th Revision (ICD-10), these groups of disorders are classified under somatoform disorders, i.e., somatoform autonomic dysfunction and persistent somatoform pain disorder.[4] In the Diagnostic and Statistical Manual of Mental Disorders, 5th Edition (DSM-5), FGIDs are classified under somatic symptom disorder.[5] There is a shift in focus across specialties toward a positive diagnosis of FGIDs, rather than diagnoses of exclusion.

BOX 1: List of functional gastrointestinal disorders (FGIDs) as per Rome IV classification.

A	*Esophageal disorders*
A1	Functional chest pain
A2	Functional heartburn
A3	Reflux hypersensitivity
A4	Globus
A5	Functional dysphagia
B	*Gastroduodenal disorders*
B1	*Functional dyspepsia:* a. Postprandial distress syndrome b. Epigastric pain syndrome
B2	*Belching disorder:* a. Excessive supragastric belching b. Excessive gastric belching
B3	*Nausea and vomiting disorders:* a. Chronic nausea vomiting syndrome b. Cyclic vomiting syndrome c. Cannabinoid hyperemesis syndrome
B4	Rumination syndrome
C	*Bowel disorders*
C1	Irritable bowel syndrome IBS with predominant constipation IBS with predominant diarrhea IBS with mixed bowel habits IBS unclassified
C2	Functional constipation
C3	Functional diarrhea
C4	Functional abdominal bloating/distention
C5	Unspecified functional bowel disorder
C6	Opioid-induced constipation
D	*Centrally mediated disorders of gastrointestinal pain*
D1	Centrally mediated abdominal pain syndrome
D2	Narcotic bowel syndrome/Opioid-induced GI hyperalgesia

Contd...

Contd...

E	*Gallbladder and sphincter of Oddi (SO) disorders*
E1	*Biliary pain:* a. Functional gallbladder disorder b. Functional biliary SO disorder
E2	Functional pancreatic SO disorder
F	*Anorectal disorders*
F1	Fecal incontinence
F2	*Functional anorectal pain:* a. Levator ani syndrome b. Unspecified functional anorectal pain c. Proctalgia fugax
F3	*Functional defecation disorders:* a. Inadequate defecatory propulsion b. Dyssynergic defecation
G	*Childhood FGIDs: Neonate/Toddler*
G1	Infant regurgitation
G2	Rumination syndrome
G3	Cyclic vomiting syndrome
G4	Infant colic
G5	Functional diarrhea
G6	Infant dyschezia
G7	Functional constipation
H	*Childhood FGIDs: Child/Adolescent*
H1	*Functional nausea and vomiting disorders:* a. Cyclic vomiting syndrome b. Functional nausea and functional vomiting c. Rumination syndrome d. Aerophagia
H2	*Functional abdominal pain disorders:* a. Functional dyspepsia b. Irritable bowel syndrome c. Abdominal migraine d. Functional abdominal pain NOS
H3	*Functional defecation disorders:* a. Functional constipation b. Nonretentive fecal incontinence

(NOS: not otherwise stated)

These are chronic disorders leading to huge economic burden and poor quality of life. The cost of unnecessary diagnostic evaluations and time spent in consultations adversely impact the meagre health services available in developing countries.[6]

Functional gastrointestinal disorders have been documented throughout the human history, not only by the physicians but also by scholars from other fields. However, until recently, these groups of disorders were neglected, possibly because of absence of obvious pathology, and specifically a lack of conceptual framework to understand and classify them.[7] Systematic assessment of FGIDs started only after the middle of the 20th century. Before this period, there were only a handful of published reports on functional GI symptoms. More than 3,000 years ago, *principle of holism* was propounded by the Greek philosophers such as Plato, Aristotle, and Hippocrates.[7] According to this, while studying any medical disease the person as a whole should be considered rather than focusing only on the diseased part. There was a shift in thinking of the illness when the *theory of dualism* was proposed by Rene Descartes in 17th century.[7] This concept of dualism, which allows a distinction between the mind and body, paved the way for scientific investigation of the human body, and new medical discoveries, because the prohibition of human dissection by the church was lifted.[7]

COMMON FUNCTIONAL GASTROINTESTINAL DISORDERS

Irritable Bowel Syndrome

Irritable bowel syndrome (IBS) is the most common FGID, found in 15% of the population. It is characterized by abdominal pain/discomfort, bloating, irregular stool form and passage. There are several *subtypes of IBS* based on the bowel habit that is predominant: (1) IBS with constipation (IBS-C), (2) IBS with diarrhea (IBS-D), (3) IBS with alternating bowel habit or mixed type (IBS-M), (4) IBS unclassified (IBS-U).[8] These presentations appear to be in a continuum, rather than discrete illness. The symptoms may change from one subtype to other in the same patient. Rome IV criteria for IBS specifies that the pain symptom should be present for 1 day/ week in past 3 months associated with two or more of the following criteria: (1) related to defecation (may be increased or unchanged by defecation), (2) associated with a change in the frequency of stool, and (3) associated with a change in the form (appearance) of stool. The criteria should be fulfilled with symptoms onset 6 months prior to diagnosis.[9]

In Asian patients, bloating is more commonly reported than pain or discomfort, and this is reported to lessen with the passage of stool or flatus. Symptoms beyond the GI system are also common in IBS patients, which may include tiredness, dysmenorrhea, headache, and dyspareunia.[10] IBS occurs in all age groups and across gender but is more common among females.[11] There is a gender difference in the predominant subtype, diarrhea is more among men, whereas, females are more likely to suffer from constipation.[12] Comorbid psychiatric disorders are common in IBS patients; anxiety, depression, and hypochondriasis are seen in more than half of them.[13,14]

Functional Dyspepsia

This is the second most common FGID and includes two conditions: (1) postprandial distress syndrome (PDS) and (2) epigastric pain syndrome (EPS), with an overlap in clinical presentation. The clinical features include fullness after meals, early satiety, epigastric pain or burning, bloating, belching, and nausea. Peptic ulcer, gastric cancer, and reflux esophagitis may also present with similar symptoms but the majority of patients with these complaints usually have functional dyspepsia.[15]

Postprandial distress syndrome includes troublesome experience of fullness after meals or has early satiety, which is severe enough to affect functioning, or completing a meal for 3 or more days/week in the past 3 months, with the duration of illness at least 6 months. *EPS* is characterized by bothersome epigastric pain or epigastric burning 1 or more days/week in the past 3 months, with at least a 6-month history.[16] Both the conditions require the absence any other systemic, metabolic, or organic disease that is likely to explain the symptoms on routine investigations including upper GI endoscopy.[17]

Functional dyspepsia is always a diagnosis of exclusion as esophagogastroduodenoscopy is required to exclude other pathologies such as peptic ulceration, esophagitis, and malignancy which can present with similar symptoms.[18,19]

Functional Abdominal Pain

Recurrent or continuous abdominal pain without any change in bowel habits, leading to socio-occupational dysfunction is characteristic of functional abdominal pain syndrome. This is not a common condition, with an estimated prevalence of 0.5–2% in the population, and is more common among females.[20]

Centrally Mediated Abdominal Pain Syndrome

The Rome IV diagnostic criteria of FGIDs have recently included two new disorders namely centrally mediated abdominal pain syndrome (CAPS) and narcotic bowel syndrome (NBS). In the earlier diagnostic Rome (III) criteria, CAPS was referred to as "functional abdominal pain syndrome".[21] It was postulated that this could be a type of neuropathic pain and shares some of its clinical characteristics such as allodynia (i.e., the nonpainful stimuli is perceived as painful), hyperalgesia (i.e., painful stimuli is perceived as being more painful), and the pain being constant and occurring spontaneously.[22] The hallmark feature of CAPS is continuous abdominal pain; this distinguishes it from the episodic and intermittent nature of the other painful FGIDs, which are also linked with GI physiological events (e.g., eating or defecation). The centrally mediated pain sometimes worsens with physiological GI events; nevertheless, the pain is present and continuous, irrespective of the GI function. There can be impaired GI function; however, the pain is a prominent feature and overshadows other symptoms. Due to this, these patients are usually distressed, and have poor quality of life and lower levels of functioning.[23]

In those with NBS, patients use an increasing dose of opioid, which corresponds to increasing pain levels, occurring in a vicious cycle. The abdominal pain recurs when the effect of narcotics wears down; this is known as the "soar and crash" phenomenon. The clinical presentation includes pain symptoms of varying intensity that are expressed verbally and nonverbally, reporting of intense symptoms, frequent health care visits, requests for repeated investigations, which overlap with somatoform pain syndrome.[24]

Anorectal Pain (Proctalgia)

Functional anorectal pain has been classified into two types in Rome III: (1) *chronic proctalgia*, which is characterized by a dull ache or a pressure sensation in the rectum and (2) *proctalgia fugax*, which is characterized by sudden, severe, short-lasting pain in anal region.[20] There can be an overlap between proctalgia fugax and chronic proctalgia, but episodes of proctalgia fugax are usually less frequent and they respond to simple reassurances.[25] Chronic proctalgia can be of two different subtypes (based on digital rectal examination findings): (1) *levator ani syndrome*, which includes tenderness on palpation of puborectalis muscle and (2) *unspecified functional anorectal pain* (no tenderness on digital palpation of the puborectalis). It is ascribed to chronic tension of the pelvic floor muscles. The term "chronic proctalgia" has been removed from the Rome IV classification system.[26] The maximum duration of pain episodes in proctalgia fugax has been revised from earlier 20 to 30 minutes, based on reports of longer duration of such attacks. This helps in distinguishing proctalgia fugax from levator ani syndrome and unspecified functional anorectal pain syndrome. Furthermore, the location of pain in proctalgia fugax is high up in the rectum in Rome IV criteria;[3] in Rome III criteria, pain in "lower rectum or anus" was also included.[1]

PATHOPHYSIOLOGY OF FUNCTIONAL GASTROINTESTINAL DISORDERS

The etiology of FGIDs is multifactorial and includes complex interaction between genetic vulnerability, physiological factors, early life experiences, and psychosocial factors.

Brain-Gut Interactions

There is a complex interaction between the gut and the brain through the enteric nervous system (ENS) and neurotransmitter signaling. It is likely that FGIDs arise from a dysregulation of the brain-gut axis. The constituents of the brain-gut axis include the CNS, autonomic nervous system (ANS), ENS, and hypothalamic-pituitary axis. The interaction between the brain and the gut is *bidirectional*. The thoughts, emotions, and perceptions have an influence on the GI sensation, intestinal motility, GI secretions, regulation of immune function, and mucosal inflammation as well as its permeability; the converse of this is also true, i.e., alterations in GI function influence emotions, thoughts, and behavior.[7,27]

In functional dyspepsia, one of the constant finding has been significant duodenal eosinophilia, which is found particularly in patients with PDS.[18] Abnormalities such as small bowel homing T cells that is suggestive of intestinal inflammation, and high circulating levels of cytokines have been reported.[18] Also, an increased circulating levels of tumor necrosis factor-α have been significantly correlated with high anxiety in these patients.[18]

Gut Microbiome

The gut microbiota is composed mostly of bacteria (Firmicutes, Bacteroidetes, Proteobacteria, Fusobacteria, and Actinobacteria species), and other organisms such as archaea, viruses, and protozoa. This gut microbiota helps in the conversion of nondigestible carbohydrates or the dietary fibers to short-chain fatty acids, in transformation of bile acids, in forming a protective barrier against the pathogenic bacteria, and modulation of both innate and the adaptive immune systems. Gut microbiota also appears to be important in the development of normal ENS and CNS.[27]

Dysbiosis, the qualitative alterations of microbiota are associated with cognitive and behavioral changes. *Small intestinal bacterial overgrowth* (SIBO), a quantitative increase in intestinal bacteria has been associated with IBS, but the association is not clear.[28,29] Bacterial fermentation of food in the lumen produces gases such as hydrogen, methane, and carbon dioxide, which may cause symptoms including abdominal distention, abdominal pain, flatulence, and bloating in patients with IBS. SIBO is more often associated with diarrhea-predominant IBS than constipation-predominant IBS.

Various psychosocial and physical stressors may alter the bacterial colonization and increases in pathogenic bacteria may lead to increased levels of cytokines and a proinflammatory state. Postinfectious gastroenteritis is a risk factor for functional dyspepsia. Functional dyspepsia is known to develop after acute bacterial, viral, or protozoal gastroenteritis, the risk is almost 2.5 times higher. Smoking is a risk factor for postinfectious functional dyspepsia, and also a risk factor for duodenal eosinophilia. Acute GI infections may lead to visceral hypersensitivity that may persist for a much longer duration after the resolution of the infection. Higher rates of FGIDs have been found after GI infections.[30,31] Other mechanisms may include increased permeability, altered motility, and persistent inflammation in susceptible individuals.

Visceral Hypersensitivity

The FGIDs with pain predominant symptoms could be related to the visceral hypersensitivity, specifically when the GI motility is not much altered, or the symptoms do not correlate with motility disturbances. It has been observed that the pain threshold is reduced in those with visceral hypersensitivity that is demonstrated using balloon distention studies of the bowel.[32] These patients could also have a higher sensitivity to even normal intestinal functions. Also, the referred visceral pain could be in unusual areas and is much higher in patients with FGID. There have been recent studies that suggest that rectal or colonic distention can induce visceral hypersensitivity even in normal subjects, and it may be much higher in those having IBS.[32] Hence, the pain experienced in patients with FGIDs may be related to the sensitization arising from chronic abnormal motor hyperactivity, trauma/injury to the viscera or GI infection.[32]

Microbiota-Gut-Brain Axis

There is a predominance of sulfate-reducing bacteria in IBS-C patients, which results in increased hydrogen sulfide production. Hydrogen sulfide might affect visceral perception in patients with FGIDs. It has been found that many bacterial probiotic strains improve the severity of symptoms and abdominal pain in IBS patients. Probiotics improve not only gut symptoms, but also have beneficial effect on anxiety, depression, and stress symptoms.

Altered Motility

An increase in GI motility is reported in patients with IBS diarrhea subtype, whereas, there is a decrease in motility with IBS constipation subtype. The pathophysiology of motility disturbances in FGIDs is not clear. There is some association between connective tissue disorders and GI symptoms. Benign joint hypermobility syndrome was found to be commonly associated with GI dysmotility.[33-35] The mechanism may include mechanical alterations and distensibility of the intestinal walls, leading to altered motility and pain perception.

Autonomic Dysfunction

Many patients with postural tachycardia syndrome present with recurrent nausea, vomiting, and abdominal pain. Autonomic dysregulation characterized by lower heart rate variability is reported to occur in IBS patients.[36]

Immune Dysfunction

In a subgroup of patients, FGIDs may occur following infections, which could be associated with a state of low-grade immune activation. It is possible that inflammation associated with these infections causes some minor alterations in the structure and function of the GI system including changes in lymphocytes, enterochromaffin cells, mast cells, and enteric nerves that are likely to be permanent and may cause or contribute to some of the FGID symptoms.[37]

Psychosocial Factors

It is well established that several early life adverse experiences such as neglect or abuse, life events in adulthood including death or separation, the perceived level of social support, and other social experiences can have effect on the physiologic and psychological responses of the individual, resulting in distress, psychiatric disorders, beliefs and coping mechanisms. The GI system responds not only to the environmental and physiological factors, but also interacts with the brain directly through the ENS, thus having a two-way interaction along the "brain-gut" axis.[38,39]

The clinical expression of abdominal pain could be affected by behavioral or social learning. Modeling of the symptoms can occur in the family, e.g., children may observe and learn the depiction of the illness behavior of their parents or neighbors. The symptoms could be maintained by positive and negative reinforcement, e.g., care and concern shown by the adults toward pain symptoms in children. It has been observed that children of IBS patients have more health-related problems that requited medical consultations as compared to children of those without IBS; these increased health-related visits are seen not only with FGIDs, but with other somatoform disorders also. Similarly, several studies have shown that when the mothers reinforce illness behaviors in children, they have more severe abdominal pain and have more absences from school than other children.[1]

The effect of psychosocial factors on FGIDs includes: (1) their impact on the GI physiology; (2) their effect on the experience of symptoms; (3) their effects on illness behavior; (4) their influence on the clinical outcome; and (5) the choice of the treatment modality. Psychological trauma has been shown to change visceral pain sensitivity as well as perception of central pain. Stress can influence gut secretions, motility, immune function and the microbiome, through hypothalamic-pituitary-adrenal (HPA) and ANS axis. Personality factors can affect the health-seeking behavior. All these psychosocial factors can affect the functioning of the gut, the experiences of pain and other symptoms, associated quality of life, effect on the occupational functioning, and the utilization and cost of health care.[40]

Dietary Factors

Fermentable oligosaccharides, disaccharides, monosaccharides, and polyols (FODMAPs) have been identified as possible triggers of symptoms in FGIDs including IBS. FODMAPs are short-chain carbohydrates that consist of small osmotically active molecules that are absorbed poorly leading to cause excessive fluid and gas accumulation, thus causing bloating, distention, and abdominal pain.[41,42] They are found in some foods which contain lactose, fructose in excess of glucose, galacto-oligosaccharides, fructans, and polyols such as sorbitol, xylitol, mannitol, and maltitol. FODMAPs are not absorbed well owing to a lack enzyme in the gut lumen which hydrolyzes the glycosidic bonds in carbohydrates, lower activity or absence of lactase enzyme on the brush border, or the presence of lower capacity epithelial transporters such as fructose, glucose transporter-2, and glucose transporter-5. The rate of fermentation also depends on the chain length of the carbohydrate.[41,42]

A unifying disease model now better explains the FGIDs, such as functional dyspepsia. It conceptualizes that GI infection, alteration of the gut microbiome or presence of a particular food allergen, can lead to an increase in permeability of duodenum, and duodenal eosinophilia with or without increased mast cells, which in turn activates a mucosal immune response. Furthermore, local duodenogastric reflex responses to the inflammation could modify the gastroduodenal function that may include impairment in fundic relaxation in some patients. In addition, cytokines such as tumor necrosis factor-α in the circulation may cause systemic effects such as anxiety symptoms.[43]

Psychiatric Comorbidity

Psychiatric disorders such as depression and anxiety are common in patients with FGIDs. In a large Swedish cohort, anxiety at baseline was associated with new-onset functional dyspepsia at the follow-up examination (OR, 7.6; 99% CI, 1.2–47.7).[44] IBS has been reported to co-occur with panic disorder in several studies.[45-47] A meta-analysis of 10 studies showed significantly higher anxiety [standardized mean difference (SMD) = 0.76; 95% CI, 0.47–0.69] and depression (SMD = 0.76; 95% CI, 0.47–0.69) levels in patients with IBS than controls.[14]

Neuroticism is also reportedly common in patients with FGIDs. It has been found that IBS score higher on trait anxiety as well as neuroticism as compared to control subjects having similar GI complaints without IBS. Negative emotionality, which is a feature of neuroticism, has been associated with altered colonic motility. Traits such as neuroticism, anxiety sensitivity, excessive worry, and increased attention to visceral sensations are recognized as common features of IBS.[48] However, there is no personality profile identified which is very specific or unique to IBS.

About 15–45% of patients with FGIDs also meet the diagnostic criteria for somatization disorder (Briquet's syndrome), which is a severe form of somatoform disorder.[49] In these patients, symptoms suggestive of other organ systems and comorbid conditions such as fibromyalgia, chronic fatigue, and chronic pain are reported, particularly those with severe and refractory symptoms. These patients are typically the "nonresponders" in several pharmacological intervention research studies. It may be surmised that these individuals might set a lower threshold for symptom reporting. These patients may have central dysregulation of their pain regulatory pathways, i.e., central sensitization.[50] Some of these pathways are activated by neurotransmitters such as serotonin, norepinephrine, and opiates, which are also associated with psychiatric disorders; psychotropic medications may be indicated for the treatment of FGIDs. This can be done as monotherapy or in combination with other pain medications, along with psychotherapeutic treatments such as cognitive-behavioral therapy (CBT) and hypnotherapy.

ASSESSMENT OF FUNCTIONAL GASTROINTESTINAL DISORDERS

A biopsychosocial approach of assessment is recommended for all patients. This is particularly relevant for treatment-resistant patients who fail to respond to the first-line medical treatment. A psychosocial history may be helpful in identifying the maintaining factors for the symptoms and thus help in reducing unnecessary consultations.

Clinical history: It includes description of symptoms in terms of severity, frequency, pattern, duration of illness, identifying possible precipitating factors before the onset (e.g., GI infection, life changes), possible factors that can potentially trigger or exacerbate the symptoms (e.g., stress, food allergy), the impact of symptoms on psychological and socio-occupational functioning (e.g., avoidance behavior, relationships, work), coping strategies used by the patients and whether it is helpful or not, general habits such as eating and sleeping patterns, personal circumstances, general interests and hobbies, and personality factors.

The assessment may be done briefly, and if needed in detail. The domains that should be included are (also mentioned are relevant screening and rating instruments): (1) depression and anxiety (Hospital Anxiety and Depression Scale or Patient Health Questionnaire-9 or Generalized Anxiety Disorder-7); (2) somatization or the general tendency to report multiple bodily symptoms (Patient Health Questionnaire); (3) health beliefs and coping (Cognitive Strategies Questionnaire-Catastrophizing or Visceral Sensitivity Index); (4) illness impact and quality of life (IBS-Quality of Life); and (5) the association between psychosocial factors and periods of worsening or improvement of symptoms.

Potential *red flags* that indicate need for early referral to a mental health professional are patients with suicidal ideations, severe depression, chronic refractory pain, severe disability, maladaptive illness behavior, idiosyncratic health beliefs, and difficulties in the physician-patient relationship.[1]

The Rome Criteria is based on the description of symptoms for classification of FGIDs. In the absence of clear pathophysiology, symptom description forms the basis of diagnostic criteria, similar to the diagnostic systems in psychiatry and rheumatology. It is based on the premise that the symptom clusters consistently occur together in patients with functional GI complaints, even though they cannot be grouped meaningfully using known structural, physiological, or biochemical changes. The Rome Criteria arose from the Manning Criteria, which was developed using discriminant analysis of GI symptoms in patients. The use of symptom-based diagnostic criteria (e.g., Rome criteria) helps avoiding unnecessary investigations in reaching a clinical diagnosis, as it no longer remains a diagnosis of exclusion, but is a form of positive diagnosis.

Investigations: Any laboratory testing or investigations in patients with FGIDs should be based on the atypical presentations such as age of onset, or on other objective data such as blood in the stool or abnormal blood reports, rather than just the patient's requests to "do something". The other considerations for testing include safety of the procedure, whether the results would alter management plan, and cost-benefit analysis.[40]

The clinical course of FGIDs is mostly chronic and requires planning regarding long-term management. The clinician should spend some time asking for the immediate reasons for each visit, the physiological and psychosocial factors that could be associated with the patient's illness behavior, and the extent of socio-occupational and functional impairment, following which the treatment can be based on the severity and nature of symptoms. All these factors can help categorize the patients into mild, moderate, and severe illness that help in planning management.[20]

Mild illness: FGID patients having mild symptoms present themselves mostly to general physicians or primary care settings. The impairment in functioning or psychological disturbance is minimal, and most of them are able to do their activities of daily living. These groups of patients are concerned about their symptoms but respond well to simple reassurances. They do not change doctors frequently and do not visit their physicians very frequently. These patients require psychoeducation about the disorder and its manifestations, simple dietary advices, and the effects and adverse effects of the medications.

Moderate illness: Those with moderate level of illness have symptoms that interfere with functioning intermittently. They present to primary care settings as well as for specialist services in secondary care centers. On close questioning precipitating events can be identified proximal to the onset of the symptoms that may include psychosocial stress or altered dietary habits. These patients do well when they are asked to monitor the symptoms and their severity in daily diaries and the psychosocial stress, which gives them some sense of mastery over their symptoms and ways to control them. Along with this, medications targeting specific symptoms which are troublesome, and psychotherapeutic measures such as relaxation training, hypnosis, and CBT may be required to reduce associated anxiety and encourage positive behaviors.

Severe illness: Patients having the severe forms of illness have symptoms that interfere with socio-occupational and daily functioning. They have severe psychological problems which occur very frequently that necessitate frequent consultations. Furthermore, they are not satisfied with one physician and frequently change doctors. In management of such cases, it is necessary to establish some therapeutic alliance and continue treatment under a single physician. Also, setting realistic treatment goals rather than promise for magical cure is needed. For example, patients can be educated that there may be some reduction in pain symptoms which can lead to improvement in functioning and quality of life, rather than saying that all pain symptoms can be controlled. Instead of focusing only on the treatment of the disease, the patients should be encouraged to learn to cope with the disorder as they are long-standing conditions. Wherever indicated, adding antidepressants may also help control chronic pain and improve associated depressive symptoms.[7]

MANAGEMENT OF FUNCTIONAL GASTROINTESTINAL DISORDERS

Approach to the Patient

Therapeutic relationship: The most important element in the treatment of patients with FGIDs is establishing a positive therapeutic relationship. The clinician needs to develop this through: (1) assessing and acknowledging the patient's beliefs, concerns, and expectations; (2) expressing empathy; (3) dealing with the misconceptions; (4) educating the patient about the illness; and (5) negotiating a treatment plan with the patient. Not all patients are willing to identify or accept the role of psychosocial factors at the beginning, and may require specific therapy. This is more likely in those with a history of childhood trauma such as sexual abuse.

Active listening: The clinician should not just passively hear what the patient says, but strive to actively listen to the complaints and encourage the patients during the consultations. A patient-centered approach is helpful, which includes eliciting and addressing the patient's concerns such as fears of a serious illness. Physicians may unwittingly discredit the patient's symptoms as unreal and imaginary, calling these as "mental" or "all in the head", not paying attention to the concerns of the patients, or just referring patients to psychiatrists without explaining the reason for the referral, may lead to therapeutic failures and patients shifting from one physician to other.

Linking GI symptoms with psychosocial factors: It is necessary to link the GI symptoms with the psychosocial factors for the patient to understand the relationship. This is easily done by asking the patient to maintain a daily record of the symptoms, the timings of bowel movements, the timing of menstrual periods, along with documentation of stressors, dietary and lifestyle changes. This information can be brought to the consultation and may provide the basis for CBT.[1,7,39]

Dietary Approaches

Food triggers for the symptoms are commonly reported in FGIDs. Lactose intolerance is commonly associated with IBS symptoms. It has been suggested that a diet with less FODMAPs may improve symptoms in patients with IBS, irrespective of the underlying cause.[41,42]

Gut Psychopharmacology

Antibiotics: Rifaximin has been the preferred antibiotic for the treatment of SIBO in IBS.[51] It is poorly absorbed bactericidal antibiotic that inhibits bacterial protein synthesis. The recommended dose in IBS is 200 mg twice daily for a period of 14 days. Empirical use of other antibiotics is not indicated in the management of FGIDs.

Prebiotics, probiotics, and synbiotics: Probiotics are living bacteria or fungi that provide a health benefit for the host. Prebiotics are nondigestible oligosaccharides, such as fructo-oligosaccharides, galacto-oligosaccharides, inulin, and lactulose, which can stimulate the growth beneficial gut bacteria selectively, specifically lactobacilli and bifidobacteria. Synbiotic is a combination of a probiotic and a prebiotic which increases the survival and activity of the probiotics in the body, and also stimulate growth of indigenous anaerobic bacteria.[52] Treatment with these groups of medications is called *bacteriotherapy*. VSL#3, a mixture of eight probiotic strains and *Lactobacillus plantarum* have been found to decrease flatulence and relieved abdominal bloating.[53] Probiotics such as *Bifidobacterium bifidum* MIMBb75 and *Escherichia coli*, Nissle 1917 have been found to be beneficial in IBS.[54,55]

Prokinetics: Several medications that stimulate GI smooth muscle and accelerate transit are included in this group.[56] Cholinergic agonists (bethanechol, neostigmine, pyridostigmine, and acotiamide) stimulate through acetylcholine but are poorly tolerated. Dopamine antagonists (metoclopramide, domperidone, and levosulpiride) accelerate gastric emptying and may be useful in functional dyspepsia. Itopride is another dopamine antagonist, which is devoid of any CNS or cardiovascular side effects. Serotonin agonists (e.g., cisapride) stimulate acetylcholine release from myenteric neurons through their action on 5-HT4 receptors. Tegaserod is a selective serotonergic agonist with clinically relevant effects but was withdrawn because of cardiac toxicity. Prucalopride increases GI motility, decreases esophageal reflux, and improves gastric emptying, and has been found to be useful in patients with refractory constipation. Selective 5-HT4 agonists (velusetrag, naronapride, and mosapride) increase colonic motility and transit, and increase spontaneous bowel movements. Macrolide antibiotics (erythromycin and azithromycin) are motilin agonists that accelerate gastric emptying time. Camicinal is a nonantibiotic prokinetic macrolide that has a similar effect. Ghrelin agonists (ulimorelin and relamorelin) increase gastric emptying and accelerate colonic motor activity and transit.[56]

Antidepressants: When the first line of treatment for FGIDs including the low-risk interventions (reassurance, pharmacological, and nonpharmacological therapies) directed at specific gut symptoms fail, treatment with antidepressants can be considered.[57] A moderate-to-severe level of illness with significant level of impairment in functioning justifies the need for an antidepressant. A risk-benefit analysis will help the clinician in deciding for an antidepressant.

Patients with severe somatization based on clinical evaluation may not tolerate the medication side effects well. This can affect treatment compliance and overall treatment effectiveness. There is some evidence to suggest that unexplained medical symptoms, as in FGIDs, may respond to antidepressants, even in patients with high degrees of somatization. Therefore, initiating an early antidepressant trial is recommended for most. Considering possibility of emergent adverse effects, specifically with tricyclic antidepressants (TCAs), it is suggested to start low and go slow. For example, amitriptyline 10 mg/day, and gradually increase the dose to 25-50 mg/day over weeks. There is evidence that the TCAs are more effective than specific serotonin reuptake inhibitors (SSRIs) across the spectrum of unexplained somatic symptoms and syndromes. Thus, the initial trial should be with a TCA. Furthermore, TCAs have effect on pain symptoms that can be beneficial for many patients.

Several classes of antidepressants have shown efficacy in improving outcomes and reducing pain symptoms in FGIDs.[58] The analgesic effect appears to have a different time course of action (within 1-2 weeks) and is independent of their effects on mood which is seen much later (3-4 weeks). Apart from the central effects on mood and pain modulation, antidepressants also impact the gut motility. TCAs with noradrenergic and anticholinergic activity prolong GI transit time, thus improving symptoms of diarrhea. In contrast, SSRIs reduce GI transit time, and improve constipation.

Almost 80% of IBS patients have shown at least a moderate response to antidepressants, and adherence to treatment is higher. A low dose of TCA (25-50 mg/day) is the initial treatment option in most patients without significant anxiety and depressive symptoms. It improves symptoms of somatization along with other GI symptoms due to its dual central and peripheral pain controlling effects. The dose of TCA may be increased if the initial response is poor, at 25 mg every 5–7 days, to 75–100 mg/day. In persons with significant anxiety or depression, an adequate trial with SSRI or serotonin-norepinephrine reuptake inhibitor (SNRI) is the preferred option. Furthermore, the sedating effect of TCAs may be helpful in FGID patients with insomnia. TCAs and SSRIs may improve global measures of well-being without having a direct correlation with pain ratings. Specifically, SSRIs improve the global measures of well-being in most of the patients, rather than direct effects on pain ratings. Adding low dose of a TCA to a daily SSRI regimen for psychiatric disorders may improve functional GI symptoms.[58]

Common reason for treatment failure with antidepressants is inadequate dosing. Although the rate at which the dosage increase should be done has no consensus, but most of the patients do well with dosage increase of TCA by 10–25 mg/day every 5–7 days. If the patient tolerates the medications but with minimal improvement, it is recommended to increase to full antidepressant dose before changing the medication. Some patients receive antidepressant doses of SSRIs from the beginning, but many patients receiving TCAs are given lower dosages. Therefore, it is recommended that in nonresponders, patients should receive these medications in full antidepressant doses. After a fair trial with an antidepressant, i.e., adequate doses (antidepressant doses or maximum tolerated doses) and adequate duration (4–6 weeks), only the medications may be changed.

The antidepressants act in FGIDs through alterations of neurotransmitter levels, specifically serotonin and norepinephrine in the brain, thus having effect on mood and pain symptoms. In addition, the peripheral effects of antidepressants on the neurotransmitters in the gut may also contribute to their therapeutic effects, specifically in disorders such as IBS. Serotonin is found in abundance in the gut wall, the blood vessels, and in the ENS. Reduction in serotonin and norepinephrine transmission in the ENS may be one of the mechanisms leading to lower transmission of pain messages to brain centers, thus restoring the normal brain-gut connections. It is likely that serotonin has important actions on GI motility, sensations, and the brain-gut connection. SSRIs and TCAs possibly increase the serotonin levels by reuptake inhibition in both gut and brain, thereby increasing the pain threshold of gut through peripheral effect and improving mood through their central effects. However, studies in FGIDs have not shown clinically significant effects on the GI physiology or symptoms with antidepressant treatment, but have shown effects on overall functioning in the patients.

Brain-Gut Psychotherapies

Psychoeducation: The patients with FGIDs should be educated about the normal gut functions, including the anatomy and physiology in simple terms. Patients with IBS may be explained regarding the alterations in muscle contractions and the increased sensitivity of the lining of the gut, and how the brain interprets the gut signals in a distorted way thus leading to increase in gut sensations and pain, which give rise to the IBS symptoms.[59]

The rationale for the use of cognitive and behavioral therapies is to change maladaptive thoughts or behaviors that maintain the symptoms and cause impairment in functioning. Psychotherapy does not modify specific IBS symptoms directly, rather it helps patients to better cope with the symptoms, improve their problem-solving skills, and enhance their functioning and quality of life.[60]

Relaxation therapy: Relaxation therapy is a simple form of therapy that can be taught easily to patients. It is based on the premise that stress contributes to symptoms of FGIDs, and relaxation training may reduce autonomic arousal, thereby reduce symptoms and induce a sense of well-being. Patients learn to identify the sources of stress and practice relaxation in these situations. *Arousal reduction training* includes specific techniques that can be taught to the patients which can help them counter the physiological effects of stress or anxiety. Some of the most common arousal reduction techniques include: (1) Jacobson's progressive muscle relaxation training or their abbreviated versions; (2) Electromyographic (EMG) biofeedback for muscle tension; (3) autogenic training; (4) mindfulness-based stress reduction; and (5) Tai chi, transcendental meditation or Sudarshan kriya yoga.[40]

Cognitive-behavioral therapy is the most widely researched psychological treatment for IBS. There is evidence supporting other therapies as well including mindfulness and hypnotherapy.[39,61]

Cognitive-behavioral therapy: The CBT is focused on replacing maladaptive coping strategies with more positive cognitions and behaviors. Psychotherapy changes illness-specific cognitions, behaviors, and anxiety to achieve reduction in symptom severity.[62] Specifically, unhelpful GI-related cognitions and GI safety behaviors reduce before anxiety during CBT treatment for IBS.[63]

Hypnotherapy: Gut-directed hypnotherapy is effective for GI symptoms of patients with IBS not only in the short-term, but the improvements are sustained over time.[64] Typically, suggestions and metaphors are used after hypnotic induction for control and normalization of GI symptoms.[59] The possible mechanisms underlying the efficacy of gut-directed hypnotherapy include psychological and physiological effects such as changes in gut motility, visceral sensitivity, immune function, central processing of signals, and ANS activity.[64]

Biofeedback: This is a form of treatment in which physiological information is conveyed back to the person in the form of a simple visual or auditory signal that helps the person to control the function. Biofeedback training includes two types of learning: (1) motor skills training, in which the patients receive an augmented feedback on a physiological response which they learn to modify and (2) sensory discrimination training, in which there is exposure to graded physiological sensations and patients learn through feedback to perceive weaker sensations accurately.[65] Biofeedback treatment has been found to be useful for several FGIDs including fecal incontinence, functional constipation, functional anorectal pain, IBS, functional dyspepsia, and aerophobia.

Factors Affecting Outcome of FGIDs

The outcome is poor in patients who do not accept pharmacotherapy or are not adherent to the prescribed medications, and those experiencing adverse effects of medications. It is important to educate the patients regarding potential benefits of medications beyond simple antidepressant effects or anxiolytic effects. Similarly, discussions regarding potential adverse effects, some of which may be transient, and measures to counter them may improve acceptance and drug adherence. Many a times including a family member while explaining the risk-benefits to the patients may be helpful.

Choosing the right medication for the treatment of FGIDs may also help. For example, in IBS patients with diarrhea predominance or pain symptoms, there may be a good response to TCAs, whereas, constipation-predominant patients do well with SSRIs. Patients with higher levels of somatization presenting with several diffuse functional symptoms should receive antidepressants, as there is usually higher functional impairment. In contrast, patients with single symptom presentations may not require high doses of medications. However, those with severe illness are also the ones who report frequent medication adverse effects, thus reducing the overall effectiveness of the antidepressants. Therefore, what constitutes "treatment responder patients" can only be known after a treatment trial. It is recommended to continue antidepressant treatment for at least 6 months, though several patients will require longer term treatment to maintain the therapeutic gain.

The overall outcomes are poor in those with objective evidence of altered GI motility, comorbid medical conditions or specific symptoms that are exacerbated by adverse effects of antidepressants. Among the antidepressants, TCAs are poorly tolerated because of adverse effects, specifically at higher doses. Patients with higher somatization and prior sensitivity to other medications do not tolerate even low doses of antidepressants. Identifying these subsets of patients early and treating with nonpharmacological interventions instead of medications may improve outcome.[58]

CONCLUSION

Functional gastrointestinal disorders are disorders of gut-brain interaction. The best way to manage these disorders is by adopting a biopsychosocial model. The basic clinical principles such as active listening, therapeutic relationship, patient-centered approach, education of the patients regarding biopsychosocial plan of care are required for proper management of these patients. With more understanding of pathophysiology, several treatment options are likely to emerge; however, they are unlikely to change the fundamental treatment principles.

REFERENCES

1. Levy RL, Olden KW, Naliboff BD, Bradley LA, Francisconi C, Drossman DA, et al. Psychosocial aspects of the functional gastrointestinal disorders. Gastroenterology. 2006;130:1447-58.
2. Mukhtar K, Nawaz H, Abid S. Functional gastrointestinal disorders and gut-brain axis: what does the future hold? World J Gastroenterol. 2019;25:552-66.
3. Schmulson MJ, Drossman DA. What is new in Rome IV. J Neurogastroenterol Motil. 2017;23: 151-63.
4. Chandran S, Prakrithi SN, Mathur S, Kishor M, Rao TS. A review of functional gastrointestinal disorders: a primer for mental health professionals. Arch Ment Health. 2018;19:70-81.
5. American Psychiatric Association. Diagnostic and Statistical Manual of Mental Disorders (DSM-5). Arlington, VA: American Psychiatric Publishing; 2013.
6. Lackner JM. The role of psychosocial factors in functional gastrointestinal disorders. Front Gastrointest Res. 2014;33:104-16.
7. Drossman DA. Functional gastrointestinal disorders: history, pathophysiology, clinical features, and Rome IV. Gastroenterology. 2016;150:1262-79.
8. Saha L. Irritable bowel syndrome: pathogenesis, diagnosis, treatment, and evidence-based medicine. World J Gastroenterol. 2014;20: 6759-73.
9. Lacy BE, Mearin F, Chang L, Chey WD, Lembo AJ, Simren M, et al. Bowel disorders. Gastroenterology. 2016;150:1393-407.
10. Gwee KA, Bak YT, Ghoshal UC, Gonlachanvit S, Lee OY, Fock KM, et al. Asian consensus on irritable bowel syndrome. J Gastroenterol Hepatol. 2010;25:1189-205.
11. Heitkemper M, Jarrett M. Irritable bowel syndrome: does gender matter? J Psychosom Res. 2008;64:583-7.
12. Adeyemo MA, Spiegel BM, Chang L. Meta-analysis: do irritable bowel syndrome symptoms vary between men and women? Aliment Pharmacol Ther. 2010;32:738-55.
13. Lydiard RB, Falsetti SA. Experience with anxiety and depression treatment studies: implications for designing irritable bowel syndrome clinical trials. Am J Med. 1999;107:65-73.

14. Fond G, Loundou A, Hamdani N, Boukouaci W, Dargel A, Oliveira J, et al. Anxiety and depression comorbidities in irritable bowel syndrome (IBS): a systematic review and meta-analysis. Eur Arch Psychiatry Clin Neurosci. 2014;264:651-60.
15. Talley NJ, Ford AC. Functional dyspepsia. N Engl J Med. 2015;373:1853-63.
16. Talley NJ, Cook DR. Functional dyspepsia. In: Lacy BE, DiBaise JK, Pimentel M, Ford AC (Eds). Essential Medical Disorders of the Stomach and Small Intestine. Switzerland: Springer; 2019. pp. 155-72.
17. Stanghellini V, Chan FK, Hasler WL, Malagelada JR, Suzuki H, Tack J, et al. Gastroduodenal disorders. Gastroenterology. 2016;150:1380-92.
18. Talley NJ. Functional dyspepsia: advances in diagnosis and therapy. Gut Liver. 2017;11:349-57.
19. Moayyedi PM, Lacy BE, Andrews CN, Enns RA, Howden CW, Vakil N. ACG and CAG clinical guideline: management of dyspepsia. Am J Gastroenterol. 2017;112:988-1013.
20. Drossman DA, Dumitrascu DL. Rome III: New standard for functional gastrointestinal disorders. J Gastrointestin Liver Dis. 2006;15:237-41.
21. Drossman DA, Hasler WL. Rome IV functional GI disorders: disorders of gut-brain interaction. Gastroenterology. 2016;150:1257-61.
22. Paine P. Centrally mediated abdominal pain syndromes. Medicine. 2019;47:354-7.
23. Keefer L, Drossman DA, Guthrie E, Simrén M, Tillisch K, Olden K, et al. Centrally mediated disorders of gastrointestinal pain. Gastroenterology. 2016;150:1408-19.
24. Drossman D, Szigethy E. The narcotic bowel syndrome: a recent update. Am J Gastroenterol Suppl. 2014;2:22-30.
25. Whitehead WE, Wald A, Diamant NE, Enck P, Pemberton JH, Rao SS. Functional disorders of the anus and rectum. Gut. 1999;45:II55-9.
26. Simren M, Palsson OS, Whitehead WE. Update on Rome IV criteria for colorectal disorders: implications for clinical practice. Curr Gastroenterol Rep. 2017;19:15.
27. Nicholson JK, Holmes E, Kinross J, Burcelin R, Gibson G, Jia W, et al. Host-gut microbiota metabolic interactions. Science. 2012;336:1262-7.
28. Ghoshal UC, Shukla R, Ghoshal U. Small intestinal bacterial overgrowth and irritable bowel syndrome: a bridge between functional organic dichotomy. Gut Liver. 2017;11:196-208.
29. Aziz I, Törnblom H, Simrén M. Small intestinal bacterial overgrowth as a cause for irritable bowel syndrome: guilty or not guilty? Curr Opin Gastroenterol. 2017;33:196-202.
30. Mearin F. Postinfectious functional gastrointestinal disorders. J Clin Gastroenterol. 2011;45:S102-5.
31. Pensabene L, Talarico V, Concolino D, Ciliberto D, Campanozzi A, Gentile T, et al. Postinfectious functional gastrointestinal disorders in children: a multicenter prospective study. J Pediatr. 2015;166:903-7.
32. Farmer AD, Aziz Q. Visceral pain hypersensitivity in functional gastrointestinal disorders. Br Med Bull. 2009;91:123-36.
33. Zarate N, Farmer AD, Grahame R, Mohammed SD, Knowles CH, Scott SM, et al. Unexplained gastrointestinal symptoms and joint hypermobility: is connective tissue the missing link? Neurogastroenterol Motil. 2010;22:252-78.
34. Botrus G, Baker O, Borrego E, Ngamdu KS, Teleb M, Martinez JL, et al. Spectrum of gastrointestinal manifestations in joint hypermobility syndromes. Am J Med Sci. 2018;355:573-80.
35. Beckers AB, Keszthelyi D, Fikree A, Vork L, Masclee A, Farmer AD, et al. Gastrointestinal disorders in joint hypermobility syndrome/Ehlers-Danlos syndrome hypermobility type: a review for the gastroenterologist. Neurogastroenterol Motil. 2017;29:e13013.
36. Adeyemi EO, Desai KD, Towsey M, Ghista D. Characterization of autonomic dysfunction in patients with irritable bowel syndrome by means of heart rate variability studies. Am J Gastroenterol. 1999;94:816-23.
37. Spiller R, Lam C. An update on post-infectious irritable bowel syndrome: role of genetics, immune activation, serotonin and altered microbiome. J Neurogastroenterol Motil. 2012;18:258-68.
38. Fadgyas-Stanculete M, Buga AM, Popa-Wagner A, Dumitrascu DL. The relationship between irritable bowel syndrome and psychiatric disorders: from molecular changes to clinical manifestations. J Mol Psychiatry. 2014;2:4.
39. Lackner JM. The role of psychosocial factors in functional gastrointestinal disorders. In: Quigley EM, Hongo M, Fukudo S (Eds). Functional and GI Motility Disorders. Basel: Karger Publishers; 2014. pp. 104-16.
40. Drossman DA, Creed FH, Olden KW, Svedlund J, Toner BB, Whitehead WE. Psychosocial aspects of the functional gastrointestinal disorders. Gut. 1999;45:II25-30.
41. Gibson PR, Shepherd SJ. Evidence-based dietary management of functional gastrointestinal symptoms: the FODMAP approach. J Gastroenterol Hepatol. 2010;25:252-8.

42. Nanayakkara WS, Skidmore PM, O'Brien L, Wilkinson TJ, Gearry RB. Efficacy of the low FODMAP diet for treating irritable bowel syndrome: the evidence to date. Clin Exp Gastroenterol. 2016;9:131-42.
43. Talley NJ, Goodsall T, Potter M. Functional dyspepsia. Aust Prescr. 2017;40:209-13.
44. Aro P, Talley NJ, Johansson SE, Agréus L, Ronkainen J. Anxiety is linked to new-onset dyspepsia in the Swedish population: a 10-year follow-up study. Gastroenterology. 2015;148:928-37.
45. Kumano H, Kaiya H, Yoshiuchi K, Yamanaka G, Sasaki T, Kuboki T. Comorbidity of irritable bowel syndrome, panic disorder, and agoraphobia in a Japanese representative sample. Am J Gastroenterol. 2004;99:370-6.
46. Lydiard RB. Increased prevalence of functional gastrointestinal disorders in panic disorder: clinical and theoretical implications. CNS Spectr. 2005;10:899-908.
47. Kaplan DS, Masand PS, Gupta S. The relationship of irritable bowel syndrome (IBS) and panic disorder. Ann Clin Psychiatry. 1996;8:81-8.
48. Muscatello MR, Bruno A, Mento C, Pandolfo G, Zoccali RA. Personality traits and emotional patterns in irritable bowel syndrome. World J Gastroenterol. 2016;22:6402-15.
49. Hausteiner-Wiehle C, Henningsen P. Irritable bowel syndrome: relations with functional, mental, and somatoform disorders. World J Gastroenterol. 2014;20:6024-30.
50. Eller-Smith OC, Nicol AL, Christianson JA. Potential mechanisms underlying centralized pain and emerging therapeutic interventions. Front Cell Neurosci. 2018;12:35.
51. Boltin D, Perets TT, Shporn E, Aizic S, Levy S, Niv Y, et al. Rifaximin for small intestinal bacterial overgrowth in patients without irritable bowel syndrome. Ann Clin Microbiol Antimicrob. 2014;13:49.
52. Ford AC, Quigley EM, Lacy BE, Lembo AJ, Saito YA, Schiller LR, et al. Efficacy of prebiotics, probiotics, and synbiotics in irritable bowel syndrome and chronic idiopathic constipation: systematic review and meta-analysis. Am J Gastroenterol. 2014;109:1547-61.
53. Chapman CM, Gibson GR, Rowland I. Health benefits of probiotics: are mixtures more effective than single strains? Eur J Nutr. 2011;50:1-7.
54. Guglielmetti S, Mora D, Gschwender M, Popp K. Randomised clinical trial: *Bifidobacterium bifidum* MIMBb75 significantly alleviates irritable bowel syndrome and improves quality of life—a double-blind, placebo-controlled study. Aliment Pharmacol Ther. 2011;33:1123-32.
55. Kruis W, Chrubasik S, Boehm S, Stange C, Schulze J. A double-blind placebo-controlled trial to study therapeutic effects of probiotic Escherichia coli Nissle 1917 in subgroups of patients with irritable bowel syndrome. Int J Colorectal Dis. 2012;27:467-74.
56. Quigley EM. Prokinetics in the management of functional gastrointestinal disorders. Curr Gastroenterol Rep. 2017;19:53.
57. Mertz HR. Irritable bowel syndrome. N Engl J Med. 2003;349:2136-46.
58. Clouse RE, Lustman PJ. Use of psychopharmacological agents for functional gastrointestinal disorders. Gut. 2005;54:1332-41.
59. Gonsalkorale WM. Gut-directed hypnotherapy: the Manchester approach for treatment of irritable bowel syndrome. Int J Clin Exp Hypn. 2006;54:27-50.
60. North CS, Hong BA, Alpers DH. Relationship of functional gastrointestinal disorders and psychiatric disorders: implications for treatment. World J Gastroenterol. 2007;13:2020-7.
61. Aucoin M, Lalonde-Parsi MJ, Cooley K. Mindfulness-based therapies in the treatment of functional gastrointestinal disorders: a meta-analysis. Evid Based Complement Alternat Med. 2014;2014:140724.
62. Windgassen S, Moss-Morris R, Chilcot J, Sibelli A, Goldsmith K, Chalder T. The journey between brain and gut: a systematic review of psychological mechanisms of treatment effect in irritable bowel syndrome. Br J Health Psychol. 2017;22:701-36.
63. Windgassen S, Moss-Morris R, Goldsmith K, Chalder T. Key mechanisms of cognitive behavioural therapy in irritable bowel syndrome: the importance of gastrointestinal related cognitions, behaviours and general anxiety. J Psychosom Res. 2019;118:73-82.
64. Peters SL, Muir JG, Gibson PR. Gut-directed hypnotherapy in the management of irritable bowel syndrome and inflammatory bowel disease. Aliment Pharmacol Ther. 2015;41:1104-15.
65. Chiarioni G, Whitehead WE. The role of biofeedback in the treatment of gastrointestinal disorders. Nat Clin Pract Gastroenterol Hepatol. 2008;5:371-82.

CHAPTER 7

Interface with Medical and Surgical Specialties

Shiva Shanker Reddy, Santosh K Chaturvedi

INTRODUCTION

Psychiatry is now significantly integrated with other medical and surgical specialties than in the past. Psychiatric disorders are highly prevalent among medically ill patients. Studies done in our country found 38.6% of psychiatric comorbidity with depressive disorder (28.2%) being the most common psychiatric diagnosis in the outpatient medically ill.[1] Several explanations have been offered for this association:

- Psychological reaction to distress imposed by a chronic medical condition, by a life-threatening condition or by the overall severity of illness
- Common etiological factor producing both medical illness and psychiatric illness or medical illness directly causing psychiatric disorder
- Bodily symptoms due to psychiatric disorders presenting to medical outpatient department (OPD) instead of psychiatric OPD
- Medically-ill patients are more prone develop psychiatric disorders than healthy people.

Many medically ill with psychiatric comorbidity will not directly seek psychiatric help due to several reasons such as lack of awareness among patients, stigma, and lack of psychiatric services. Other important issues are psychiatric disorders in medically ill are underdiagnosed and undertreated due to several reasons such as physicians inability to pick up the psychiatric symptoms, not sensitive to psychological matters, lack of proper referral services to psychiatrist. The psychiatric symptoms will also interfere in the medical and surgical management of patients such as complying with doctor's recommendations, obtaining consent for procedures, and risk to patient and staff. So, the association between psychiatric disorders and medical illness is complex. The comorbidity has detrimental implications for the patient's health outcome, quality of life, and medical treatment. In this chapter, we discuss about the various psychiatric issues that arise in physical ill patients and the complex interplay between physical and psychological factors. We also discuss about various subspecialties in this field and role of psychiatrist. The role of psychiatry in the interface of medical and surgical specialties is related to:

- Psychological reactions to medical diseases and surgical procedures
- Disturbances resulting from medical disorders affecting brain function, acute or chronic organic brain syndromes
- Medical complications of maladaptive behavior, drug abuse, obesity, anorexia
- Emotional disorders manifested by somatic symptoms with no organic basis such as chronic pain or fatigue which present with medical symptoms to begin with

- Physiologic concomitants of emotional states, such as the classical psychophysiological medical disorders
- Psychosomatic diseases
- Physical illnesses presenting as emotional or psychological problem, e.g., myxedema, thyrotoxicosis
- Psychological adverse drug reactions to drugs used for medical illnesses.

INTERFACE WITH MEDICAL SPECIALTIES

The interface between psychiatry and medical specialties is very vast. It starts from the etiopathogenesis of a medical illness due to psychological and emotional problems, to psychiatric consequences of medical diseases, especially those which are chronic or life threatening. This has a lot to do with psychiatric side effects of medications and procedures, as well as drug interactions between drugs for medical treatment and psychopharmacological agents. Some of the interfaces have developed into superspecialties such as:

- *Psycho-oncology:* Psychiatric aspects of cancer
- *Psychonephrology:* Psychiatric aspects of renal diseases
- *Psychocardiology:* Psychiatric aspects of heart diseases
- *Psycho-ophthalmology:* Psychiatric aspects of eye diseases
- *Psychogynecology:* Psychiatric aspects of gynecological disorders
- *Neuropsychiatry:* Psychiatric aspects of neurological diseases.

However, psychosurgery is not psychiatric aspects of surgery, psychopathology is not psychiatric aspects of pathology, and orthopsychiatry is not psychiatric aspects of orthopedics.

Here we discuss about various psychiatric issues seen in noncommunicable diseases, infectious diseases, autoimmune diseases, and endocrine disorders.

NONCOMMUNICABLE DISEASES

Noncommunicable diseases (NCDs) are a group of conditions/diseases, which are noninfectious and nontransmissible among people. The common NCDs include diabetes, hypertension (HTN), ischemic heart diseases (IHDs), and chronic kidney diseases. In India, NCDs are estimated to account for 53% of all deaths and 44% of disability-adjusted life-years lost in 2005.[2] Psychiatric illnesses are important group of comorbidities among patients with NCDs. Among the cross-sectional studies, the prevalence of depressive, anxiety, somatoform symptoms in NCDs found as 29.1%, 19.1%, and 35.1%, respectively.[2] In diabetic patients, depression was found to be present in 27.6%.[3] In a another study done on cardiac illness patients, moderate-to-severe level of depression was found in 51.36% of females and 38.45% of males; and moderate-to-severe level of anxiety was found in 57.13% of females and 38.45% of males.[4] From the above studies, it is clear that psychiatric disorders are more prevalent in people with NCDs. The higher occurrence can be direct result of direct disease process, reaction to chronic illness or both are caused by single etiological factor which might be common gene polymorphism. There are common risk factors for mental illness and chronic NCDs such as stress, irregular sleep habits, sedentary lifestyle, and substance use so they share a bidirectional relationship. Often presence of mental illness in person with NCD makes the management of chronic disease difficult and challenging as these patients will have difficulty in having lifestyle modification, regular checkups, and compliance to medication. This was shown in a meta-analysis where postmyocardial infarction patients with a clinical diagnosed depressive disorder had found to have a 2.0- to 2.5-fold increased risk of new cardiovascular events and cardiac mortality.[5] So, it is important to screen for the common mental illness in patients with NCDs and also treatment of psychiatric comorbidity.

INFECTIOUS DISEASES

Infectious organisms are implicated in causing psychiatric disorders. Psychiatric symptoms can occur as part of the clinical manifestations of several systemic and central nervous system infections.[6] On the other hand, psychological stress can affect the function of the immune system and increase infectious diseases susceptibility. Even a small focus of chronic infection can result in organic psychiatric disorder with symptoms of subtle cognitive dysfunction, irritability, depression, psychosis, and delirium. Febrile illness (e.g., urinary tract infection), septicemia, and encephalitis can lead to delirium. Dementia can be caused by infections such as human immunodeficiency virus (HIV), neurosyphilis, postencephalitis syndromes, and Lyme disease. The prevalence of psychiatric disorder in patients with epilepsy with neurocysticercosis was 68% as compared to 44% in patients with only epilepsy.[7] In HIV-positive patients, there is psychiatric comorbidity as high as 90%.[8] The relation between infectious diseases and psychiatric disorders can be categorized as:

- *Infectious diseases causing psychiatric symptoms:* Psychiatric symptoms can be the initial presenting symptoms (as in viral encephalitis), or could be part of the clinical picture (such as psychosis or mood symptoms in brucellosis or toxoplasmosis).
- *Infectious diseases with possible etiological role for major psychiatric disorders:* Influenza virus and HSV with possible etiological role for schizophrenia.[9]
- Psychiatric symptoms due to adverse effects of drugs used for treatment of the infectious disease, e.g., mefloquine, interferons (INFs), cycloserine, and efavirenz.
- *Primary psychiatric disorders can increase the risk of contracting infection:* High-risk behaviors in patients with mania and schizophrenia may lead to increased risk of infection.
- Psychiatric symptoms as a reaction to chronic and serious infections, e.g., HIV can lead to depression, anxiety or adjustment reactions.

The above discussion emphasizes on early identification of the underlying etiology for organic/secondary psychiatric symptoms and early treatment of the primary conditions that could be the cause of psychiatric symptoms.

AUTOIMMUNE AND INFLAMMATORY DISEASES

The positive correlation between the medical conditions and psychiatric illness suggests the presence of an underlying inflammatory process affecting the brain. Studies have shown that peripheral cellular and humoral immunological abnormalities are more prevalent in psychiatric patients relative to healthy controls. Common systemic autoimmune diseases which present with psychiatric symptoms are systemic lupus erythematosus (SLE), antiphospholipid syndrome (APS), autoimmune thyroiditis, multiple sclerosis (MS), and rheumatoid arthritis (RA). The term lupus cerebritis refers to the neuropsychiatric manifestations that appear due to SLE. The prevalence of neuropsychiatric manifestations in SLE has the following order (from most to least prevalent): cognitive dysfunction, headache, mood disorder, cerebrovascular disease, seizures, polyneuropathy, anxiety disorder, and psychosis.[10] In a systematic review in 2012 found depression (in up to 39% of patients) and cognitive dysfunction (up to 80%)

as most common psychiatric symptoms in SLE.[11] The neuropsychiatric symptoms in APS are similar to those seen in SLE with most common psychiatric symptom being cognitive impairment.[12] Hashimoto's thyroiditis usually presents either as change in personality or as depression. Alternatively, it may present as myxedema madness where patients have restlessness, hallucinations, and persecutory delusions. MS is inflammatory demyelinating condition which is associated with psychiatric symptoms.[13] The lifetime prevalence rate of psychiatric disorders in MS are approximately 50%, as compared to a rate of 10-15% in the general population and most frequent symptoms are dysphoria (79%), agitation (40%), anxiety (40%), irritability (35%) and rates of suicide are also significantly higher in those with MS.[14] In a study of relapsing-remitting patients with MS in remission, 95% reported significant psychiatric symptoms. RA affects 0.5-1% of the general population and is 2- to 3-fold more common among women. The frequency of depression and anxiety disorders among patients with RA ranges from 14 to 42%. Among female patients with RA who committed suicide, 90% had a depressive disorder.[15] Patients with RA who experience depression report significantly higher levels of pain, greater number of painful joints, and poorer functional ability.[16] Pediatric autoimmune neuropsychiatric disorders associated with streptococcal infections (PANDAS) is a condition associated with childhood obsessive-compulsive disorders (OCDs) and tic disorders triggered by group A β-hemolytic *Streptococcus pyogenes* infection.[17] There are another group of autoimmune diseases called synaptic autoimmune encephalitides or limbic encephalitis which present with psychiatric symptoms. In these conditions, symptoms evolve over days to weeks and include psychiatric manifestations as diverse as irritability, depression, hallucinations, and personality disturbances, with neurocognitive changes in the form of short-term memory loss, sleep disturbances, and seizure.[18] Cases of autoimmune encephalitis many times come to psychiatrist due to the nonspecific nature of symptoms or with only psychiatric symptoms initially. The treatment of autoimmune diseases involves immunosuppressant's mostly corticosteroids which again may cause or contribute to the behavioral problems. Autoimmune diseases have relapsing and remitting course each time there is a relapse and there is also recurrence of psychiatric symptoms. The management of these patients includes keeping the autoimmune disease under control and symptomatic management of psychiatric presentations.

ENDOCRINE DISORDERS

Psychiatric symptoms and syndromes are common in patients with endocrine disorders. Thyroid disorders are among the most frequent endocrine disorders in India. Psychiatric manifestations of hypothyroidism include cognitive deficits (impaired memory, psychomotor slowing, reduced attention span), vegetative symptoms (hypersomnia, sleep apnea, fatigue, lethargy, apathy, anergia, low libido), mood symptoms (depression, mood instability, mania, anxiety), and rarely psychosis (myxedemic madness).[19] Psychiatric manifestations seen in hyperthyroidism include anxiety, apathy, fatigue, cognitive deficits, emotional lability, hypomania or mania, irritability, and psychosis.[20] Hyperadrenalism (Cushing's syndrome) most commonly results from exogenous corticosteroids, but may also be the result of adrenocorticotropic hormone (ACTH) secretion by a pituitary tumor (Cushing's disease), or corticosteroid secretion by an adrenal tumor. In addition to somatic consequences—including diabetes, HTN, muscle weakness, obesity, and osteopenia—psychiatric symptoms are common in hyperadrenalism and may actually appear before physical signs. Depression is most common, but anxiety, hypomania/mania, psychosis, and cognitive dysfunction are all common.[21] Hyperprolactinemia may be caused by pituitary adenoma, pregnancy, antipsychotics. These patients may experience reduced libido, depression, and anxiety along physical manifestations.[22] Hyperparathyroidism (HPT) is well recognized endocrine disease producing psychiatric symptoms. Early symptoms of HPT include vague neurotic symptoms such as lack of spontaneity, initiative, emotional lability, and depression. Chronic hypercalcemia is known to produce cognitive deficits but there is a poor correlation between severity of hypercalcemia and psychiatric manifestations.[23]

PSYCHIATRIC ISSUES IN SURGICALLY ILL

Psychiatric disorders are quite common in surgical patients. A large proportion of psychopathology in surgical patients is either undiagnosed or misdiagnosed and not optimally treated. In the preoperative period, anxiety and health-related phobias, such as fear of anesthesia, needles, sight of blood, and contamination from blood transfusions, are common in surgical patients. Approximately 8–10% of adults have unreasonable fears of needles that may interfere with treatment. In the preoperative period, surgeons sometimes request psychiatric consultation regarding informed consent and assessment of the patient's decision-making capacity. During the postoperative period, common issues include complications related to alcohol abuse, dependence, and withdrawal; pain management, postoperative delirium and continuing psychotropic in patient with past psychiatric illness. Anxiety disorders, depression, bipolar disorder, schizophrenia, and personality disorders may all flare up during the postoperative period. In a 2-year prospective study in 221 consecutive inpatients undergoing cataractomy found that the incidence of delirium at 1.8%.[24] In a study done to known the type of psychiatric referrals in tertiary care, multispecialty hospital in medicosurgical patients found that organic psychosis constitutes (25.5%), nonorganic psychosis constitutes (11.2%), neurosis included (24.8%) other disorders (substance abuse disorders and adjustment reaction) (21.5%), and "nil psychiatric" (17%).[25] Delirium was included in organic psychosis category. Postoperative delirium is very common, particularly in elderly patients undergoing hip replacement, major abdominal surgery, or cardiac surgery. Up to 40% of elderly orthopedic surgery patients experience delirium.[26] Traumatic brain injury (TBI) is another surgical problem in which almost half of people later be diagnosed with neuropsychiatric disorders. TBI commonly is implicated in cognitive deficits, mood disorders, organic personality disorders, and rarely psychosis.[27]

SPECIALTY AREAS: PSYCHO-ONCOLOGY

Psycho-oncology is presently defined as the subspecialty of cancer dealing with two psychological dimensions:
1. The psychological reactions of patients with cancer and their families at all stages of disease and the stresses on staff
2. The psychological, social, and behavioral factors that contribute to cancer cause and survival.

The common psychological and emotional responses to cancer arise from knowledge of life-threatening diagnosis, its prognostic uncertainty, and fears about death and dying. The emotional responses are also due to physical symptoms such as pain, nausea, lymphedema, and unwanted effects of medical, surgical, and radiation treatments. The stigma due to cancer and its consequences adds to the negative reactions to the disease.[28] In the Indian setting, 38–53% of cancer patients were found to have identifiable the Diagnostic and Statistical Manual of Mental Disorders, Third Edition, Revised (DSM-III-R) psychiatric disorder. In a large study including 903 cancer patients attending a hospice, a general hospital, and the neurosurgery department of the National Institute of Mental Health and Neurosciences (NIMHANS), psychiatric disorders were identified in 48%, of which 44% had adjustment disorders. One of the most difficult and challenging roles of a psychiatrist in cancer care is dealing with issues related to communication skills of health professionals. Health professionals dealing with cancer patients find it difficult to disclose diagnosis to cancer patients and their relatives. Psychiatrists are called upon to train cancer specialists in skills of breaking bad news. Dealing with "collusion" is another challenging situation. In a study done regarding awareness of their diagnosis, in 294 newly admitted cancer patients at an oncology center in South India found 54% of patients were aware that they had cancer and were able to discuss their diagnosis and 46% of patients reported nonawareness of diagnosis.[29] Dealing with collusion and breaking collusion sensitively is important to maintain trust and communication between patient and family members without the conspiracy of silence. It also has been reported that antidepressants are grossly underused in cancer patients, for fear of addiction/dependence, caution against adverse side effects, drug interactions and thinking that depression is natural reaction. The principles of management include sensitive to breaking of bad news, providing information in accord with person's wishes, permitting expression of emotions and feelings, clarification of concerns and problems, involving patient in decisions about treatments, and appropriate use of psychotropic.

PSYCHODERMATOLOGY

Psychodermatology or psychocutaneous medicine encompasses disorders prevailing on the boundary between psychiatry and dermatology. Connecting the two disciplines is a complex interplay between neuroendocrine and immune systems that has been described as neuroimmunocutaneous system (NICS). The interaction between nervous system, skin, and immunity has been explained by release of mediators from NICS. It has been reported that psychologic stress perturbs epidermal permeability barrier homeostasis, and it may act as precipitant for some inflammatory disorders such as atopic dermatitis and psoriasis.[30] Approximately 30–40% patients seeking treatment for skin disorders have an underlying psychiatric or a psychological problem that either causes or exacerbates a skin complaint.[31] The prevalence of active suicidal ideation among the patients with psoriasis and acne was 5.6–7.2%.[32] Ample evidence in literature suggests that the course of many skin disorders is affected by stress and psychological events.[33] Psychocutaneous disorders classified into three types:
1. Psychosomatic disorders are those in which the course of a given skin disease is affected by the psychological state of a patient. These disorders are often precipitated or exacerbated by emotional stress and/or anxiety in a significant number of cases, e.g., psoriasis, atopic dermatitis.
2. Primary psychiatric disorders where the primary pathology is in psyche and skin

complaints are self-induced or secondary. Psychiatric disorders with dermatological symptoms such as delusional parasitosis, trichotillomania, skin excoriation, and OCD.
3. Secondary psychiatric disorders caused by disfiguring skin conditions such as ichthyosis, acne conglobata, vitiligo which can lead to states of fear, depression or suicidal thoughts.[34]

Once the disorder has been diagnosed, management requires a dual approach, addressing both dermatologic and psychologic aspects. Majority of psychocutaneous disorders can be treated with cognitive-behavioral psychotherapy, psychotherapeutic stress and anxiety management techniques, and psychotropic drugs.[35] The cooperation of the dermatologist and a psychiatrist in the management of these patients is of utmost importance. Medication is used where there is primary psychiatric condition causing skin manifestation in liaison with dermatologist.

PAIN, PALLIATIVE CARE AND END OF LIFE ISSUES

Palliative care deals with expertise in understanding the psychosocial dimensions of human experience to the care of dying patients and support of their families. Palliative care is specialized medical care for people with serious illnesses. This care is focused on providing patients with relief from the symptoms, pain, and stress of a serious illness irrespective of the diagnosis. The goal is to improve quality of life for both the patient and the family. With this holistic and all-encompassing view of pain, Saunders advocated for a more person-centered and comprehensive approach to address not just the nociceptive components of a patient's pain, but the emotional, spiritual, social, and experiential dimensions.[36] More specifically, psychiatric syndromes, such as depression, anxiety, and delirium, are common in palliative care settings. In hospice patients, roughly 50% will experience symptoms of depression; approximately 70% will experience clinically significant anxiety. Psychiatric conditions are often difficult to differentiate in the setting of serious illness, due to symptom overlap with medical conditions.[37] The Psychiatrist working in palliative care should focus on increasing the quality of life using psychological interventions and psychotropic wherever appropriate. There are studies reporting about underusing, undertreating the pain and psychiatric symptoms in palliative care. Psychiatrist as a part of palliative care focuses on comprehensive pain management as well as increasing the quality of life of the patients. Psychiatrist also does interventions such as reducing the fear of dying and preparing the family for bereavement.[38]

PSYCHONEPHROLOGY

Psychonephrology is subspecialty that deals with the psychological impact of kidney disease and focuses particularly on patients receiving kidney transplants or dialysis treatment. Patients on forms of dialysis and those who receive kidney transplants face many stresses connected with their illness and forms of treatment. These stresses may result in a variety of psychiatric disorders.[39] The most common psychiatric complications occurring as a result of renal failure are depression and anxiety. Many observational studies have demonstrated that dialysis patients have higher suicide rates than the normal healthy population. Delirium is another common phenomenon observed in dialysis patients due to electrolyte imbalances that may occur after a dialysis run termed as the dialysis disequilibrium syndrome. Dialysis dementia is a term used to describe a rapidly progressive form of dementia, now considered rare, associated with aluminum toxicity in end-stage renal disease (ESRD) patients.[40] The management of these patients includes individual, group therapy and psychotropic. Many patients on dialysis do well if individual psychotherapy is administered during the dialysis sessions. It is also important to remember that pharmacokinetics of medications used to treat these patients requires special consideration of the route of elimination, whether or not the medication is dialyzable.[41] There are many challenges in treating these patients such as denial of their problems, multiple comorbidities, noncompliance, and change in pharmacokinetics of many drugs. The management of these patients involves multidisciplinary team.

MEDICAL ISSUES IN PSYCHIATRIC PATIENTS

A number of reviews and studies have shown that people with severe mental illness (SMI), have an excess mortality, being two or three times as high as that in the general population.[42] About 60% of this excess mortality is due to physical illness. Evidence suggests that persons with SMI are, compared to the general population, at increased risk for overweight [i.e., body mass index (BMI) = 25–29.9, unless Asian: BMI = 23–24.9], obesity (BMI ≥ 30, unless Asian: BMI ≥ 25).[43] People with schizophrenia have a 2.8–3.5 increased likelihood of being obese, those with major depression or bipolar disorder have a 1.2–1.5 increased risk.[44,45] The metabolic syndrome (MetS) is highly prevalent among treated patients with schizophrenia. Depending on used MetS criteria, gender, ethnicity, country, age groups, and antipsychotics treatment, percentages vary considerably (between 19.4 and 68%).[46] MetS rates in patients with bipolar disorder and schizoaffective disorder have been reported to be 22–30% and 42%, respectively.[47,48] The prevalence of diabetes mellitus (DM) in people with schizophrenia as well as in people with bipolar disorder and schizoaffective disorder is 2- to 3-fold higher compared with the general population.[49,50] The risk of DM in people with depression or depressive symptoms is 1.2–2.6 times higher compared to people without depression.[51] The prevalence of cardiovascular risk disease (CVD) in people with schizophrenia and bipolar disorder is approximately 2- to 3-fold.[52] People with depression have a 50% greater risk of CVD, this is besides the fact that depression is an independent risk factor for aggravating morbidity and mortality in coronary heart disease.[53] The prevalence of HIV positivity in people with SMI is generally higher than in the general population (1.3–23.9%).[54] The prevalence rates of hepatitis B virus (23.4%) and hepatitis C virus (19.6%) in SMI patients found to be approximately 5 and 11 times the overall estimated population rates.[55] From the above discussion, it is clear that people with mental illness are at risk physical illness (noninfective or infective). There are several reasons for this association which includes:

- Poor nutrition
- Reduced physical activity
- Poor self-care and hygiene
- More often involved in high-risk sexual behavior and substance use
- Adverse effect of psychotropic
- Genetic factors where people with certain polymorphisms are at higher risk for mental illness and physical illness.

ROLE OF PSYCHIATRIST IN THE MEDICAL AND SURGICAL INTERFACE

There is major role of psychiatrist in dealing with psychosocial issues in medicosurgical specialties. It starts with identifying the

high-risk groups in medical ill patients. This includes:
- Elderly patients who have multiple physical illness
- Patients with certain autoimmune conditions such as SLE, Hashimoto's thyroiditis, limbic encephalitis
- Patients with chronic medical illness such as diabetic mellitus
- Specific infections such as tuberculosis, retroviral disease
- Patients with terminal illness
- Patients undergoing amputations and postoperative patients
- Patients who are taking multiple medication and medication which can cause psychiatric symptoms, e.g., antituberculosis treatment (ATT), antiretroviral therapy (ART), corticosteroids.

Whenever a psychiatrist was called to see medical ill patient or send to psychiatric clinic, he should see the patient in systemic manner. This includes identifying the patient with his hospital reference number, reading the referral note, going through the case record or documents, taking history form reliable informant, inquiring for pain and distress, making temporal correlation of events, doing bedside cognitive tasks, and coming to diagnosis. Many a times patient may not have syndromal diagnosis, they just may have subthreshold symptoms or specific symptoms such as pain, anger dyscontrol, sleep-related problems. The management includes using appropriate psychotropic starting at low dose and monitoring for side effects. Along with medication psychological interventions should be done. In situations where mental capacity of patients requires assessment, psychiatrist should assess patient for his orientation, comprehension, his understanding of his illness, and nature of treatment offered to him. Psychiatrist should also involve in educating the staff and doctors about communication skills for example breaking bad news about diagnosis or prognosis of disease and identifying the psychological illness at earliest.

REFERENCES

1. Thappa J, Kaur H, Thappa S, Banal R, Chowhan A. Psychiatric morbidity in patients attending medical OPD at Govt. Medical College Jammu. Research Gate; 2008.
2. Kulkarni V, Chinnakali P, Kanchan T, Rao A, Shenoy M, Papanna MK. Psychiatric co-morbidities among patients with select non-communicable diseases in a coastal city of South India. Int J Prev Med. 2014;5:1139-45.
3. Guruprasad KG, Niranjan MR, Ashwin S. A study of association of depressive symptoms among the type 2 diabetic outpatients presenting to a tertiary care hospital. Indian J Psychol Med. 2012;34:30-3.
4. Choudhary R, Kumar P, Wander GS, Mishra BP, Sharma A. (2014). Psychiatric manifestations among cardiac patients: a hospital-based study. [online] Available from: http://medind.nic.in/daa/t14/i2/daat14i2p253.pdf [Last accessed June, 2021].
5. van Melle JP, de Jonge P, Spijkerman TA, Tijssen JG, Ormel J, van Veldhuisen DJ, et al. Prognostic association of depression following myocardial infarction with mortality and cardiovascular events: a meta-analysis. Psychosom Med. 2004;66:814-22.
6. Nicolson GL, Haier J. Role of chronic bacterial and viral infections in neurodegenerative, neurobehavioral, psychiatric, autoimmune and fatiguing illnesses: Part 1. BJMP. 2009;2(4):20-8.
7. Srivastava S, Chadda RK, Bala K, Majumdar P. A study of neuropsychiatric manifestations in patients of neurocysticercosis. Indian J Psychiatry. 2013;55:264-7.
8. Satapathy R, Krishna MN, Babu AM, Vijayagopal M. A study of psychiatric manifestations of physically asymptomatic HIV-I seropositive individuals. Indian J Psychiatry. 2000;42:427-33.
9. Meyer U, Feldon J. Neural basis of psychosis-related behaviour in the infection model of schizophrenia. Behav Brain Res. 2009;204:322-34.
10. Hanly JG. ACR classification criteria for systemic lupus erythematosus: limitations and revisions to neuropsychiatric variables. Lupus. 2004;13:861-4.

11. Meszaros ZS, Perl A, Faraone SV. Psychiatric symptoms in systemic lupus erythematosus: a systematic review. J Clin Psychiatry. 2012;73: 993-1001.
12. Furmańczyk A, Komuda-Leszek E, Gadomska W, Windyga J, Durlik M. Catastrophic antiphospholipid syndrome. Pol Arch Med Wewn. 2009;119:427-30.
13. Diaz-Olavarrieta C, Cummings JL, Velazquez J, Garcia de la Cadena C. Neuropsychiatric manifestations of multiple sclerosis. J Neuropsychiatry Clin Neurosci. 1999;11:51-7.
14. Politte LC, Huffman JC, Stern TA. Neuropsychiatric manifestations of multiple sclerosis. Prim Care Companion J Clin Psychiatry. 2008;10:318-24.
15. Timonen M, Timonen M, Viilo K, Hakko H, Särkioja T, Ylikulju M, et al. Suicides in persons suffering from rheumatoid arthritis. Rheumatology (Oxford). 2003;42:287-91.
16. Katz PP, Yelin EH. Prevalence and correlates of depressive symptoms among persons with rheumatoid arthritis. J Rheumatol. 1993;20:790-6.
17. Moretti G, Pasquini M, Mandarelli G, Tarsitani L, Biondi M. What every psychiatrist should know about PANDAS: a review. Clin Pract Epidemiol Ment Health. 2008;4:13.
18. Kayser MS, Dalmau J. The emerging link between autoimmune disorders and neuropsychiatric disease. J Neuropsychiatry Clin Neurosci. 2011;23:90-7.
19. Geracioti TD. Identifying hypothyroidism's psychiatric presentations. Curr Psychiatry. 2006;5(11):98-117.
20. Geracioti TD. Identifying hyperthyroidism's psychiatric presentations. Curr Psychiatry. 2006;5(12):84-92.
21. Pivonello R, Simeoli C, De Martino MC, Cozzolino A, De Leo M, Iacuaniello D, et al. Neuropsychiatric disorders in Cushing's syndrome. Front Neurosci. 2015;9:129.
22. Byerly M, Suppes T, Tran QV, Baker RA. Clinical implications of antipsychotic-induced hyperprolactinemia in patients with schizophrenia spectrum or bipolar spectrum disorders: recent developments and current perspectives. J Clin Psychopharmacol. 2007;27: 639-61.
23. Coker LH, Rorie K, Cantley L, Kirkland K, Stump D, Burbank N, et al. Primary hyperparathyroidism, cognition, and health-related quality of life. Ann Surg. 2005;242:642-50.
24. Chaudhury S, Mahar RS, Augustine M. Post-cataractomy delirium: a two year prospective study. Indian J Psychiatry. 1992;34:154-8.
25. Avasthi A, Sharan P, Kulhara P, Malhotra S, Varma VK. Psychiatric profiles in medical-surgical populations: need for a focused approach to consultation-uaison psychiatry in developing countries. Indian J Psychiatry. 1998;40:224-30.
26. Galanakis P, Bickel H, Gradinger R, Von Gumppenberg S, Förstl H. Acute confusional state in the elderly following hip surgery: incidence, risk factors and complications. Int J Geriatr Psychiatry. 2001;16:349-55.
27. Chaudhury S, Pande V, Saini R, Rathee SP, Dev S, Lyons I, et al. Neuropsychiatric sequelae of head injury. Indian J Neurotrauma. 2005;2:13-21.
28. Chaturvedi SK. Psychiatric oncology: cancer in mind. Indian J Psychiatry. 2012;54:111-8.
29. Chandra PS, Chaturvedi SK, Kumar A, Kumar S, Subbakrishna DK, Channabasavanna SM, et al. Awareness of diagnosis and psychiatric morbidity among cancer patients—a study from South India. J Psychosom Res. 1998;45:257-61.
30. Garg A, Chren MM, Sands LP, Matsui MS, Marenus KD, Feingold KR, et al. Psychological stress perturbs epidermal permeability barrier homeostasis: implications for the pathogenesis of stress-associated skin disorders. Arch Dermatol. 2001;137:53-9.
31. Picardi A, Abeni D, Melchi CF, Puddu P, Pasquini P. Psychiatric morbidity in dermatological outpatients: an issue to be recognized. Br J Dermatol. 2000;143:983-91.
32. Gupta MA, Gupta AK. Depression and suicidal ideation in dermatology patients with acne, alopecia areata, atopic dermatitis and psoriasis. Br J Dermatol. 1998;139:846-50.
33. Humphreys F, Humphreys MS. Psychiatric morbidity and skin disease: what dermatologists think they see. Br J Dermatol. 1998;139:679-81.
34. Yadav S, Narang T, Kumaran MS. Psychodermatology: a comprehensive review. Indian J Dermatol Venereol Leprol. 2013;79: 176-92.
35. Basavaraj KH, Navya MA, Rashmi R. Relevance of psychiatry in dermatology: present concepts. Indian J Psychiatry. 2010;52:270-5.
36. Fairman N, Irwin SA. Palliative care psychiatry: update on an emerging dimension of psychiatric practice. Curr Psychiatry Rep. 2013;15:374.
37. Irwin SA, Ferris FD. The opportunity for psychiatry in palliative care. Can J Psychiatry. 2008; 53:713-24.
38. Sharma H, Jagdish V, Anusha P, Bharti S. End-of-life care: Indian perspective. Indian J Psychiatry. 2013;55:S293-8.

39. Levy NB. What is psychonephrology? J Nephrol. 2008;21 (Suppl 13):S51-3.
40. Tamura MK, Yaffe K. Dementia and cognitive impairment in ESRD: diagnostic and therapeutic strategies. Kidney Int. 2011;79:14-22.
41. De Sousa A. Psychiatric issues in renal failure and dialysis. Indian J Nephrol. 200;18:47-50.
42. Brown S. Excess mortality of schizophrenia: a meta-analysis. Br J Psychiatry. 1997;171:502-8.
43. Citrome L, Vreeland B. Schizophrenia, obesity, and antipsychotic medications: what can we do? Postgrad Med. 2008;120:18-33.
44. Krishnan KR. Psychiatric and medical comorbidities of bipolar disorder. Psychosom Med. 2005;67:1-8.
45. Simon GE, Ludman EJ, Linde JA, Operskalski BH, Ichikawa L, Rohde P, et al. Association between obesity and depression in middle-aged women. Gen Hosp Psychiatry. 2008;30:32-9.
46. De Hert MA, van Winkel R, Van Eyck D, Hanssens L, Wampers M, Scheen A, et al. Prevalence of the metabolic syndrome in patients with schizophrenia treated with antipsychotic medication. Schizophr Res. 2006;83:87-93.
47. Basu R, Brar JS, Chengappa KN, John V, Parepally H, Gershon S, et al. The prevalence of the metabolic syndrome in patients with schizoaffective disorder—bipolar subtype. Bipolar Disord. 2004;6:314-8.
48. Garcia-Portilla MP, Saiz PA, Benabarre A, Sierra P, Perez J, Rodriguez A, et al. The prevalence of metabolic syndrome in patients with bipolar disorder. J Affect Disord. 2008;106:197-201.
49. Bushe C, Holt R. Prevalence of diabetes and impaired glucose tolerance in patients with schizophrenia. Br J Psychiatry. 2004;47:S67-71.
50. McIntyre RS, Konarski JZ, Misener VL, Kennedy SH. Bipolar disorder and diabetes mellitus: epidemiology, etiology, and treatment implications. Ann Clin Psychiatry. 2005;17:83-93.
51. Brown LC, Majumdar SR, Newman SC, Johnson JA. History of depression increases risk of type 2 diabetes in younger adults. Diabetes Care. 2005;28:1063-7.
52. Osborn DP, Levy G, Nazareth I, Petersen I, Islam A, King MB. Relative risk of cardiovascular and cancer mortality in people with severe mental illness from the United Kingdom's General Practice Research Database. Arch Gen Psychiatry. 2007;64:242-9.
53. Ruo B, Rumsfeld JS, Hlatky MA, Liu H, Browner WS, Whooley MA. Depressive symptoms and health-related quality of life: the Heart and Soul Study. JAMA. 2003;290:215-21.
54. Volavka J, Convit A, Czobor P, Douyon R, O'Donnell J, Ventura F. HIV seroprevalence and risk behaviors in psychiatric inpatients. Psychiatry Res. 1991;39:109-14.
55. Rosenberg SD, Goodman LA, Osher FC, Swartz MS, Essock SM, Butterfield MI, et al. Prevalence of HIV, hepatitis B, and hepatitis C in people with severe mental illness. Am J Public Health. 2001;91:31-7.

CHAPTER 8

Interface with Dermatology

Shubh Mohan Singh, Tarun Narang, Dalton N

INTRODUCTION

The skin is the largest organ of the body and carries out a host of important functions. Like all other organs, it is influenced and in turn influences various organ systems of the body in health and disease. Embryologically the skin is derived from the same substrate as the central nervous system (CNS).

What makes the skin important beyond its immediate importance as an organ of the body essential for functioning and survival are the following important facts. The first is that skin is readily visible to the observer unlike other organs that usually require specialized techniques or instruments to assess and examine. Thus, all pathologies are usually readily accessible. The second and more important quality of skin is its influence on human self-image, self-esteem and its influence on human relations. Indeed, the skin defines us as what we are. We use qualities of the skin such as color and notions of beauty to automatically classify people into desirable and undesirable. This is true for humans from infancy onward. Thus, stigmata on skin are often disproportionately influential on the human psyche than obscure pathologies elsewhere.[1] A quick look at human history reveals that qualities such as color and appearance have defined humanity since times immemorial. While appearance and color for instance have often been symbols of affiliation and identity, some of the greatest crimes in history of humanity have also been carried out for the same reasons. Qualities such as skin color are major determinants of perceived attractiveness, suitability for marriage, etc., as is exemplified in the popularity of skin whitening products in many societies.[2]

In contemporary times, the spread of technology and advances in medicine mean that self-image is more important and malleable than ever. It is intuitive that the skin is major determinant of self-esteem. Another important quality of visible skin lesions is the phenomenon of stigma. Historically, stigmata meant an unconcealable mark on the skin that served as a mark of discredit. Deeply stigmatizing conditions have traditionally been disfiguring and visible disorders such as leprosy.[3]

Finally, many skin disorders are chronic, relapsing conditions. As such they carry all the burden inherent in chronic diseases in addition to being visible and stigmatizing. Thus, it is not surprising that there is a significant interface between the soma (the skin in this case) and the psyche. This is not unexpected as the skin and CNS have the same embryological basis.

The interface of psychiatry and dermatology is dependent on the setting. There are various psychiatric disorders that can present with or have dermatological complaints as significant manifestations. On the other hand, various dermatological conditions can also have psychiatric implications. These can occur in the form of psychiatric comorbidities or as iatrogenic manifestations such as exemplified by side effects of medications used in dermatological conditions which have psychiatric or psychological manifestations.[4]

As per the mandate provided to the authors, this chapter is an overview of this area with an idea to provide the reader with an up-to-date understanding of the various interfaces between psychiatry and dermatology with an examination of how the knowledge of the above can translate into better health care. This chapter is primarily geared toward psychiatrists and thus in the interests of brevity, less emphasis has been put on various diagnostic criteria of psychiatric disorders and more on the various clinical manifestations and concepts of this interface. The disorders are treated as per the diagnostic criteria laid down in accepted nosological systems such as the International Classification of Diseases, Tenth Revision (ICD-10) and the Diagnostic and Statistical Manual of Mental Disorders, Fifth Edition (DSM-5).

INTERFACE OF PSYCHIATRY AND DERMATOLOGY

This section will examine the ways and situations in which the interface between psychiatry and dermatology can occur. As this is a very vast topic and each section can merit a chapter in itself, only the salient points will be discussed. An outline is provided in **Table 1**.

Psychiatric Disorders and Dermatological Implications

Practically any psychiatric disorder can have a coexisting dermatological disorder. Dermatological disorders may arise from factors, such as poor hygiene due to chronic psychiatric symptoms or because of metabolic disorders such as diabetes, that are common in people suffering from psychiatric disorders.

TABLE 1: Interface of psychiatry and dermatology.		
Psychiatric disorders and dermatological implications	Psychiatric disorders with dermatological manifestations understandable on basis of psychopathology	• Substance abuse disorders • Delusional disorders • Obsessive-compulsive disorder • Somatoform disorders • Habit, impulse disorders • Factitious disorders • Eating disorders • Personality disorders • Neurodevelopmental disorders • Skin-picking disorders • Body-focused repetitive behaviors • Dermatological manifestations of psychotropic drug use
	Skin disorders more common in certain psychiatric disorders	Skin infections most common
Dermatological disorders and psychiatric implications	Dermatological disorders and psychiatric comorbidities	Depression and anxiety disorders most common
	Psychiatric side effects of drugs used in dermatological practice	Mood changes (uncommon)
	Dermatological conditions that are influenced by psychological factors	Psoriasis, vitiligo, etc.

However, certain psychiatric disorders are known to have typical dermatological manifestations. Some dermatological disorders are supposed to be influenced by psychological factors as well. In this section, we shall examine some of these conditions.

The importance of dermatological manifestations in psychiatric disorders is twofold. Firstly, many patients have classical and specific lesions that are associated with specific syndromes. However, these are often first seen by dermatologists. Secondly, while skin manifestations may seem minor when compared to the overall corpus of morbidity, these do contribute to overall impairment in quality of life.

Psychiatric Disorders with Cutaneous Manifestations including Treatment Emergent Side Effects

In this section, we will examine the psychiatric disorders that have specific and well-described dermatological manifestations; these disorders are sometimes referred to as primary psychocutaneous disorders.[1] These can arise as a part of the common pathophysiology or more commonly as a result of the behavioral aspects of the psychiatric disorder. Some of the more important entities are described here.

Substance abuse disorders: The dermatological manifestations of substance abuse are commonly seen in relation to chronic intravenous drug use.[5,6] These may include among other manifestations acute or delayed local complications, hypersensitivity reactions, cutaneous manifestations of systemic infections or becoming the site of toxigenic infections. Track marks, deep necrotic ulcers at the sites of skin popping, sooting tattoos due to use of hot needles are some of the characteristic cutaneous stigmata that may help in identifying/suspecting intravenous (IV) drug abuse **(Fig. 1)**.

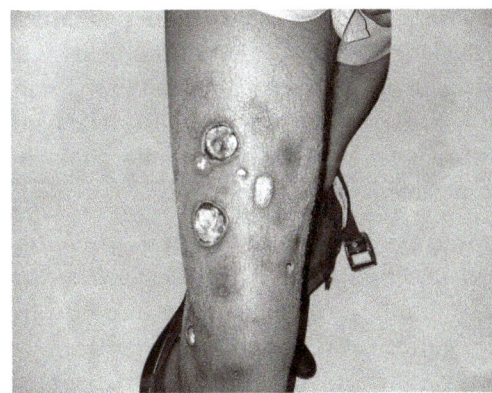

Fig. 1: Necrotic deep ulcers on the thigh in a patient with pentazocine addiction.

Delusional disorders: Delusional parasitosis or Ekbom's disease is the most common monosymptomatic hypochondriacal psychosis in dermatology, classified as a delusional disorder, somatic type in DSM-5 criteria. This is characterized by a fixed false belief that a patient is infested with some living organisms or inanimate materials in the absence of any objective proof.[7] Patients with delusional infestations experience symptoms of formication such as crawling, biting or stinging (pins and needle sensation) with a strong belief of being infested with a parasite and may attempt to pick the imaginary organism from the body site. Self-picking may lead to the findings on examination such as excoriations, erosions, prurigo-like lesions and even deep ulcers. The patients keep collecting the specimens from the skin by repetitive picking as proof of infestation, known as "matchbox sign", "ziplock sign" or "specimen sign". Before making a diagnosis of delusional parasitosis, it is very important to rule out other causes of formication such as scabies, pediculosis, cerebrovascular, and CNS causes such as dementia, meningitis, encephalitis, neurosyphilis endocrine disorders, drugs, vitamin B_{12} deficiency. The possible infestants include insects, fungi, inanimate objects or even larger animals and mammals.

Morgellons disease is another variant of delusional belief where the fixed belief is in terms of fibers being embedded in the skin, or being extruded out. Musculoskeletal pain, arthritis, fatigue, and poor memory may be associated.[8]

Obsessive-compulsive disorder—dermatological obsessive-compulsive disorders: The skin manifestations in these patients are a result of obsession with something or a thought and repetitive skin directed compulsive behavior. The common disorders include trichotillomania **(Fig. 2)**, compulsive skin picking, neurotic excoriations **(Fig. 3)**, onychotillomania **(Fig. 4)**, rhinotillexomania (frequent nose digging), lip licking **(Fig. 5)**, frequent handwashing leading to cumulative insult or allergic contact dermatitis and fungal infection of hands/nails.[9]

Somatoform disorders including body dysmorphic disorder: Body dysmorphic disorder, previously known as dysmorphophobia or dermatological nondisease, is a somatoform disorder characterized by an excessive preoccupation of the patient with an imaginary or minimal physical defect in appearance like mild acne or scars or sometimes they may feel that their faces are asymmetrical or they look more aged. Individuals having this condition are very distressed leading to embarrassment, depression, and suicidal ideation. Body dysmorphic disorder is probably increasing

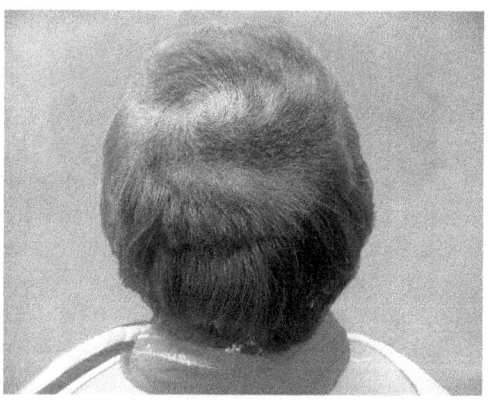

Fig. 2: Trichotillomania.

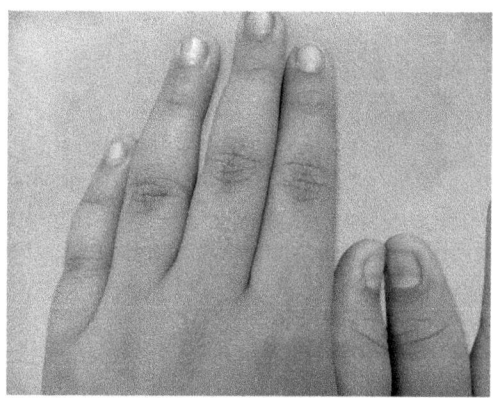

Fig. 4: Onychotillomania.

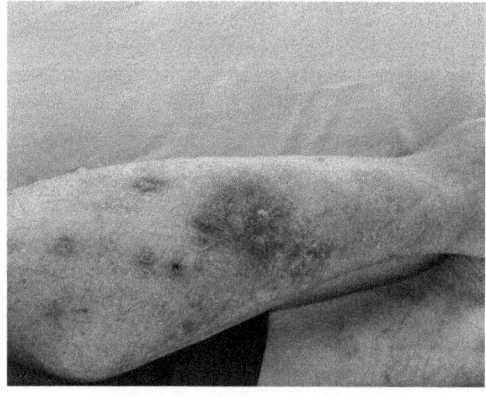

Fig. 3: Neurotic excoriations.

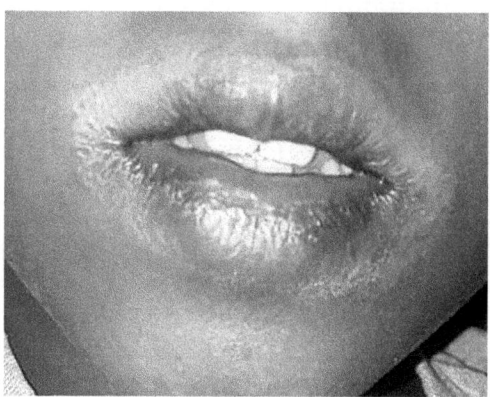

Fig. 5: Lip-lick cheilitis.

due to ever increasing dependence on social media. Males and females are equally affected and males may present with a focus on hair, genitals, and body build. The characteristic feature in these patients is excessive thinking approximately 3-8 hours/day about the alleged defect in appearance. These patients visit the healthcare practitioners frequently to find a solution for their minor or imagined flaws and are often dissatisfied with results. These patients are often seen doctor shopping and they will never be satisfied with the results of treatments or procedures done by the doctors they had earlier visited.[10]

Habit and impulse disorders, tic disorders including trichotillomania: Trichotillomania is an impulse control disorder characterized by a repetitive pulling of hair resulting in hail loss. Most of these cases visit a pediatrician or dermatologist first and are diagnosed as alopecia areata (AA) or sometimes tinea capitis (fungal infection of scalp hair) before being referred to psychiatrists. The prevalence of trichotillomania ranges from 1 to 4% with average age of onset around 10-17 years and a female preponderance. Associated psychiatric conditions include anxiety, depression, dementia, adjustment disorder, and rarely substance abuse. Scalp is generally the most common site affected, however, any region of body with hair such as eyebrows or eyelashes can also be involved. Although the patients or the attendants are never forthcoming with the history of self-pulling of hair but sometimes there is a characteristic history of increasing tension and urge to pull the hair which is relieved after hair pulling. On examination, irregular patches of nonscarring and scarring alopecia are seen over the scalp, site of which depends on the patient's handedness. Hairs are broken at different lengths with split ends[11] **(Fig. 6)**.

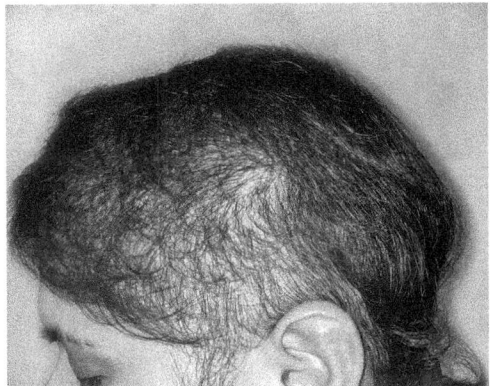

Fig. 6: Trichotillomania.

Factitious dermatitis: Factitial dermatitis is a condition whereby the patients induced dermatitis or other skin changes such as ulceration in order to satisfy a conscious or unconscious desire to assume the sick role. It is particularly common in women and in those with an underlying psychiatric diagnosis or external stress.[12] These include dermatitis artefacta (DA), dermatitis simulata, dermatological pathomimicry and additionally Munchausen syndrome, Munchausen by proxy and malingering. The psychiatric disorders associated with it are borderline personality disorder, dependency, and manipulative behavior. Artifactual lesions can also be produced as a result of malingering or in the case of Munchausen's by proxy, be produced in children or even pets.[13]

Dermatitis artefacta is one of the most common factitious disorders seen in dermatology outpatient and the patient may present with various types of lesions such as abrasions, bullae, ulcers, and burns over accessible sites. Peak age of onset is around 20 years with a female preponderance with an equal sex incidence in children. Patients with DA often have a history of abuse or neglect during childhood and is associated with other psychological comorbidities. The two characteristic features of DA are the physical

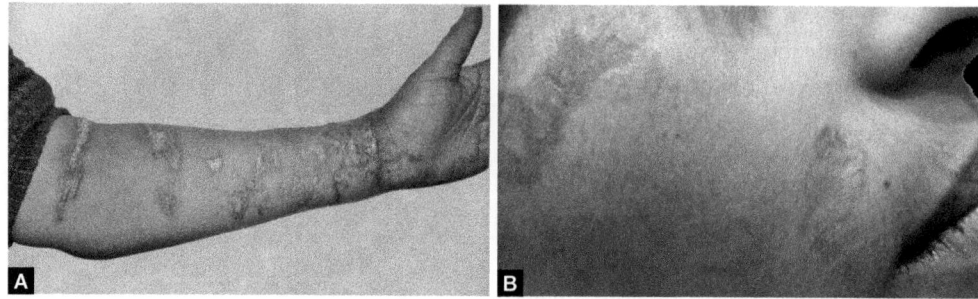

Figs. 7A and B: Dermatitis artefacta.

signs and fabricated story that accompanies these signs. These patients classically present with a hollow history with vague evolution of lesions and often unsatisfactory previous treatment. The lesions of DA are usually symmetrical and present over accessible sites with bizarre-shaped ulcers or erosions and zigzag or geometrical borders **(Figs. 7A and B)**. Other lesions which can be seen, include erythema, purpura, eczematous lesions over commonly affected sites such as face, upper and lower extremities, and hands. Self-induced chemical injuries may show a "drip sign".

Eating disorders: Both anorexia nervosa and bulimia can manifest with prominent and specific skin manifestations[14,15] such as alopecia, xerosis, dry and lusterless skin, carotenoderma, nail dystrophies, angular cheilitis, bald tongue, etc. Russell sign or knuckle callosities found on the dorsal aspect of dominant hand due to repeated insertion of hand into mouth and friction with upper teeth is one of the characteristic signs of eating disorders.

Personality disorders: Individuals with certain personality disorders namely borderline personality disorder and antisocial personality disorders are prone to characteristic self-injurious behavior.[16] This behavior may be an outlet for psychic distress, as a call for help or for manipulative reasons. Whatever be the reason, this is usually a repetitive pattern of behavior that is characterized by nonfatal injuries mostly caused by superficial cuts. The cuts are usually in the accessible parts of the body. An episode of such behavior may be brought about stress or frustration due to any reason. The scars are usually characteristic. While suicide is rare, occasionally such self-injurious behavior may become serious either by accident or by design.[17]

Neurodevelopmental disorders—intellectual disabilities including syndromes, autism: Self-induced injuries like head are commonly observed in children with mental retardation and sometimes the severity of these injuries such as head banging and self-biting is inversely proportional to the intelligence quotient (IQ) of the child. Genetic or metabolic syndromes such as Cornelia de Lange syndrome, the Lesch–Nyhan syndrome, and familial dysautonomia are metabolic disorders associated with mental retardation and excessive self-mutilation. Many patients lose a considerable amount of tissue from the tongue, lips, and fingers. In the Lesch–Nyhan syndrome, it may be the most troublesome feature for parents or caretakers.

Midface toddler excoriation syndrome (MiTES) is a recently described syndrome which is seen in patients with congenital insensitivity to pain or hereditary autonomic sensory neuropathy, it is characterized by severe, chronic, scarring, self-inflicted, midface

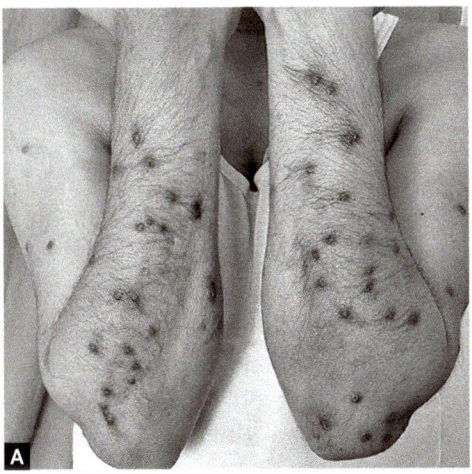 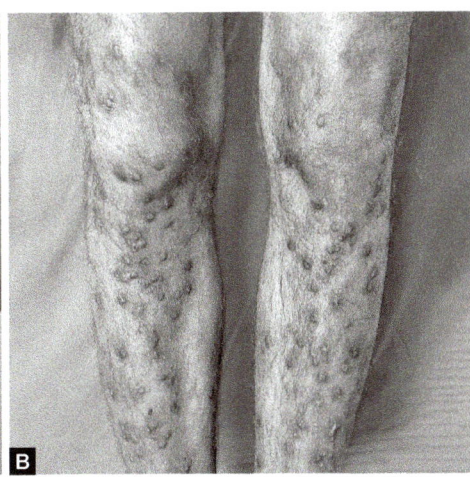

Figs. 8A and B: Prurigo nodularis.

excoriations, commencing in infancy. MiTES resembles fabricated and induced illness and may often be misdiagnosed as factitious disorder or even child abuse but a knowledge of this syndrome and careful observation of child with abnormal repetitive behaviors such as constant rubbing or scratching the area and subsequent genetic analysis help to confirm or refute the diagnosis.[18]

Some newer disorders: Some newer disorders are being described and have also found their way into nosological systems, notably the DSM-5. Two of them are described here.

Skin-picking disorder: Neurotic excoriations or skin-picking disorder is characterized by cutaneous lesions occurring because of an uninhibited urge to scratch, pick or rub the skin excessively in the absence of any primary cutaneous disease **(Figs. 8A and B)**. The most common site affected is face, with a general tendency to pick the damaged areas such as acne, scars or insect bites. The skin lesions can sometimes be indistinguishable from itchy skin disorders such as eczema or prurigo nodularis; however, they may be heterogeneous, with newer lesions being angulated crusted erosions with scabs while older lesions have depigmented center with peripheral hyperpigmentation **(Fig. 5)**. Patients having this disorder usually acknowledge the self-inflicted nature of the lesions and may have associated psychiatric disorders such as mood and anxiety disorder. Various precipitating factors include stress, anxiety, or depression. Females are more commonly affected. Onset is usually between 30 and 50 years of age. A thorough history and examination is essential to rule out dermatologic causes and primary psychiatric conditions such as DA and delusional infestations.[19]

Body-focused repetitive behavior (BFRB): This is a general term for a group of related compulsive disorders such as skin biting or picking, cheek, nail biting (onychophagia), onychotillomania, cuticle picking, tongue lip biting (morsicatio buccarum, linguarum and labiorum), and nose picking (rhinotillexomania). These behaviors usually occur when the patient is sedentary or involved in activities like watching TV, reading or studying. Pathogenesis includes genetic, temperamental, environmental factors as well as personal and family stressors.[20] Trichotillomania and skin picking (dermatillomania), though essentially repetitive behaviors, are classified separately by DSM-5.

Dermatitis para-artefacta syndrome refers to disorders of impulse control, almost similar to BFRBs, but here the patient manipulates a pre-existing skin condition, often without awareness. They readily agree to the same, when questioned. The various conditions include acne excoriée, factitial cheilitis, scab picking, etc.[21] **(Figs. 9 and 10)**.

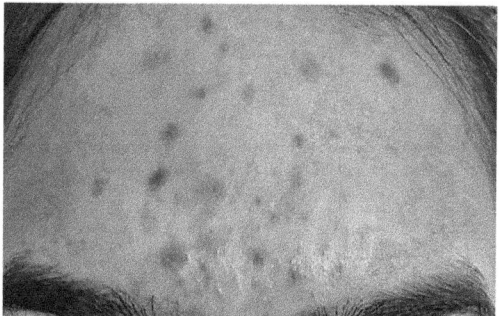

Fig. 9: Acne excoriée.

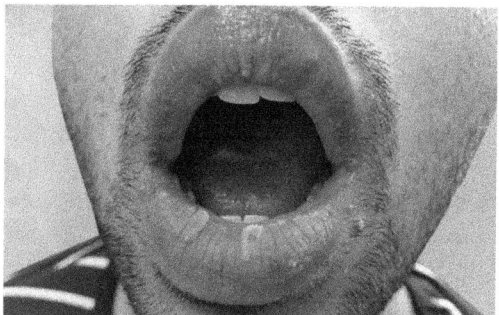

Fig. 10: Exfoliative cheilitis.

Dermatological manifestations of psychotropic drug use: Most adverse dermatological reactions to psychotropic use are idiosyncratic, unpredictable and may reflect a genetic or constitutional vulnerability on part of the patient.[22] Adverse cutaneous effects can range from mild to severe and life-threatening.[23] Some of the common and benign skin reactions are hyperpigmentation which is generally seen with chlorpromazine and drug-induced alopecia seen with valproate and lithium. Serious or life-threatening drug reactions such as Stevens–Johnson syndrome, toxic epidermal necrolysis and drug hypersensitivity syndrome **(Figs. 11A and B)** are reported commonly with valproate, carbamazepine or antiepileptics. Lithium is associated with triggering or exacerbation of psoriasis, and acneiform eruptions. Even apparently safe drugs such as quetiapine may be involved in serious dermatological side effects.[24,25]

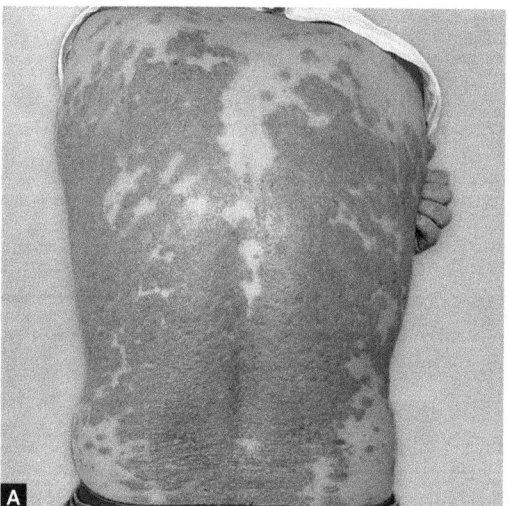
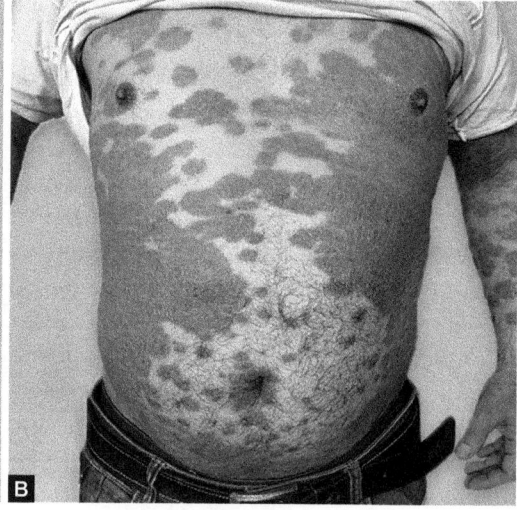

Figs. 11A and B: Drug hypersensitivity syndrome (DHS).

Dermatological Disorders Commonly Prevalent in Patients with Psychiatric Disorders

Infective and noninfective dermatoses are often diagnosed in patients with psychiatric disorders. These may reflect various etiological pathways. These include factors resulting from chronic severe mental illness such as poor hygiene, malnutrition, and neglect which may predispose to infective dermatoses. Many patients in mental hospitals were often tonsured to prevent the spread of lice infestation. However, such sights are now mercifully rare. Many patients with psychiatric disorders are often diagnosed with metabolic abnormalities such as diabetes and dyslipidemias. These conditions are also known to predispose to infective dermatoses. Finally, the co-occurrence of dermatological conditions in psychiatric disorders may also reflect deeper predisposing factors such as compromised immunological function. Various surveys have been carried out which are briefly discussed here. Results indicate that the prevalence of any skin disorders in patients with psychiatric diagnoses has been reported to be 71.5% and infective dermatoses have been reported at 48%.[26] Parasitic infections were especially common in patients with schizophrenia. Similar results were reported and the importance of diabetes as a predisposition to skin infections was mentioned.[27] A high prevalence of fungal infections and comorbidity with diabetes and hypertension were reported in a sample of patients with psychiatric disorders and known dermatological disorder.[28] The presentation of typical washerwoman's hands as seen in patients who wash excessively is well known.[29]

These surveys are methodologically not as robust as they might have been. However, they do indicate that various infective and noninfective dermatoses are common in patients with psychiatric disorders.

Dermatological Disorders and Psychiatric Implications

Dermatological disorders have a high comorbidity with psychiatric disorders and also show significant levels of psychological distress. We examine the different scenarios and possible mechanisms in this section.

Dermatological Conditions and Associated Psychiatric Disorders including Treatment Emergent Side Effects

Psychiatric comorbidity is associated with most of the skin disorders but most of the times it is temporary and the psychological condition improves drastically with the improvement of dermatological condition. However, in chronic skin disorders, it becomes a part of the dermatoses and eventually may even be one of the factors associated with the exacerbation or recalcitrance of the skin condition. For example, a case of psoriasis continues to suffer from the stigma, depression, and anxiety even after psoriasis improves and he is in a constant fear that it will come back again.[30]

The psychiatric comorbidities are an outcome of emotional distress of living with disfiguring dermatoses such as psoriasis, acne, vitiligo, AA, ichthyosis, eczema or hidradenitis suppurativa, etc. A recent multicenter study found rates of depression, anxiety, and suicidal ideation to be 10.1%, 17.2%, and 12.7%, respectively, in patients with dermatological disorders compared with 4.3%, 11.1%, and 8.3% in controls.[31] The psychosocial aspects of psoriasis are extensively studied and it associated with marked impairment in physical and mental functioning which is comparable to cancer, chronic lung disease, hypertension, and type 2 diabetes.[21] Population-based studies have shown that patients with psoriasis have increased risk of depression with an odds ratio of 2.09 (95% CI 1.41–3.11) and a higher risk of suicidality with a hazard ratio of 1.44 (95% CI 1.32–1.57) as compared to the general population.[32] The quality of life of all the patients of psoriasis should be assessed irrespective of the Psoriasis Area Severity Index (PASI) or psoriasis severity and patients who have poor quality of life can further be evaluated in depth for the presence of psychiatric comorbidities such as depression, anxiety, or suicidal ideation.

Vitiligo is a disfiguring skin disease characterized by depigmented lesions on the skin. Although it is considered a cosmetic problem by most healthcare professionals, it has a significant psychosocial impact on patients' lives especially in people with dark skin. People with vitiligo may suffer stigmatization or be ashamed of their body and have a negative self-image and low self-esteem which may be devastating for their social life.[33]

Atopic dermatitis (AD) is a common itchy skin condition characterized by redness, scaling and oozing from the skin, it is commonly observed in childhood but in some patients the condition may start during adulthood or may persist till adult life. Many patients with AD develop secondary psychological problems due to the appearance of their skin and severe intractable pruritus. AD is associated with high levels of stigmatization, social withdrawal, anxiety, and depression among patients and their caregivers. In children, AD causes irritability, clingy behavior, sleep disturbance, anxiety, and depression. It affects the family members as well who suffer from depression, sleep deprivation, and loss of work and this eventually disrupts the physical and mental health of the family.

Alopecia areata is characterized by patchy hair loss which may sometimes progress to involve the entire scalp (alopecia totalis) or the entire body (alopecia universalis). Psychological distress can trigger the onset of AA and the resultant hair loss has its negative consequences in the form of difficulty in coping with stress, depression, anxiety, adjustment disorder, paranoid disorder, and negative self-esteem.[34] The impairment of quality of life in AA is similar to other chronic dermatologic diseases such as AD and psoriasis. Similar results have been reported for recently described disorders such as prurigo nodularis.[35]

Drugs commonly used in dermatological disorders can have significant side effects which may be clinically relevant from the psychiatric point of view. A major class of drugs that are known to have effects on the psychological state of an individual are steroids. This is especially so when these are started or their dose is increased or these are given parenterally in high doses as is sometimes required.[36] Drugs such as isotretinoin should probably be used with caution in patients with a history of depression even though evidence is not conclusive.[37]

Dermatological Conditions that are Observed to be Influenced by Psychological Factors

Certain skin conditions are triggered by or can fluctuate in clinical severity according to emotional state of the individual. The psyche or the emotional status may influence the dermatological condition or dermatoses in the following ways; it may lead to triggering, aggravation or maintenance of the dermatoses, may be the factor responsible for resistance to the treatment or sometimes even facilitate the cure. This category includes conditions such as psoriasis, AD, vitiligo, AA, acne, telogen effluvium, and urticaria.[38,39] Many patients with these disorders report flares in response to stress or anxiety, and others find that their disease worsens when they are sad or depressed. The role of stress is well established in dermatoses such as psoriasis,

AD, and AA, but in disorders such as urticaria, vitiligo, acne, lichen planus, and herpes simplex, the role of stress is known but not proven.[40] One of the most common complaints or symptoms in dermatology patients is pruritus, and its intensity or severity correlates strongly with depression, anxiety, and stress that the patient experiences.[41,42] The patient may not reveal this at the first visit; thorough and repeated history helps to unravel the link between the psychosocial stressors and disease exacerbation or symptom worsening.

The principal mediators of stress-induced cutaneous changes are corticotropin-releasing hormone (CRH) CRH, adrenocorticotropic hormone (ACTH), cortisol, catecholamines, prolactin, substance P, nerve growth factor (NGF), interleukins, and cytokines which induce a series of physiological and behavioral changes that may eventually result in inflammation, pruritus, and aging. Acute stress triggers innate and adaptive cellular immune responses, which may help in fighting bacterial or viral infections and sometimes even killing tumor cells but it is associated with collateral tissue damage as well. The response changes when this stress becomes persistent and the body or mind does not get time to repair and the acute inflammatory response is replaced with humoral inflammatory response which has a proallergic and proautoimmune effect.[43]

Atopic dermatitis and psoriasis are the skin conditions where the role of stress of psychopathological factors has been studied extensively and proven. The prevalence of AD and psoriasis has increased significantly and genetic factors cannot explain this increase in the prevalence of inflammatory skin conditions, environmental factors, and psychosocial factors such as stress may also be playing an important role in this. High-quality data from research studies has proven that stress plays a critical role in the pathogenesis of psoriasis. Psoriasis begets stress and stress begets psoriasis, neuroimmunomodulators such as substance P, calcitonin gene-related peptide, vasoactive intestinal peptide, and NGF are potent regulators of neurogenic inflammation that trigger or induce flares of both AD and psoriasis through a stress-mediated mechanism.

Dermatoses which are present on uncovered parts of the body or which cannot be hidden like lesions on the face are associated with more psychological distress than the ones which can be hidden by clothes. The importance of our face cannot be undervalued as it affects our social and sexual life and may even play an important role in the economic success of an individual. Common facial dermatoses such as acne, rosacea, flushing, and seborrheic dermatitis are considered to be influenced or triggered by emotional factors. The main culprit is stress, but depression and anxiety may play a role, among other factors. Some patients may experience a vicious cycle: their facial dermatosis is triggered or worsened by stress, and in turn, the exacerbation itself is a major stressogenic stimulus.

CONCLUSION AND CLINICAL IMPLICATIONS

The interface of dermatology and psychiatry is reflective of the important role that the skin plays in the human existence and more importantly in how humans are perceived by others and the quality of their relationships. Thus, the skin is not just a covering for the soma but the medium through which the psyche is expressed. There is a wide variety of ways in which the psyche and the skin can interact. A healthcare professional working in this area needs to be aware of the fact that a patient with psychiatric disorder can have specific and reproducible skin manifestations that can be helpful in clinching a diagnosis or there may be clinically relevant adverse events. On the other hand, patients with skin disorder often have high degree of psychiatric comorbidity, this relationship may be specific or general. There is a need to have more robust epidemiological data and to try to tease the mechanisms of this interaction. There is also a need for easy screening methods for detection of psychiatric disorders in dermatological patients.[44]

Another important aspect is management. Whereas all disorders have to be treated as per merit, there is a trend toward the use of more nonpharmacological methods that may improve eventual outcomes in disorders such as psoriasis.[45]

The great degree of comorbidity underscores the importance of a closer liaison between the psychiatrist and the dermatologist. Many patients may simply be missed or have reluctance to be assessed by another specialist due to the effort involved. One way of overcoming this problem is to have specialized psychocutaneous clinics.[46] In the absence of this, dermatologists and psychiatrists with an interest in psychodermatology can develop this specialty as is happening in various other centers. This will go a long way in alleviating avoidable distress and improve the quality of life in this group of patients.

REFERENCES

1. Basavaraj KH, Navya MA, Rashmi R. Relevance of psychiatry in dermatology: present concepts. Indian J Psychiatry. 2010;52(3):270-5.
2. Shroff H, Diedrichs PC, Craddock N. Skin color, cultural capital, and beauty products: an investigation of the use of skin fairness products in Mumbai, India. Front Public Health. 2017;5:365.
3. Sermrittirong S, Van Brakel WH. Stigma in leprosy: concepts, causes and determinants. Lepr Rev. 2014;85(1):36-47.
4. Jafferany M, Pastolero P. Psychiatric and psychological impact of chronic skin disease. Prim Care Companion CNS Disord. 2018;20(2):17nr02247.
5. Del Giudice P. Cutaneous complications of intravenous drug abuse. Br J Dermatol. 2004;150(1):1-10.
6. Lee KC, Ladizinski B. Mucocutaneous manifestations of illicit drug use. Int J Dermatol. 2014;53(8):1048-51.
7. Narang T, Singh SM, Kavita. Delusional infestation with fungus. Indian J Dermatol Venereol Leprol. 2012;78(5):645-6.
8. Aung-Din D, Sahni DR, Jorizzo JL, Feldman SR. Morgellons disease: insights into treatment. Dermatol Online J. 2018;24(11):13030/qt38x1k82r.
9. Lampel HP, Powell HB. Occupational and hand dermatitis: a practical approach. Clin Rev Allergy Immunol. 2019;56(1):60-71.
10. Fang A, Matheny NL, Wilhelm S. Body dysmorphic disorder. Psychiatr Clin North Am. 2014; 37(3):287-300.
11. Grant JE, Chamberlain SR. Trichotillomania. Am J Psychiatry. 2016;173(9):868-74.
12. Lavery MJ, Stull C, McCaw I, Anolik RB. Dermatitis artefacta. Clin Dermatol. 2018;36(6):719-22.
13. Narang T, Kanwar AJ, Kumaran MS, Singh SM. Munchausen by proxy in a family. Indian J Dermatol Venereol Leprol. 2012;78(6):748-50.
14. Strumia R. Skin signs in anorexia nervosa. Dermatoendocrinol. 2009;1(5):268-70.
15. Strumia R. Bulimia and anorexia nervosa: cutaneous manifestations. J Cosmet Dermatol. 2002;1(1):30-4.
16. Gerson J, Stanley B. Suicidal and self-injurious behavior in personality disorder: controversies and treatment directions. Curr Psychiatry Rep. 2002;4(1):30-8.
17. Herpertz S. Self-injurious behaviour. Psychopathological and nosological characteristics in subtypes of self-injurers. Acta Psychiatr Scand. 1995;91(1):57-68.
18. Srinivas SM, Gowda VK, Owen CM, Moss C, Hiremagalore R. Mid-face toddler excoriation syndrome (MiTES): a new paediatric diagnosis. Clin Exp Dermatol. 2017;42(1):68-71.
19. Lochner C, Roos A, Stein DJ. Excoriation (skin-picking) disorder: a systematic review of treatment options. Neuropsychiatr Dis Treat. 2017;13:1867-72.
20. Sampaio DG, Grant JE. Body-focused repetitive behaviors and the dermatology patient. Clin Dermatol. 2018;36(6):723-7.

21. Novak TG, Duvančić T, Vucić M. Dermatitis artefacta: case report. Acta Clin Croat. 2013;52(2):247-50.
22. Drake LA, Dinehart SM, Farmer ER, Goltz RW, Graham GF, Hordinsky MK, et al. Guidelines of care for cutaneous adverse drug reactions. American Academy of Dermatology. J Am Acad Dermatol. 1996;35(3 Pt 1):458-61.
23. Mitkov MV, Trowbridge RM, Lockshin BN, Caplan JP. Dermatologic side effects of psychotropic medications. Psychosomatics. 2014;55(1):1-20.
24. Mattoo SK, Shah R, Rajagopal R, Biswas PS, Singh SM. Quetiapine: relatively safe in overdose? Indian J Psychiatry. 2009;51(2):139-40.
25. Bujor CE, Vang T, Nielsen J, Schjerning O. Antipsychotic-associated psoriatic rash—a case report. BMC Psychiatry. 2017;17:242.
26. Moftah NH, Kamel AM, Attia HM, El-Baz MZ, Abd El-Moty HM. Skin diseases in patients with primary psychiatric conditions: a hospital based study. J Epidemiol Glob Health. 2013;3(3):131-8.
27. Mookhoek EJ, Van De Kerkhof PC, Hovens JE, Brouwers JR, Loonen AJ. Skin disorders in chronic psychiatric illness. J Eur Acad Dermatol Venereol. 2010;24(10):1151-6.
28. George A, Girisha BS, Rao S. A perspective study of cutaneous manifestations in primary psychiatric disorders in a tertiary care hospital. Indian J Psychiatry. 2018;60(2):213-6.
29. Fontenelle LF, Mendlowicz MV, Versiani M. Clinical subtypes of obsessive-compulsive disorder based on the presence of checking and washing compulsions. Braz J Psychiatry. 2005;27(3):201-7.
30. Singh SM, Narang T, Dogra S, Verma AK, Gupta S, Handa S. Psychiatric morbidity in patients with psoriasis. Cutis. 2016;97(2):107-12.
31. Dalgard F, Gieler U, Tomas-Aragones L, Lien L, Poot F, Jemec GB, et al. The psychological burden of skin diseases: a cross-sectional multicenter study among dermatological out-patients in 13 European countries. J Invest Dermatol. 2015;135(4):984-91.
32. Rapp SR, Feldman SR, Exum ML, Fleischer AB, Reboussin DM. Psoriasis causes as much disability as other major medical diseases. J Am Acad Dermatol. 1999;41(3 Pt 1):401-7.
33. Cupertino F, Niemeyer-Corbellini JP, Ramos-E-Silva M. Psychosomatic aspects of vitiligo. Clin Dermatol. 2017;35(3):292-7.
34. Mulinari-Brenner F. Psychosomatic aspects of alopecia areata. Clin Dermatol. 2018;36(6):709-13.
35. Dhawan L. Study of psychiatric comorbidity and associated factors in patients with prurigo nodularis. Postgraduate Institute of Medical Education and Research, Chandigarh, India; 2015.
36. Singh SM, Narang T, Dogra S, Handa S. Self-perceived emotional side effects of systemic corticosteroid therapy in dermatology patients. Indian J Dermatol Venereol Leprol. 2015;81(6):655.
37. Magin P, Pond D, Smith W. Isotretinoin, depression and suicide: a review of the evidence. Br J Gen Pract. 2005;55(511):134-8.
38. Yadav S, Narang T, Kumaran MS. Psychodermatology: a comprehensive review. Indian J Dermatol Venereol Leprol. 2013;79(2):176-92.
39. Gupta MA. Psychosocial aspects of common skin diseases. Can Fam Physician. 2002;48:660-70.
40. Pavlovsky L, Friedman A. Pathogenesis of stress-associated skin disorders: exploring the brain-skin axis. Curr Probl Dermatol. 2007;35:136-45.
41. Schut C, Mollanazar NK, Kupfer J, Gieler U, Yosipovitch G. Psychological interventions in the treatment of chronic itch. Acta Derm Venereol. 2016;96(2):157-61.
42. Kuo CL, Chen CY, Huang HL, Chen WL, Lee HC, Chang CY, et al. Increased risk of major depression subsequent to a first-attack and non-infection caused urticaria in adolescence: a nationwide population-based study. BMC Pediatr. 2014;14:181.
43. Peters EM. Stressed skin?—a molecular psychosomatic update on stress-causes and effects in dermatologic diseases. J Dtsch Dermatol Ges. 2016;14(3):233-52; quiz 253.
44. Singh SM, Narang T, Dogra S, Verma AK, Gupta S, Handa S. Screening for depressive disorders in outpatients with mild to moderate psoriasis: a study from North India. Indian J Dermatol Venereol Leprol. 2015;81(2):148-50.
45. Singh SM, Narang T, Vinay K, Sharma A, Satapathy A, Handa S, et al. Clinic-based group multi-professional education causes significant decline in psoriasis severity: a randomized open label pilot study. Indian Dermatol Online J. 2017;8(6):454-9.
46. Goyal N, Shenoi S, Prabhu SS, Sreejayan K, Munoli R, Rai S. Psychodermatology liaison clinic in India: a working model. Trop Doct. 2018;48(1):7-11.

CHAPTER 9

Interface with Cardiology

G Prasad Rao, Amulya Koneru, V Sriramya

INTRODUCTION

The relationship of our emotions and psyche to the heart and heart disease is intriguing. There exists interplay between the heart and the mind. The relationship between psychiatric illness and cardiac disorder is complex and not yet fully understood. However, literature in this area has demonstrated that disease in one system does affect the other system. Because of the high mortality and morbidity associated with cardiovascular disease, presence of the illness has been shown to impact patient's mental well-being. Conversely, certain aspects of behavior and psychiatric illness can result in cardiovascular system changes and worsen cardiac outcomes. Cardiovascular diseases (CVDs) are the leading cause of death in India amounting to 24.8% of total deaths (age 25–69 years). Comorbidity poses a treatment challenge for cardiology and psychiatry. Treatment, whether medical, surgical, or psychiatric, is also complicated given patients' disease states, medication side effects, and drug-drug interactions and metabolic syndrome.

The presence of depression as a risk for coronary artery disease (CAD) incidence, morbidity, and mortality has been well understood. Behavioral risk factors for coronary disease, such as smoking, failure to exercise, and failure to adhere to treatment and lifestyle recommendations, are clearly exacerbated by depression or anxiety and hence, these patients will benefit from psychiatric intervention.

Anxiety or anxiety disorders independently predict sudden cardiac death in the general population as well as future cardiac events in patients with CVD. The treatment of psychiatric disorders in patients with CVD can be challenging because of the cardiovascular side effects of many psychotropic medications as well as the potential of multiple drug-drug interactions. Moreover, many medications for CVD have psychiatric side effects. Clinicians who treat patients with cardiac and psychiatric illnesses must understand the intricate relationship between these two systems in order to provide optimal patient care. In this chapter, the first section deals with interaction between cardiac diseases, psychiatric illness, and psychosocial factors. The second section details the psychiatric complications of cardiac procedures and medications.

PSYCHOSOCIAL FACTORS AND CARDIOVASCULAR DISEASE

Although traditional risk factors explain a substantial amount of CVD risk, psychological factors have also been shown to predict adverse CVD outcomes. Multiple psychological factors have been examined as potential risk factors for CVD and generally fall into one of the three broad domains:
1. Negative affective states including depression, anxiety, anger, and distress

2. Personality factors such as type A behavior pattern, hostility, and type D personality
3. Social factors including socioeconomic status (SES) and poor social support.

THE RELATIONSHIP OF NEGATIVE AFFECT AND CARDIOVASCULAR DISEASE

Depression

Depression appears to be the most common psychiatric disorder in patients with CAD, acute myocardial infarction (AMI), and unstable angina. Prevalence of depression in cardiac illness is often two to three times higher than the rates found in general population. Minor forms of depression are found in up to two-third of patients in hospital after an acute attack of MI with major depressive episodes generally being found in almost 15% of CVD patients. Depression is even more prevalent in chronic heart failure patients with the prevalence being related to the severity of the illness, ranging from 10% in asymptomatic patients to 40% in those with severe functional impairment, with an average prevalence rate of 20–25%.

Often, depressive symptoms are attributed to underlying cardiac disease or a "normal" psychological reaction to the illness. Depression increases the risk of development and progression of CVD. A dose–response relationship appears to exist between the severity of depressive symptoms after acute MI or unstable angina and the risk of death over 5-year follow-up, even after controlling for other prognostically significant factors. The multicenter Canadian Cardiac Randomized Evaluation of Antidepressant and Psychotherapy Efficacy (CREATE) trial found that in 284 patients with major depression and CAD, citalopram plus clinical management was more effective for remission of depression than placebo or clinical management alone. Interpersonal therapy (IPT) for depression conferred no advantage over clinical management alone. Poor response to antidepressant treatment after a heart attack may predict a higher risk for cardiac events and death. Nonresponse to antidepressant treatment is associated with significantly higher risk for cardiac death than in the group that responded to antidepressant treatment.

Given the increased risk of heart disease and related death in depression, does treating depression in these populations decrease the risk of cardiac morbidity and mortality? Two clinical trials sought to answer this question by studying patients following MI.

The Sertraline Antidepressant Heart Attack Randomized Trial (SADHART) was a randomized, double-blind, placebo-controlled trial of sertraline versus placebo examining 369 subjects with major depressive disorder (MDD) hospitalized for unstable angina or acute MI. Originally designed to evaluate the safety of sertraline in this group, the study did not have sufficient power to detect a statistically significant difference in major cardiac events. Absolute numbers demonstrated that sertraline was superior to placebo in a lower rate of recurrent major adverse cardiac events.

The Enhancing Recovery in Coronary Heart Disease (ENRICHD) trial also examined how treating depressive symptoms in post-MI patients affected mortality. In this study, patients were randomized to cognitive-behavioral therapy (CBT) or usual care if they were depressed or determined to have poor social support after their cardiac event. The CBT group received 6–10 sessions over a 6-month period and mortality was assessed after 30 months. The intervention was found to not be effective in reducing mortality rates. Interestingly, in this study, while the prescription of sertraline was not randomized, mortality in those patients who took sertraline was only 7.4%, as compared to 15.3% in patients without antidepressant treatment and 10.6% in patients on tricyclic antidepressants. Sertraline had no effect on risk of recurrent non-fatal MI.

Other studies suggest that treatment with selective serotonin reuptake inhibitors (SSRIs) improves cardiovascular outcomes in patients with coronary disease. A study examined prophylaxis against depression in patients following cerebrovascular accidents. Not only did this study show a statistically significant decrease in depression in sertraline-treated patients, but it also found this group to have a two-third reduction in cardiovascular adverse events over the following year.

Further study is essential to elucidate how treating depression in patients with heart disease improves cardiovascular morbidity and mortality.

Mechanism

Dysregulation of the hypothalamic–pituitary–adrenal (HPA) axis is closely tied to sympathetic activity and has been shown to occur among individuals with depression and other psychosocial risk factors. Chronic stimulation from this central output induces multiple pathophysiologic responses, including increased sympathetic nervous system activity causing heightened autonomic activity, insulin resistance, hypertension, exaggerated inflammatory response, platelet activation, endothelial dysfunction, and somatic effects, among others. Depression in particular has been shown to result in hypercortisolemia, blunted HPA activity, and diminished feedback control, which may in turn increase the progression of atherosclerosis. There is preliminary data to suggest that HPA dysregulation may be associated with increased risk of CVD death.

Anxiety

Anxiety has also been associated with increased cardiac mortality. Although anxiety appears to be associated with increased risk of CHD, it is also often comorbid with depression. Prevalence of anxiety disorders in individuals with CVD ranges from 10 to 30% depending on the type of anxiety disorder. Although studied less than depression, anxiety is common in patients with CAD. Anxiety may drive both hypervigilant and avoidant behaviors (nonadherence to medications and doctor visits). The latter type of behavior can have negative consequences on the health status of patients and is frequently a precipitant for psychiatric consultation. Anxiety symptoms have been found to be elevated in 5–10% of patients with chronic heart disease. Anxiety is associated with an increased risk of sudden cardiac death.

Bipolar Disorder

Bipolar disorder is a chronic episodic illness. It has been strongly associated with cardiovascular illness. CVD is the leading cause of death in bipolar disorder, there being an almost five-fold increased risk of CVD in this population as compared to the general population. Research has found that bipolar disorder accelerates CVD and atherosclerosis in young people. The symptoms occurring during an episode such as increased use of substances such as alcohol, smoking, cocaine, heroin, and amphetamines often contribute to precipitating or worsening of cardiac symptoms. There is an increased risk of metabolic syndrome, either due to poor lifestyle factors or use of psychotropic drugs. Biological factors that underscore a link between bipolar illness and CVD include increased inflammation, decreased oxidative stress, anomalous microvascular structure and physiology, and reduced levels of BDNF (brain-derived neurotrophic factor). Poor compliance to medication, delay in regular screening, and interventions for cardiac illness in these patients contribute to the higher morbidity and mortality rates in them.

Schizophrenia

Coronary heart disease is the leading cause of death in patients with schizophrenia, with more than two-third of the patients succumbing to it. Their lifespan is also decreased by almost 20% when compared to the general population. Poor lifestyle factors such as poor nutrition, smoking, decreased exercise, poor social and family support, and poor adherence to treatment often contribute to the mortality rates. Psychotropic drugs often lead to metabolic syndrome, thus increasing the risk of CVD. People with chronic mental illness are more often than not marginalized and hence healthcare services are often delayed in this group owing to stigma and poor understanding of psychiatric illnesses in primary care physicians. There has been a genetic link that has been found between schizophrenia and CVD. A few single nucleotide polymorphisms or SNPs have been found to be common between schizophrenia and CVD, with common links including waist–hip ratio, body mass index, systolic blood pressure, and lipoprotein and triglyceride levels.

Sexual Dysfunction

Heart disease patients often suffer from sexual dysfunction in silence, and physicians neglect to inquire about this aspect of their patients' lives. Physical factors, such as comorbid peripheral vascular disease, diabetes, medication side effects, and impaired cardiac output, can result in sexual dysfunction. Use of phosphodiesterase-5 inhibitors for erectile dysfunction might have cardiac side effects, especially in patients already suffering from CVD. Psychological factors also can play a large role. Depression and anxiety may result in loss of interest and desire in sexual activity or fear of causing a heart attack during sexual intercourse. Coital angina is however rare in patients who do not have angina during strenuous physical activity.

TYPE A BEHAVIOR PATTERN, ANGER, AND HOSTILITY

The relationship between a behavior pattern characterized by easily aroused anger, impatience, aggression, competitive striving, and time urgency (type A) and coronary heart disease dominated studies in psychosomatic cardiology in the 1970s and 1980s. Several large prospective epidemiological studies found the type A pattern to be associated with a nearly two-fold increased risk of incidents such as MI and coronary disease-related mortality. A clinical trial randomized survivors of acute MI to usual care versus usual care with type-A behavior modification. After >4 years, the behavior modification group was found to have a significant reduction in recurrent MI.

Acute and Chronic Mental Stress

The relationship of psychosocial stress and CVD can be considered in two broad categories: Acute stressors, or triggers, and chronic stress. Acute mental stress impacts CVD physiology by increasing the risk for arrhythmias, myocardial ischemia, and MI, which may be proximally measured by physiological reactivity to mental stress in a laboratory and in real-life situations. Acute stressors may include situations such as catastrophic events (war, earthquakes, etc.), intense sporting events (e.g., World Cup soccer), and acute physical activity (e.g., exercise or sexual activity).

Chronic factors, in contrast, may be associated with CVD through chronic physiologic changes, such as persistently elevated blood pressure and coagulation factors. Chronic stressors may include work-related stress, marital dissatisfaction, neighborhood factors (crowding, etc.), and lower SES. Acute mental stress is provoked by tasks such as public speaking and mental arithmetic, and has been shown to be associated with elevation in heart rate, blood pressure, and sympathetic activation in people with and without coronary heart disease. Acute mental stress may also cause coronary vasospasm and resulting ischemia. Emotional stress is purported to be a trigger for approximately 20–30% of acute coronary events.

The INTERHEART study retrospectively examined >11,000 patients with a first MI and matched them to >13,000 controls from >50 countries. The study showed that a high level of work, home, and financial stress in conjunction with major life events over the past year were associated with increased risk of MI.

A meta-analysis of studies with interventions including stress management and health education conducted in cardiac rehabilitation settings found a reduction in recurrent MI of 29% and death of 34% at 2–10-year follow-up.

SOCIAL FACTORS AND CARDIOVASCULAR DISEASE

Social factors, including social support and SES, have also been linked with CVD outcomes. Social support may act as a buffer against negative life events, serving a protective function. Several forms of social support have been identified in the existing literature: Structural support refers to the size, type, and density of one's social network, and the frequency of contact one has with this network. Functional support, sometimes referred to as tangible support, refers to the support provided by one's social structure. Low social support was associated with a 1.5- to 2-fold increased risk of CVD in both healthy and cardiac populations.

IMPLICATIONS FOR MEDICATION MANAGEMENT

Treatment of patients with both psychiatric and cardiac illness can be complicated due to the cardiac complications of psychotropic medications.

Psychiatric Side Effects of Cardiac Drugs

Some cardiac medications are known for psychiatric side effects. Digoxin and lidocaine toxicities can result in delirium. Digoxin is also classically associated with visual hallucinations of yellow rings around objects. Depression is associated with several cardiac medications including α-blockers, methyldopa, reserpine, clonidine, and amiodarone (via thyroid effects). Although β-blockers are possibly associated with depression, sexual dysfunction and fatigue are more problematic symptoms. Angiotensin-converting enzyme inhibitors may cause derangements in mood.

Cardiac Side Effects of Psychiatric Medications

Antidepressants

Tricyclic antidepressants have been shown to increase mortality in post-MI patients and should not be used as first-line agents in depressed patients with heart disease. These medications have several effects on the cardiovascular system, including orthostatic hypotension, cardiac conduction delay, and ventricular arrhythmias in overdose. Nortriptyline and desipramine are better tolerated if tricyclics are required. They tend to cause less orthostatic hypotension than the tertiary-amine tricyclic medications, such as amitriptyline.

Selective serotonin reuptake inhibitors have very little effect on the cardiac system. In the SADHART study, sertraline did not have an effect on heart rate, blood pressure, arrhythmias, ejection fraction, or cardiac conduction. SSRIs can cause a clinically insignificant slowing of heart rate (1–2 beats per minute). Clinicians should take this reaction into consideration when these medications are being used in conjunction with β-blockers.

Other antidepressants are less well studied. Mirtazapine and bupropion may occasionally cause hypertension. Monoamine oxidase inhibitors (MAOIs) cause hypotension, orthostatic hypotension, and, if a tyramine-free diet is not strictly followed, may result in hypertensive crises. As a result, MAOIs are rarely used in patients with heart disease.

Antipsychotics

The most significant cardiac side effects of antipsychotics are orthostatic hypotension and QT interval prolongation. This must be considered when treating chronically psychotic patients with heart disease or patients with delirium in cardiac care settings. Orthostatic hypotension is caused by α-adrenergic blockade and is common with low potency typical (e.g., chlorpromazine) and atypical (e.g., quetiapine) antipsychotics. Although less common, cardiac arrest due to ventricular tachyarrhythmia, specifically torsades de pointes, can occur at low doses of antipsychotics and in populations other than schizophrenic patients. Thioridazine is the most common antipsychotic medication associated with torsades de pointes and sudden cardiac death.

Haloperidol is frequently used to treat delirium and agitation. Although this medication is associated with QT prolongation, it has been shown to be safe and effective in smaller doses in a 24-hour period. Risk factors for torsades de pointes include QT interval prolongation of >500 milliseconds, family history of sudden death, female sex, hypokalemia, hypomagnesemia, and low ejection fraction. Close electrocardiographic monitoring is prudent.

The US Food and Drug Administration issued a mandate requiring manufacturers of atypical antipsychotics to add a black box warning noting that these drugs are associated with an increased risk of death in elderly patients with behavioral dyscontrol associated with dementia. Causes of these deaths were either heart-related events (sudden cardiac death, heart failure) or infections (pneumonia).

As a general rule, when using these medications, the potential risks and benefits must be considered and discussed with patients and their families.

IMPACT OF PSYCHOSOCIAL INTERVENTIONS AND PSYCHOTHERAPY ON CARDIOVASCULAR DISEASE

When learning of the presence of medical illness, patients have unique physiological responses, including sadness, denial, anxiety, and anger. These are natural reactions and do not interfere with the ability to function or experience pleasure. However, these reactions can be maladaptive and lead to problems. For example, patients whose denial of illness allows them relief from anxiety or fear may demonstrate nonadherence to treatment recommendations. Psychotherapy can play an important role in helping patients understand their cognitive distortions and an eventual positive behavioral responses.

Few studies have examined the effectiveness of psychotherapeutic interventions in patients with heart disease. The ENRICHD trial examined the effect of CBT on measures of social support and depression in patients who had a recent MI. Results showed a modest benefit of CBT compared to the usual-care group. The Recurrent Coronary Prevention Project showed that a CBT-like type-A behavior modification protocol in post-MI patients had a strong benefit on type-A behavior. IPT, which is geared toward patients with specific interpersonal issues including interpersonal disputes, grief following loss, interpersonal deficits, and social role transitions, was studied in the Canadian Cardiac Randomized Evaluation of Antidepressant and Psychotherapy Efficacy (CREATE) trial. The use of citalopram and IPT in depressed post-MI patients was examined. Although the trial documented efficacy of citalopram, there was no evidence of a benefit of IPT over general clinical management during the 12-week course of the study. The SADHART trial was a randomized, double blind, placebo-controlled, 24-week trial of sertraline for MDD among patients hospitalized for acute MI. Results showed improvement in depressive symptoms among participants treated with sertraline, but only in patients with more severe depression. The MIND-IT study of antidepressant therapy for MI showed similar results. Stress management interventions among cardiac patients have shown somewhat better results. In the Stockholm Women's Intervention Trial for Coronary Heart Disease (SWITCHD), 257 women were randomized to a group-based psychosocial intervention or usual care following a CVD event [MI, coronary artery bypass graft (CABG), or percutaneous coronary intervention]. The intervention was initiated 4 months after hospitalization. Results showed that women in the treatment group were nearly three times less likely to die during the follow-up than usual care participants.

METABOLIC SYNDROME

The metabolic syndrome consists of a cluster of metabolic abnormalities associated with obesity and that contributes to an increased risk of cardiovascular disease and type 2 diabetes. The syndrome is diagnosed when a patient has three or more of the following five risk factors: Abdominal obesity, high triglyceride levels, low high-density lipoprotein (HDL) cholesterol level, hypertension, and elevated fasting blood glucose level. Second-generation antipsychotic medications have been implicated as a cause of metabolic syndrome. Treatment involves weight loss, exercise, and use of statins and antihypertensives as needed to lower lipid levels and blood pressure, respectively.

PSYCHIATRIC DISORDERS IN CORONARY ARTERY DISEASE AND HEART DISEASES

Depression

The rate of MDD has been reported to be three-fold higher among patients with CAD compared to the general population. The course of depression in those with CVD is usually chronic and recurrent, and it is often comorbid with anxiety symptoms. Younger patients, females, and those with a prior history of depression have been reported as more likely to develop depression in the context of CVD. Depression tends to exacerbate, prolong, and amplify cardiac symptoms and CAD patients with depression have more severe symptoms than nondepressed patients.

There are various reasons for CAD patients having high depression. Both depression and coronary vascular disease share many risk factors. These include diabetes mellitus (DM), hypertension, cigarette smoking, obesity, and elevated homocysteine levels.

Cholesterol and Depression

Chronically lower levels of cholesterol are associated with depression. Clinical recovery from depression is associated with increase in cholesterol to normal levels.

Mechanism

Low cholesterol causes less binding to albumin thus leading to more free albumin which binds to tryptophan causing less serotonin levels in the brain, thus being a causative factor for depression.

Congestive Cardiac Failure

Point prevalence of depression is 20% in patients with congestive cardiac failure (CCF). According to REMATCH study, a study comparing left ventricular assist device versus medical therapy in chronic, end-stage CCF patients found mean baseline BDI (Beck Depression Inventory) score of 16 with more than two-third subjects having a score >10 (threshold for depression).

Similarly, studies done in ambulatory patients with dilated cardiomyopathy, using hospital depression and anxiety scale, the scores on anxiety symptoms were higher when compared to general population.

Arrhythmias

Patients with supraventricular tachycardia often experience anxiety, especially when they are paroxysmal in nature. Paroxysmal supraventricular tachycardia (PSVT) occurs in young and middle-aged adults and may manifest with symptoms of shortness of breath, chest discomfort, and apprehension. Because these features may overlap with those of generalized anxiety symptoms and panic attacks, there is a significant risk of misdiagnosis. Patients who experience life-threatening rhythm disturbances are prone to secondary adjustment, mood, and anxiety disorders.

Hypertension

The main psychiatric consequence of hypertension seems to be long-term neurocognitive impairment and increased risk of dementia. Treatment that successfully controls blood pressure reduces the risk. There is evidence that dihydropyridine calcium channel blockers reduce the risk of dementia of probable Alzheimer disease, as well as vascular or mixed dementia, and improve or maintain cognitive function in patients with impaired cognition.

Valvular Heart Disease

In panic disorder, mitral valve prolapse is detected in 10–25% of patients. The subjective experience of valve prolapse (e.g., fluttering and chest pressure) may be a trigger for panic sensations.

Also, obsessive-compulsive disorders (OCDs), tic disorders, and Tourette syndrome have probable autoimmune pathology that is similar to those leading to glomerulonephritis and rheumatic heart disease.

Coronary Bypass Surgery

Depressive symptoms are present in almost 40% of CABG patients.

Mild-to-moderate depression occurs in approximately one-third of patients following coronary bypass surgery but may remit within weeks to months.

Cognitive Impairment after Coronary Bypass Graft Surgery

Persistent, subtle memory and cognitive impairment may occur after CABG. The associations between cognitive and effective disturbances after coronary bypass are attributable to small vessel cerebrovascular changes seen in many elderly persons with depression. These events were predicted by older age, proximal aortic atherosclerosis, and prior history of neurological disease. Nonspecific impairment in intellectual function occurred in 2.6%, and seizures occurred in 0.4%.

Patients on Defibrillators

Patients on defibrillators report of various unpleasant experiences such as like being kicked in the chest. These patients often report of symptoms of anxiety disorder, depression, and post-traumatic stress disorder (PTSD). Patient who complained of sudden shocks during the follow-up period report reduced mental well-being, physical functioning, and anxiety.

Valve Replacement

A high prevalence of delirium occurs in early postcardiotomy patients. Delirium can be attributed to toxic or metabolic processes in many cases.

Prolonged exposure to the intensive care unit (ICU) environment with sleep deprivation, sensory stimulation, and simultaneous monotony led to the phenomenon of delirium following a lucid interval (so-called ICU psychosis).

Three main categories of patients are at risk: Patients with severe congestive heart failure, patients receiving antiarrhythmic agents for tachyarrhythmias early after MI, or cardiac surgery.

CONCLUSION

There is a very complex and complicated interplay between cardiac disorders and psychiatric illness with often intricate reciprocal relationships between the two. People with psychiatric illnesses have often undiagnosed cardiac disorders leading to high mortality and morbidity rates while higher rates of mental illness have been found in patients suffering from CVD. Multidisciplinary approach with involvement of primary care physicians, psychiatrists, cardiologists, cardiovascular surgeons and paraclinical staff is needed for a comprehensive management of comorbid conditions.

SUGGESTED READING

1. Berkman LF, Blumenthal J, Burg M, Carney RM, Catellier D, Cowan MJ, et al. Effects of treating depression and low perceived social support on clinical events after myocardial infarction: the Enhancing Recovery in Coronary Heart Disease Patients (ENRICHD) Randomized Trial. JAMA. 2003;289(23):3106-16.
2. ENRICHD Investigators. Enhancing Recovery in Coronary Heart Disease (ENRICHD) study intervention: rationale and design. Psychosom Med. 2001;63(5):747-55.
3. Filho AS, Maciel BC, Romano MMD, Lascala TF, Trzesniak C, Freitas-Ferrari MC, et al. Mitral valve prolapse and anxiety disorders. Br J Psychiatry. 2011;199(3):247-8.
4. Glassman AH, Shapiro PA. Depression and the course of coronary artery disease. Am J Psychiatry. 1998;155(1):4-11.
5. Goldstein BI. Bipolar disorder and the vascular system: mechanisms and new prevention opportunities. Can J Cardiol. 2017;33(12):1565-76.
6. Hare DL, Toukhsati SR, Johansson P, Jaarsma T. Depression and cardiovascular disease: a clinical review. Eur Heart J. 2014;35(21):1365-72.
7. Hennekens CH, Hennekens AR, Hollar D, Casey DE. Schizophrenia and increased risks of cardiovascular disease. Am Heart J. 2005;150(6):1115-21.
8. Katerndahl DA. The association between panic disorder and coronary artery disease among primary care patients presenting with chest pain: an updated literature review. Prim Care Companion J Clin Psychiatry. 2008;10(4):276-85.
9. Larsen BA, Christenfeld NJS. Cardiovascular disease and psychiatric comorbidity: the potential role of perseverative cognition. Cardiovasc Psychiatry Neurol. 2009;2009:791017.
10. Lesperance F, Frasure-Smith N, Koszycki D, Laliberte' MA, Van Zyl LT, Baker B, et al. Effects of citalopram and interpersonal psychotherapy on depression in patients with coronary artery disease: the Canadian Cardiac Randomized Evaluation of Antidepressant and Psychotherapy Efficacy (CREATE) trial. JAMA. 2007;297(4):367-79.
11. Lett HS, Blumenthal JA, Babyak MA, Sherwood A, Strauman T, Robins C, et al. Depression as a risk factor for coronary artery disease: evidence, mechanisms, and treatment. Psychosom Med. 2004;66(3):305-15.

12. Luutonen S, Holm H, Salminen JK, Risla A, Salokangas RK. Inadequate treatment of depression after myocardial infarction. Acta Psychiatr Scand. 2002;106(6):434-9.
13. Ormel J, Von Korff M, Burger H, Scott K, Demyttenaere K, Huang YQ, et al. Mental disorders among persons with heart disease–results from the world mental health surveys. Gen Hosp Psychiatry. 2007;29(4):325-34.
14. O'Connor CM, Jiang W, Kuchibhatla M, Silva SG, Cuffe MS, Callwood DD, et al. Safety and efficacy of sertraline for depression in patients with heart failure: results of the SADHART-CHF (Sertraline Against Depression and Heart Disease in Chronic Heart Failure) trial. J Am Coll Cardiol. 2010;56(9):692-9.
15. Phillips AC, Batty GD, Gale CR, Deary IJ, Osborn D, MacIntyre K, et al. Generalized anxiety disorder, major depressive disorder, and their comorbidity as predictors of all-cause and cardiovascular mortality: the Vietnam experience study. Psychosom Med. 2009;71(4):395-403.
16. Sadock B, Sadock V, Ruiz P, Kaplan H. Kaplan & Sadock's Comprehensive Textbook of Psychiatry, 1st edition. Philadelphia: Wolters Kluwer Health/Lippincott Williams & Wilkins; 2009.
17. Sardinha A, de Araújo CGS, de Oliveira e Silva AC, Nardi AE. Prevalence of psychiatric disorders and health-related anxiety in cardiac patients attending a cardiac rehabilitation program. Arch Clin Psychiatry (São Paulo). 2011;38(2):61-5.
18. Skala JA, Freedland KE, Carney RM. Coronary heart disease and depression: a review of recent mechanistic research. Can J Psychiatry. 2006;51(12):738-45.
19. Smith P, Blumenthal J. Psychiatric and behavioral aspects of cardiovascular disease: epidemiology, mechanisms, and treatment. Revista Española de Cardiología (English Edition). 2011;64(10):924-33.

Interface with Sexuality and Sexual Disorders

TS Sathyanarayana Rao, Abhinav Tandon, Shivanand Manohar

"The temperate man holds a mean position with regard to pleasures. He enjoys neither the things that the licentious man enjoys most (he positively objects to them) nor wrong pleasures in general, nor does he enjoy any pleasure violently; he is not distressed by the absence of pleasures, nor does he desire them— or if he does, he desires them in moderation, and not more than is right, or at the wrong time, or in general with any other qualification."
—**By Aristotle in the Nicomachean Ethics, Book III, Chapter XI**

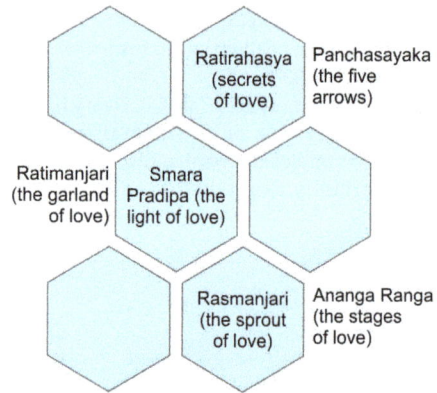

Fig. 1: The old Indian works on sexuality summarized by Burton.

SEXUALITY IN ANCIENT INDIA

Interest in the study of sexual medicine is as old as human existence. The earliest literature on sexuality can be traced to ancient Indian texts. Sexuality was combined with art and literature to educate the society. The Vedas elaborate on the moral aspects of sexuality. Vātsyāyana's classic work "Kamasutra" is still considered to be the most elaborate and detailed literature on sex. He has scientifically and boldly dealt with matters related to sex. *Subhashitha* from Vishnusharma's Panchathanthra indicates the necessity for adequate and health nutrition for normal sexual functioning. In Ayurveda (Caraka Samhita),[1] "Vajikarana" or "Virility Therapy" concerns with improving premature ejaculation, use of aphrodisiacs, virility, and improving health of progeny. A number of other authors have dealt with different aspects of sexuality and sexual functioning in the ancient times. Padmashri wrote on expression of love; Jyotirisa wrote "Panchasayaka," which elaborates on aphrodisiacs, cosmetic treatment of breasts, menstruation, impregnation, and sterility. "Ratirahasya" is a medieval Indian sex manual written by Kokkoka, which gives a fourfold classification of women, erogenous zones, days on which woman can be easily aroused. The old Indian works on sexuality were summarized by Burton as mentioned in **Figure 1**.[2]

SEXUALITY

According to World Health Organization (WHO) working definition (2006): "Sexuality is a central aspect of being human throughout life and encompasses sex, gender identities and roles, sexual orientation, eroticism, pleasure, intimacy and reproduction. Sexuality involves four factors (i) Sexual identity; (ii) Gender identity; (iii) Sexual orientation and (iv) Sexual behavior. Gender identity refers to a person's personal sense of belonging to a particular gender. It is expressed in terms of clothing, behavior of the person and personal appearance. Sexuality identity refers to what a person thinks of self, in terms of whom he or she is attracted to. Sexuality is experienced and expressed in thoughts, fantasies, desires, beliefs, attitudes, values, behaviors, practices, roles and relationships. While sexuality can include all of these dimensions, not all of them are always experienced or expressed. Sexuality is influenced by the interaction of biological, psychological, social, economic, political, cultural, ethical, legal, historical and religious and spiritual factors." Sexuality is a multidimensional concept, is socially constructed, and is shaped by gender and sexual norms and inequalities. The multiple dimensions of sexuality include sensuality, intimacy, sexual behaviors and practices, sexual orientation and gender identity, sexual and reproductive health, and power and agency in sexual relations. Sensual implies to devotedness to the fulfilment of the bodily appetites especially sexual, free indulgence in carnal pleasures and luxuriousness. Every human interaction offers the possibility of love, "a strong feeling of deep affection."[3] Love is a total submission of self and dedication to the beloved, like a saint insanely in love with God, with promise and trust to take responsibility for the soul and body.[4] Sternberg[5] has described three components of love: Intimacy, passion, and commitment. Intimacy does not necessarily mean sex and it is very much possible for two friends to be truly intimate without any sexual connection. Passion encompasses the drives that lead to romance, physical attraction, and sexual commitment. Commitment encompasses in short term, the decision to love and in long term, decision to maintain love. The interaction between these three components produce different kinds of loving experience.[6]

Sexuality is an important component of the personality and physical, intellectual, psychosocial well-being of all the individuals. However, to define what is "normal" or "healthy," a patient-centered approach has been adopted. Hence, a sexual problem is said to exist when an individual presents with a complaint about emotional or physical aspect of sexual functioning. Unless specified, sexual inadequacy refers to dysfunction in sexual functioning, by which Masters and Johnson in 1970 implied, some specific disruption of the "SEXUAL RESPONSE CYCLE."[7,8]

THE SEXUAL RESPONSE CYCLE

Masters and Johnson proposed the four phase model of human sexual response which can be abbreviated as the "EPOR Model."

E: Excitation phase characterized by somatic and psychogenic stimuli leading to increasing sexual tension and subjective sense of pleasure.

P: Plateau phase, characterized by intensified sexual tension and sexual pleasure.

O: Orgasmic phase—during this phase, there is involuntary pleasurable climax with peaking of sexual pleasure and release of sexual tension.

R: Resolution phase is characterized by a sense of well-being and relaxation; men have a refractory period for subsequent orgasm, whereas women can have multiple orgasms.

With subsequent research by Robinson and Helen Kaplan, the above model got modified into the DEOR model. Here "D" stands for the "Desire phase" which is influenced by sexual drive and fantasies and is the conscious desire to have sex.[9] The "Plateau phase" has been merged with the "Excitation phase" as it is considered to be the final stage of the "Excitation phase."[10] The "Desire phase" depends on the psychological makeup and is influenced by the biological characteristics of the individual. The "Excitation phase" begins with psychological or physiological (or both) stimulation and leads to penile tumescence and enlargement of testes in males and vaginal lubrication, hard clitoris, formation of orgasmic platform (vagina becomes barrel shaped with constriction in outer one-third), thickening of labia minora, increase in breast size in females, and nipple erection in both sexes. There is increase in heart rate, respiratory rate, and blood pressure. In the "Orgasmic phase," sexual pleasure peaks and there is rhythmic contraction of perineal muscles and reproductive organs; inevitable ejaculation triggers orgasm in males, whereas in females, there are involuntary contractions of uterus and lower third of vagina.

Resolution phase is characterized by disengorgement of blood from the genital organs; following orgasm a general feeling of well-being and muscular relaxation occur (resolution is rapid following orgasm). However, if orgasm does not occur, resolution may take up to 6 hours and may be associated with irritability[8] and other psychobehavioral symptoms.

NEUROBIOLOGY OF SEXUAL RESPONSE CYCLE

Human sexual response cycle is mediated by neurotransmitters and hormones. Neurotransmitters such as serotonin, acetylcholine, and nitric oxide (NO) and hormones such as testosterone acting in specific brain structures such as hypothalamus, limbic system, and cortex mediate sexual response cycle.

Sexual desire is mediated by emotions originating from the limbic system. Activation of amygdala can lead to penile erection, sensations of extreme pleasure, and sexual feelings. Amygdala is known to produce sex-specific behaviors. Visual sexual stimulation produces greater activation of amygdala in males when compared to females. An increased density of enkephalins and opiate receptors gives amygdala the ability to produce feelings of pleasure and motivate individuals for pleasure seeking behavior.[11-13]

Brainstem exerts both excitatory and inhibitory influence over sexual impulses from the spinal cord. Ejaculation is the forceful expulsion of semen and seminal fluid from the epididymis, vas deferens, seminal vesicles, and prostate into the urethra. Normal antegrade ejaculation includes three steps: Emission (under sympathetic control; T10-L2), ejection (under parasympathetic control; S2-4), and orgasm (occurs due to cerebral processing of sensory stimuli from pudendal nerve).[14]

In females, vulva forms the external genitalia and includes the mons pubis, major and minor lips, clitoris, glans, vaginal orifice, vestibule of vagina, and the internal system includes part of the vagina, uterus, fallopian tubes, and ovaries. Masters and Johnson have described the clitoris as the primary female sexual organ. Thrusting of the penis stimulates the clitoris via traction on the minor lips and leads to orgasm. Ernst Graefenberg in 1950 described an area of around 0.5-1 cm in the anterior wall of vagina surrounding the female urethra, known as the G spot; it is considered equivalent of prostate in males. Stimulation of this area is highly pleasurable and leads to orgasm in females.

Nerves from the autonomic nervous system (ANS) innervate the sexual organs; parasympathetic nerves (S2, 3, 4) mediate reflex erections and a thoracolumbar sympathetic system mediates psychological impulses. Both sympathetic and parasympathetic system are involved in relaxing cavernosal smooth muscles which is aided by NO. In females, the sympathetic system causes contraction of smooth muscles of vagina, urethra, and uterus during orgasm. The autonomic nervous system is influenced by external events such as stress and also by biological mediators (internal events) of sexual functioning.[15]

Erection involves dopamine (increases), serotonin (minimal change), norepinephrine (decreased activity at α and increased activity at β), and modulation of acetylcholine. Dopamine antagonists cause erectile dysfunction (ED), whereas dopamine agonists enhance erection and libido. α1 blockade may lead to priapism and β blockade may lead to impotence.[16] Multiple neurotransmitters such as dopamine, norepinephrine, serotonin, acetylcholine, oxytocin, GABA (gamma amino butyric acid) and NO are involved in ejaculation.[17]

During ejaculation and orgasm, there is increased activity of norepinephrine at α1 receptors. α1 blockers may lead to impaired ejaculation and serotonergic agents may impair potency.

Serotonergic system largely plays inhibitory role in all phases of sexual response cycle. Serotonin's effects in the central nervous system are determined by the specific receptors activated. 5-hydroxytryptamine (5HT)-type 2 and 5-HT3 receptors inhibit sexual activity, while 5HT1 receptors stimulate sexual activity. Dopamine plays a significant role in sexual response cycle, through its involvement in mesolimbic pathway and reward system. Activation of nucleus accumbens and medial preoptic hypothalamic region by dopamine is essential for sexual motivation. Activation of paraventricular nucleus of hypothalamus by dopamine is essential for penile erection.[18-21]

Testosterone is associated with libido in both men and women; in men, it is inversely related to stress and lifestyle factors with highest levels seen in the morning (normal range 270–1,100 ng/dL). Estrogen, testosterone, and progesterone promote sexual desire; oxytocin enhances sexual activity in both sexes and promotes orgasm. Prolactin inhibits arousal; androgens are said to increase libido in females but this still needs further confirmation.[22-24]

SEXUALITY AS A SOCIAL CONSTRUCT

Sexuality is a primary instinct of human species, enabling pleasure and survival. Various biopsychosocial factors can help us understand the etiopathogenesis of sexual disorders. Race, ethnicity, religion, socioeconomic factors, interpersonal relationships, social stigma, and personality of an individual interact in complex ways to influence the sexuality of an individual.

The Spectrum Concept of Sexuality

The spectrum concept of sexuality allows for better understanding of individuals based on their gender identity and orientation.[25] Sexual fluidity and gender identity are concepts related to modern sexology. Sexuality includes a continuum of behaviors and fantasies beyond procreation. It may be difficult to put individuals strictly under the category of either homosexual or heterosexual, as certain individuals have a fluid sexual orientation; which may lie on a spectrum at one end of which is homosexual orientation and on the other end heterosexual with bisexuality lying somewhere in the middle.[25]

"The living world is a continuum in each and every one of its aspects"
—**Sexual Behavior in the Human Male (1948)**

Sexual orientation includes four components as mentioned in **Figure 2**.[25-27]

It was Kinsey who studied sexual orientation and its grading 70 years ago.[28] Research has shown that sexual attraction toward same

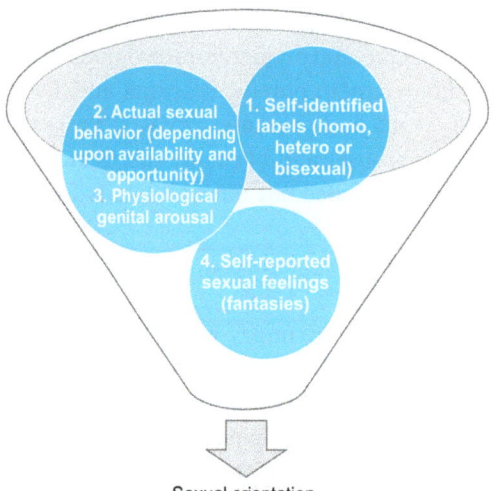

Fig. 2: The four components of sexual orientation.

TABLE 1: Sexual identity and same sex contact as per the study done by Chandra et al. between 2006 and 2008.

Sexual identity/ same sex contact	Percentage
Homosexual	• 2–4% of males • 1–2% of females
Bisexual	• 1 and 3% of males • 2–5% of females
Same sex contact	• 4–6% of males • In females, 4% in General Social Survey and 11–12% in the 2002 and 2006–2008 National Survey of Family Growth

or opposite sex is not consistent over time. In the study titled "Sexual Behaviour in the Human Male" published in 1948, Alfred Kinsey and colleagues suggested that people did not fit exclusively into categories, as far as sexual orientation is concerned. Commonly known as "The Kinsey Scale," it rates an individual on the basis of sexual orientation from 0 to 6. (0 being exclusively heterosexual and 6 being exclusively homosexual). It also has a category X which refers to no socio-sexual contact (e.g., 2 rating refers to an individual who is predominantly heterosexual but more than incidentally homosexual).[28] Kinsey's sample was taken by quota sampling method (with face-to-face interviews; 5,300 white males and 5,940 white females) from young college educated adults; hence it does not represent the lower socioeconomic strata. In 1979, Gebhard and Johnson reassessed Kinsey's data to eliminate sample bias and concluded that among noninstitutionalized individuals 9.9% of males and 3.7% of females had extensive homosexual experience.[29] A study by Chandra et al. between 2006 and 2008, collected data from a national sample of 13,495 males and females and tried to differentiate between sexual attraction, sexual behavior, and sexual identity. The results have been mentioned in **Table 1**.[30]

In 1978, Fritz Klein published a book called "The Bisexual Option." In this book, Klein explained a sexual orientation grid that rates seven aspects of sexual orientation/identity: Sexual attraction, sexual behavior, sexual fantasies, emotional preference, social preference, self-identification, and homosexual/heterosexual lifestyle, which are rated from 1 (heterosexual) to 7 (homosexual), based on Kinsey scale.[28]

In 1981, Michael Storms explained sexuality by considering that X-axis corresponded to homosexuality and Y-axis corresponded to heterosexuality. A value of zero on both axis would mean total asexuality as shown in **Figure 3**.[31] All three models can be studied while considering sexuality along a spectrum, and different ways in which sexual orientation can be assigned to a particular individual, usually by self.[32]

"Many persons do not want to believe that there are gradations in these matters from one to the other extreme."

—**Sexual Behavior of the Human Female (1953)**

A study on categorical versus spectrum nature of sexual orientation found strong correlation among the five indicators: Sexual identity, percentage of sexual attraction, infatuation, fantasy, and genital contact and romantic relationship toward males or females. Sexual orientation was helpful in predicting each indicator, though major discrepancies were also noticed. Sexual identity and orientation correlated strongly toward the ends of the sexual spectrum.[33]

Sexual fantasies, actual sexual acts, and sexual orientation may not necessarily be in unison. This depends upon the availability of a partner. For example in same-sex institutions, a male with a heterosexual orientation may need heterosexual fantasies for arousal, while performing acts with a male partner.[25] Pansexuality refers to emotional, romantic, or sexual attraction toward another person irrespective of his or her sexual and gender identity. Pansexuality may be classified as a separate sexual orientation or under bisexuality.

Asexuality Spectrum

Asexuality can also be explained along a spectrum. Individuals on the asexual spectrum are referred to as "ace-spec." Many asexuals have two orientations: A romantic one and a sexual one. A person may have no sexual attraction but still be able to form a romantic relationship. An asexual person (or demisexual or Gray-A) may form any of the romantic relationships with another person as mentioned in **Flowchart 1**.

As per the split attraction model for every sexual orientation/expression, there is a romantic counterpart **(Figs. 4A and B)**. An individual may be asexual but does feel romantic attraction. Similarly an individual may be aromantic but may be able to feel sexual attraction. Hence, sexual and romantic orientation are two different entities which may influence an individual independently.

BDSM (Bondage and discipline; dominance and submission; sadism and masochism) are a set of consensual sexual practices by individuals from across the sexual spectrum including homosexual, bisexual, heterosexual, transgender, and cisgender individuals.[34]

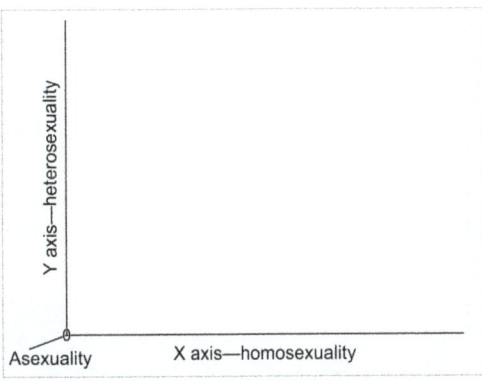

Fig. 3: Michael Storms model of sexuality

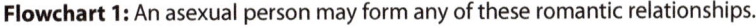
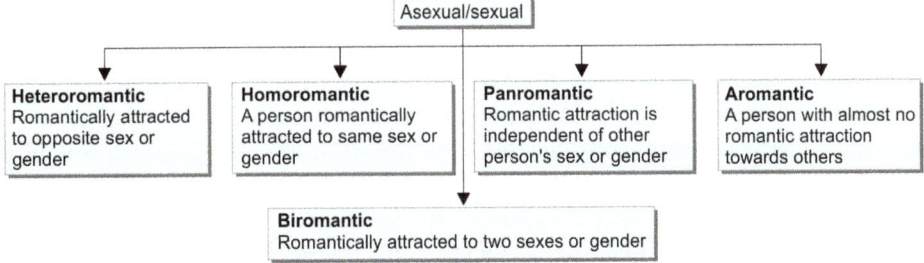

Flowchart 1: An asexual person may form any of these romantic relationships.

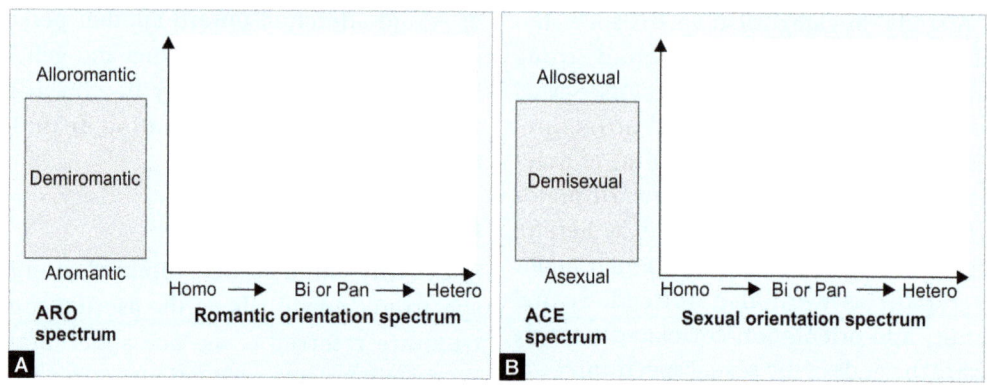

Figs. 4A and B: The split attraction model.

SEXUAL DYSFUNCTION

In order to simplify, several authors have conceptualized sexual problems arising from illness as primary, secondary, or tertiary. Primary refers to dysfunction that is organic in nature directly related to the illness, secondary sexual dysfunction relates to physical changes that cause indirect impairment such as fatigue, weakness, bowel and bladder incontinence, and tertiary sexual dysfunction refers to psychological impact of the illness such as depression, fear, and low self-esteem.[35,36]

Common sexual inadequacies include hypoactive or inhibited sexual desire which is characterized by persistently decreased or absent sexual fantasies or desire for sexual activity. Sexual aversion disorders are characterized by persistent aversion to all genital sexual contact with a sexual partner. Sexual arousal disorders also known as inhibited sexual excitement may be seen in both males and females. Male erectile disorders characterized by (1) persistent partial or complete failure to maintain an erection through completion of the sex act or (2) persistent lack of pleasure during sex. Female sexual arousal disorders characterized by either (1) partial or complete failure to maintain the lubrication in response to sexual excitement during completion of the sex act or (2) persistent lack of pleasure during sex. For the diagnosis, the problem must be present in 20–30% of occasions. In Diagnostic and Statistical Manual of Mental Disorders, Fifth Edition (DSM-5), female desire and arousal disorder have been combined, as it is difficult to delineate between desire and arousal disorders.[37]

Orgasmic disorders include inhibited female orgasm and inhibited male orgasm. Inhibited female orgasm is characterized by persistent inhibition of orgasm after an adequate sexual excitement phase. Inhibited male orgasm is characterized by persistent delay or absence of ejaculation following an adequate phase of sexual excitement. The most common male sexual dysfunction is premature ejaculation. It is characterized by recurrent ejaculation with minimal sexual stimulation before the man wishes it to occur. As per DSM-5, the time duration has been specified as 1 minute. Other sexual problems include dyspareunia, vaginismus, and Dhat syndrome. Dhat syndrome is a culture bound syndrome seen in India and the subcontinent and is characterized by neurotic features of asthenia, anxiety, depression, and hypochondria usually in young individuals who attribute the symptoms to loss of semen, in nocturnal emission, "bad dreams," semenuria, masturbation, or sexual intercourse. Fear and ignorance are the core features of this syndrome.[38-45]

Gender identity disorders and paraphilias differ broadly from sexual inadequacies. An abnormality in one's sense of being masculine or feminine is the problem in gender identity disorders. Recurrent sexual urges or fantasies involving either nonhuman objects, humiliation of oneself or ones partner or children, or other nonconsenting persons are the characteristic of sexual perversions or paraphilias. DSM-5 which was released in May 2013 has defined sexual dysfunctions as "a heterogeneous group of disorders that are typically characterized by a clinically significant disturbance in a person's ability to respond sexually or to sexual pleasure." Subtypes include lifelong versus acquired and generalized versus situational. Also partner's and individual vulnerability factors; relationship factors; psychiatric comorbidity; cultural and general medical factors need to be considered. DSM-5 has specified the threshold for making a diagnosis at 75%; that is to say that a sexual dysfunction is said to be present if the problem persists for three-fourth or more occasions.

SEXUAL FUNCTIONING AND MENTAL ILLNESS

Persons with severe mental illness (SMI) are associated with lower overall frequency of sexual activity (30–70%) and below than average occurrence of marital and long-term relationships. Around one-third and one-half of patients with SMI undergoing treatment are reported to be sexually active. Women with SMI when compared to men are more likely to be sexually active which may be associated with unprotected, high-risk sexual behavior,[46] homosexual activity, and concurrent sexual partnerships.[47] Persons with SMI have difficulty maintaining long-term sexual relationships through marriage.[48] The stigma of mental illness results in people with SMI getting sexually isolated and they are considered socially undesirable for marriage due to cultural stereotypes portraying them as dangerous.[49,50]

Often partners find it difficult to cope with symptoms of psychiatric disorder in the partner which may lead to a break in the relationship. Only mania is associated with high rates of sexual "promiscuity," other psychiatric illnesses generally decrease libido; similar is the case with most psychotropic drug which have a negative impact on sexual functioning.[51] People in treatment programs are usually prohibited from sexual activity and in institutions, sexual expression of any kind is invariably discouraged.[52]

People with mental health problems have lower self-esteem and they may lack many of the social skills to succeed in romantic partnerships.[53] To avoid rejection, they may withdraw themselves socially reducing contact with potential partners.[54] People with SMI especially women are likely to face abuse in sexual relationships.[55]

The prevalence of sexual dysfunctions is higher in persons with mental disorders and in those treated with psychotropic medications. Sexual dysfunction has been reported in as many as 30–60% of patients with schizophrenia who are on treatment with antipsychotic medications,[56] in up to 78% of individuals with depression treated with antidepressants[57] and up to 80% in patients suffering from anxiety disorders.[58] Sexual dysfunction in schizophrenia may be due to personality-related issues with lack of intimacy, paranoid behavior, and infidelity. Blunted affect, anhedonia, and antipsychotics (typical > atypical) also contribute to sexual dysfunction. A study conducted in 2003[35] concluded that 82% of men and 96% of women with schizophrenia have at least one sexual dysfunction. Male patients reported less desire for sex and female patients reported less enjoyment which was associated with negative symptoms and general psychopathology.

Loss of sexual interest is commonly seen in unipolar (up to 72%) and bipolar (77%) depression.[36] ED and premature ejaculation is noted in up to 90% cases,[59] and reduced nocturnal penile tumescence in up to 40% cases has been observed. Treatment emergent inhibition of orgasm, impairment in desire and arousal, and less sexual satisfaction has been reported, especially with selective serotonin reuptake inhibitors (in 34-78% cases).[60] Paroxetine has the highest rate of sexual dysfunction, especially delayed ejaculation, while bupropion has the lowest.

High level of anxiety is known to be associated with sexual dysfunction. Social phobia in men is reported to be associated with premature ejaculation, impairment in sexual enjoyment, and subjective sexual satisfaction.[61] Women have more impairment in desire, arousal, sexual activity, and subjective satisfaction.[62]

Post-traumatic stress disorder (PTSD) is known to affect sexual functioning (in up to 80% cases).[63] Anorexia nervosa patients are associated with less sexual interest, impaired sexual function, and fear of intimacy.[64] Pelsser[65] has described individuals with borderline personality who have sexual promiscuity, sexual avoidance, higher levels of sexual assertiveness, greater erotophilic attitudes, greater sexual preoccupation, and sexual dissatisfaction. Zeiss[66] reported 52% of Alzheimer's patients to have ED which is thought to be extremely distressing to the spouse. Common sexual problems are reduction in sexual drive or sexual apathy, increased libido,[67] sexually inappropriate behaviors, disrupted sexual relations with spouse, and inability to give consent for sexual activity.[68] Nonconsensual sexual abuse is common in adolescents with mental retardation which may include either exposure to sexual material, fondling, exhibitionism, oral sex, or sexual intercourse. More than 90% will experience sexual abuse at some point in their lives. About 39-68% of girls and 16-30% of boys will be sexually abused before their 18th birthday.

PSYCHOSOMATIC DISEASES AND SEXUAL FUNCTIONING

Sexuality is the ultimate union of the body and the mind, the inseparable relationship between the body and the mind, though known from ancient times, has been acknowledged in the modern medicine only in the recent times. Many diseases are fully described based on their effects on specific organs, but the impact on sexuality has not been emphasized.[69]

Sexual dysfunction may be one of the devastating aspects of neurological illness. Neurological illness such as epilepsy, traumatic brain injury, spinal cord injury, and multiple sclerosis can affect all phases of the sexual response cycle, which may include inability to process sexual stimuli to arousal dysfunction and anorgasmia.[70-72]

Endocrine disorders are common in people with sexual dysfunction. Testosterone has primary role in different phases of sexual cycle in both men and women.[22] Hyperprolactinemia causes decreased libido in men.[73]

Erectile dysfunction is associated with diabetes mellitus and ED is a marker of cardiovascular dysfunction. Drugs used to control diabetes may also cause ED, but changes in the drugs causes improvement only in the early stages. Loss of sexual desire has been proven consequence of diabetes mellitus in both men and women.[74-76]

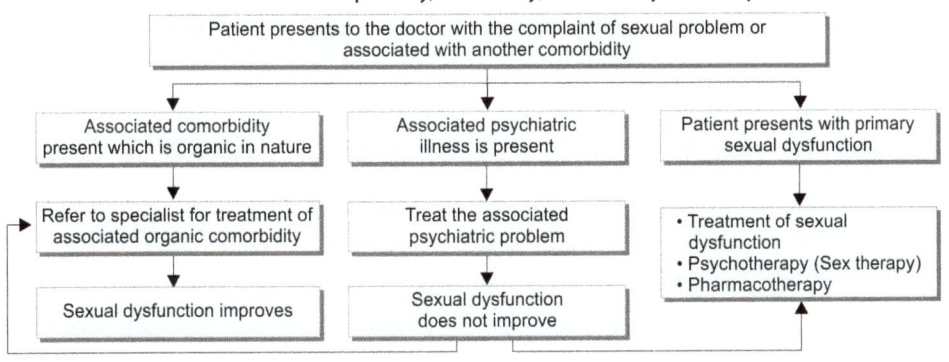

Flowchart 2: Treatment of primary, secondary, and tertiary sexual dysfunction.

Sexual dysfunction is highly prevalent in cardiovascular diseases. Recent studies have suggested impairment in penile blood flow causing ED, predicts major cardiovascular adverse events in patients free of clinical atherosclerosis. This predictive value is independent of severity of hypertension and levels of testosterone.[77]

Arterial hypertension is a systemic disorder characterized by altered vascular resistance and cardiac index. Hypertension causes endothelial dysfunction by shear stress within the vessel wall leading to reduced vasodilation and problems with erection and vulvar/vaginal congestion. The close association between hypertension and sexual dysfunction may lead, one to conclude that adequate treatment of hypertension may lead to favorable outcome in sexual functioning. To the contrary, antihypertensive drugs such as nonselective beta blockers, angiotensin-converting enzyme inhibitors, methyldopa, and thiazide diuretics are associated with sexual dysfunction.[78]

Thirty percent of men with coronary artery disease have sexual dysfunction. Woman with diagnosed coronary artery disease have impairment in desire, orgasm, arousal, and number of intercourse.[79]

There is significant decline in sexual functioning in stroke patients. Some studies report that 20–75% of people with stroke have sexual dysfunction. Post-stroke sexual dysfunction can be explained based on autonomic dysfunction, consequence of imbalance between sympathetic overactivity, and parasympathetic hypoactivity.[80]

Psoriasis is a chronic inflammatory condition of skin which also affect joints. Sexual dysfunction in psoriasis appears to stem from physical disfigurement. Patients with psoriatic lesions in areas of sexual interest (ASI) had more sexual dysfunction than patients who were free of lesions in these areas.[81,82]

Rheumatoid arthritis is an autoimmune inflammatory condition affecting all the joints leading to various degrees of disability. Hip and knee immobility causes difficulty in performing sexual acts. Pain, negative body image, morning stiffness, and increased fatigue dampen sexual desire. Vaginal dryness is associated with Sjögren syndrome and it causes dyspareunia.[83]

Flowchart 2 summarizes the treatment of sexual dysfunction.[84]

CONCLUSION

Sexuality involves the whole experience of a person's sense of self, person's ability to form relationships with others and feeling about themselves. Sexuality has a significant impact on quality of life. People of all ages and abilities involve in sexual intimacy as a means of connecting with partners and also to enhance the sense of well-being. Sexuality is considered to be along a spectrum at one end of which is homosexuality and at the other end heterosexuality. Asexuality can also be explained along a spectrum. Life-threatening illness often precludes discussion on sexual health. Even after recovery practitioners persistently fail to acknowledge about sexual dysfunction. This is due to lack of knowledge about sexual dysfunction and treatment among healthcare professionals. First step in treating sexual dysfunction is becoming aware of its association with almost every diseased organ system. Patients willingly discuss about sexual problems, if the healthcare professional touches the topic. By identifying and treating sexual dysfunction, practitioners will not only help to enhance patients' quality of life but also make complicated treatment more bearable. Even among healthy, the sexual dimension makes an individual healthier and well and ultimately brings in better quality of life.

REFERENCES

1. Acharyaukhamba Sanskrit Samsthan. Trikamji VY (Ed). Agnivesha, Charaka Samhita, with Ayurveda-Dipika Commentary of Chakrapanidatta, 5th edition. Varanasi: Cha; 2001.
2. Somasundaram O, Raghav V. The Ratirahasya—Kukkoka: Secrets of love. J Psychosexual Health. 2019;1(3-4):283-5.
3. Hornby AS, Crowther J (Eds.) Oxford Advanced Learner's Dictionary of Current English, 5th edition. Cambridge: Oxford University Press; 1996. pp. 699-700.
4. Chandwani A. Kama Sutra elixir of love. Brijbasi Art Press Ltd.; 2006.pp.43-66.
5. Sternberg R. A triangular theory of love. Psychol Rev. 1986;93:119-35.
6. Stanway A. The Art of Sexual Intimacy: A Guide For Lovers. London: Headline Book Publishing; 1993. pp. 6-17, 32-51, 72-138.
7. Masters WH, Johnson V. Human Sexual Response. Boston: Little, Brown & Co; 1966.
8. Masters WH, Johnson V. Human Sexual Inadequacy. London: Churchill; 1970.
9. Kaplan H. Disorders of Sexual Desire. New York: Simon and Schuster; 1979.
10. Robinson P. The Modernization of Sex. Ithaca, NY: Cornell University Press; 1976.
11. Georgiadis J, Holstege G. Human brain activation during stimulation of the Penis. J Comp Neurol. 2005;493:33-8.
12. Hamann S, Herman R, Nolan C, Wallen K. Men and women differ in amygdala response to visual sexual stimuli. Nature Neurosci. 2004;7(4):325-6.
13. Zimmer C. The brain: where does sex live in the brain? From top to bottom. Discover Magazine; 2019.
14. Rowland D, McMahon CG, Abdo C, Cheh J, Jannini E, Waldinger MD, et al. Disorders of orgasm and ejaculation in men. J Sex Med. 2010;7(2):1668-86.
15. Rao TSS, Rao VS, Guptha AR, Raman R, Urs O, Basavaraju M, et al. A study on desire disorders in women. Indian J Psychiatry. 2003;45(Suppl):86.
16. Sadock BJ, Sadock VA. Human sexuality. In: Kaplan & Sadock's Synopsis of Psychiatry: Behavioral Sciences/Clinical Psychiatry, 10th edition. Philadelphia: Lippincott Williams & Wilkins; 2007. pp. 680-717.
17. McMahon CG, Abdo C, Incrocci L, Perelman M, Rowland D, Waldinger M, et al. Disorders of orgasm and ejaculation in men. J Sex Med. 2004;1(1):58-65.
18. Graf H, Walter M, Metzger CD, Abler B. Antidepressant-related sexual dysfunction: perspectives from neuroimaging. Pharmacol Biochem Behav. 2014;121:138-45.
19. Stahl SM. The psychopharmacology of sex, part 2: effects of drugs and disease on the 3 phases of human sexual response. J Clin Psychiatry. 2001;62(3):147-8.
20. Stahl SM. The psychopharmacology of sex, Part 1: Neurotransmitters and the 3 phases of the human sexual response. J Clin Psychiatry. 2001;62(2):80-1.
21. Just MJ. The influence of atypical antipsychotic drugs on sexual function. Neuropsychiatr Dis Treat. 2015;11:1655-61.
22. Corona G, Isidori AM, Aversa A, Burnett AL, Maggi M. Endocrinologic control of men's sexual desire and arousal/erection. J Sex Med. 2016;13(3):317-37.
23. Davis SR, Worsley R, Miller KK, Parish SJ, Santoro N. Androgens and female sexual function and dysfunction-Findings from the Fourth

International Consultation of Sexual Medicine. J Sex Med. 2016;13(2):168-78.
24. Worsley R, Santoro N, Miller KK, Parish SJ, Davis SR. Hormones and female sexual dysfunction: Beyond estrogens and androgens: findings From the Fourth International Consultation on Sexual Medicine. J Sex Med. 2016;13:283-90.
25. Ventriglio A, Bhugra D. Sexuality in the 21st century: Sexual fluidity. East Asian Arch Psychiatry. 2019;29:30-4.
26. Mustanski BS, Chivers ML, Bailey JM. A critical review of recent biological research on human sexual orientation. Annu Rev Sex Res. 2002;13:89-140.
27. Wilson G, Rahman Q. Born Gay: The Psychobiology of Sex Orientation. London: Peter Owen; 2005.
28. Kinsey AC, Pomeroy WR, Martin CE. Sexual behavior in the human male, 1948. Am J Public Health. 2003;93:894-8.
29. Gebhard PH, Johnson AB. The Kinsey Data: Marginal Tabulations of 1938-1963; Interviews Conducted by the Institute for Sex Research. Philadelphia: WB Saunders; 1979.
30. Chandra A, Mosher WD, Copen C, Sionean C. Sexual behavior, sexual attraction, and sexual identity in the United States: Data from the 2006–2008 National Survey of Family Growth. National Health Statistics Reports; no. 36. Hyattsville, MD: National Center for Health Statistics 2011.
31. Brennan D. What Is the Sexuality Spectrum. WebMD Editorial Contributors: Medically Reviewed on June 29, 2021.
32. Tanne JH. Fritz Klein. BMJ. 2006;333(7557):47. Available at: https://www.ncbi.nlm.nih.gov/pmc/articles/PMC1488768/
33. Savin-Williams RC. An exploratory study of the categorical versus spectrum nature of sexual orientation. J Sex Res. 2014;51(4):446-53.
34. Turley EL, Butt T. BDSM -Bondage and discipline; dominance and submission; sadism and masochism. The Palgrave Handbook of the Psychology of Sexuality and Gender. Berlin: Springer; 2015. pp. 24-41.
35. Macdonald S, Halliday J, MacEwan T, Sharkey V, Farrington S, Wall S, et al. Nithsdale schizophrenia surveys 24: Sexual dysfunction. Br J Psychiatry. 2003;182:50-6.
36. Casper RC, Redmond DE, Katz MM, Schaffer CB, Davis JM, Doslow SH. Somatic symptoms in primary affective disorder. Arch Gen Psychiatry. 1985;42:1098-104.
37. American Psychiatric Association. Diagnostic and Statistical Manual of Mental disorders (DSM 5). Washington DC: American Psychiatric Association; 2013.
38. Chadda RK. Dhat syndromes: Is it a distinct clinical entity? A study of illness behaviour characteristics. Acta Psychiatr Scand. 1995;91: 136-39.
39. Behere PB, Natraj GS. Dhat syndrome: the phenomenology of a culture bound sex neurosis of the orient. Indian J Psychiatry. 1984;26:76-8.
40. Gregoire A. ABC of sexual health: assessing and managing male sexual problems. BMJ. 1999;318:315-7.
41. Rao TSS, Darshan MS, Tandon A, Raman R, Karthik KN, Saraswathi N, et al. Suttur study: an epidemiological study of psychiatric disorders in south Indian rural population. Indian J Psychiatry. 2014;56(3):238-45.
42. Rao TSS, Darshan MS, Tandon A. An epidemiological study of sexual disorders in South Indian rural population. Indian J Psychiatry. 2015;57(2):150-7.
43. Rao TSS, Ismail S, Darshan MS, Tandon A. Sexual disorders among elderly: an epidemiological study in south Indian rural population. Indian J Psychiatry. 2015;57(3):236-41.
44. Grover S, Avasthi A, Gupta S, Dan A, Neogi R, Behere PB, et al. Comorbidity in patients with Dhat syndrome: A nationwide multicentric study. J Sex Med. 2015;12(6):1398-401.
45. Grover S, Avasthi A, Gupta S, Dan A, Neogi R, Behere PB, et al. Phenomenology and beliefs of patients with Dhat syndrome: A nationwide multicentric study. Int J Soc Psychiatry. 2016;62(1):57-66.
46. Buckley PF, Robben T, Friedman L, Hyde J. Sexual behavior in persons with serious mental illness: patterns and clinical correlates. In: Buckley PF (Ed). Sexuality and Serious Mental Illness. Amsterdam: Harwood Academic Publishers; 1999. pp. 1-20.
47. Cournos F, Karen M, Heino MB, Jeannine RG, Ilan M. HIV Risk activity among persons with severe mental illness: Preliminary findings. Hosp Community Psychiatry. 1993;44(11):1104-6.
48. Dickerson FB, Clayton HB, Kreyenbuhl J, Goldberg RW, Fang LJ, Dixon LB. Sexual and reproductive behaviors among persons with mental illness. Psychiatr Serv. 2004;55(11):1299-301.
49. Wright ER, Gronfein WP, Owens TJ. Deinstitutionalization, social rejection, and the self-esteem of former mental patients. J Health Soc Behav. 2000;41(1):68-90.
50. Phelan JC, Link GB, Stueve A, Pescosolido B. Public conceptions of mental illness in 1950 and

1996: What is mental illness and is it to be feared? J Health Soc Behav. 2000;41(2):188-207.
51. John B. Pharmacosexology: the effects of drugs on sexual function: A review. J Psychoactive Drugs. 1982;14(1-2):5-44.
52. Miller LJ, Finnerty M. Sexuality, pregnancy and childrearing among women with schizophrenia-spectrum disorders. Psychiatr Serv. 1996;47(5):502-6.
53. Libet JM, Lewinsohn PM. Concept of social skill with special reference to the behavior of depressed persons. J Consult Clin Psychol. 1973;40(2):304-12.
54. Link BG, Cullen FT, James F, John FW. The social rejection of former mental patients: Understanding why labels matter. Am J Sociol. 1987;92:1461-500.
55. Goodman LA, Dutton MJ, Mark H. Prevalence and impact of sexual and physical abuse in women with severe mental illness. In: Harris M, Newark NJ (Eds). Sexual Abuse Trauma among Women with Severe Mental Illness. Philadelphia: Gordon and Beach Publishers; 1997. pp. 277-99.
56. Peuskens J, Sienaert P, De Hert M. Sexual dysfunction: the unspoken side effect of antipsychotics. Eur Psychiatry. 1998;13:23s-30s.
57. Osvath P, Fekete S, Voros V, Vitrai J. Sexual dysfunction among patients treated with antidepressants: a Hungarian retrospective study. Eur Psychiatry. 2003;18:412-4.
58. Kaplan HS. Anxiety and sexual dysfunction. J Clin Psychiatry. 1988;49:21-5.
59. Feldman HA, Goldstein I, Hatzichristou DG, Krane RJ, McKinlay JB. Impotence and its medical and psychosocial correlates: results of the Massachusetts Male Aging Study. J Urol. 1994;151:54-61.
60. Montejo-González AL, Llorca G, Izquierdo JA, Ledesma A, Bousoño M, Calcedo A, et al. SSRI-induced sexual dysfunction: fluoxetine, paroxetine, sertraline, and fluvoxamine in a prospective, multicenter, and descriptive clinical study of 344 patients. J Sex Marital Ther. 1997;23:176-94.
61. Figueira I, Possidente E, Marques C, Hayes K. Sexual dysfunction: a neglected complication of panic disorder and social phobia. Arch Sex Behav. 2001;30:369-77.
62. Bodinger L, Hermesh H, Aizenberg D, Valevski A, Marom S, Shiloh R, et al. Sexual function and behavior in social phobia. J Clin Psychiatry. 2002;63:874-9.
63. Kotler M, Cohen H, Aizenberg D, Matar M, Loewenthal U, Kaplan Z, et al. Sexual dysfunction in male posttraumatic stress disorder patients. Psychother Psychosom. 2000;69:309-15.
64. Raboch J, Faltus F. Sexuality of women with anorexia nervosa. Acta Psychiatr Scand. 1991; 84:9-11.
65. Pelsser R. Separation anxiety and intrusion anxiety in borderline personality. Information Psychiatrique. 1989;65:1001-9.
66. Zeiss AM, Davis HD, Wood M, Tinklenberg JR. The incidence and correlates of erectile problem in patient with Alzheimer's disease. Arch Sex Behav. 1990;19(4):325-31.
67. Cummings J, Victoroff J. Noncognitive neuropsychiatric syndromes in Alzheimer's disease. Neuropsychiatry Neuropsychol Behav Neurol. 1990;3(2):140-58.
68. Davis, HD, Zeiss A, Tinklenburg JR. 'Till death to us part': intimacy and sexuality in marriage of Alzheimer's patient. J Psychosoc Nurs Ment Health Serv. 1992;30(11):5-10.
69. Clayton A, Ramamurthy S. The impact of physical illness on sexual dysfunction. Adv Psychosom Med. 2008;29:70-88.
70. Demirkiran M, Sarica Y, Uguz D, Yerdelen D, Aslan K. Multiple sclerosis patient with or without sexual dysfunction; are there any differences. Mult Sclera. 2006;12(2):209-14.
71. Sander AM, Maestas KL, Pappadis MR, Hammond FM, Hanks RA. Multicenter study of sexual functioning in spouses/partners of persons with traumatic brain injury. Arch Phys Med Rehabil. 2016;97(5):753-9.
72. Rees PM, Fowler CJ, Maas CP. Sexual function in men and women with neurological disorders. Lancet. 2007;369(9560):512-25.
73. Zeitlin SI, Rajfer J. Hyperprolactinemia and erectile dysfunction. Rev Urol. 2000;2(1):39-42.
74. Hackett G, Krychman M, Baldwin D, Bennett N, El-Zawahry A, Graziottin A, et al. Coronary heart disease, diabetes, and sexuality in men. J Sex Med. 2016;13(6):887-904.
75. Holloway V, Wylie K. Sex drive and sexual desire. Curr Opin Psychiatry. 2015;28(6):424-9.
76. Rao TSS, Nagpal M, Raman R. A pilot study of prevalence of female sexual dysfunction in type 2 diabetes patients presenting to a tertiary care hospital in South India. Indian J Psychiatry. 2014;56(Suppl):S34.
77. Ioakeimidis N, Vlachopoulos C, Rokkas K, Kratiras Z, Angelis A, Samentzas A, et al. Dynamic penile peak systolic velocity predicts major adverse cardiovascular events in hypertensive patients with erectile dysfunction. J Hypertens. 2016;34(5):860-8.

78. Thomas HN, Evans GW, Berlowtiz DR, Chertow GM, Conroy MB, Foy CG, et al. Antihypertensive medications and sexual function in women: Baseline data from the Systolic Blood Pressure Intervention Trial (SPRINT). J Hypertens. 2016;34(6):1224-31.
79. Salavati A, Mehrsai A, Allameh F, Alizadeh F, Namdari F, Hosseinian M, et al. Is serum uric acid level correlated with erectile dysfunction in coronary artery disease patients?. Acta Med Iran. 2016;54(3):173-5.
80. Al-Qudah ZA, Yacoub HA, Souayah N. Disorders of the autonomic nervous system after hemispheric cerebrovascular disorders: an update. J Vasc Interv Neurol. 2015;8(4):43-52.
81. Molina-Leyva A, Almodovar-Real A, Carrascosa JCR, Molina-Leyva I, Naranjo-Sintes R, Jimenez-Moleon JJ. Distribution pattern of psoriasis, anxiety and depression as possible causes of sexual dysfunction in patients with moderate to severe psoriasis. An Bras Dermatol. 2015; 90(3):338-45.
82. Rao TSS, Basavaraj KH, Das K. Psychosomatic paradigms in psoriasis: psoriasis stress and mental health. Indian J Psychiatry. 2013;55(4): 313-5.
83. Almeida PH, Castro Ferreira CD, Kurizky PS, Muniz LF, Mota LM. How the rheumatologist can guide the patient with rheumatoid arthritis on sexual function? Rev Bras Reumatol. 2015; 55(5):458-63.
84. Avasthi A, Grover S, Rao TSS. Clinical practice guidelines for management of sexual dysfunction. Indian J Psychiatry. 2017;59(Suppl 1):S91-115.

CHAPTER 11

Interface with Ethics and Culture

Savita Malhotra, Srinivas Balachander

ABSTRACT

The universal core ethical principles of beneficence, autonomy, justice, and nonmaleficence, have had their roots in Western philosophy and ideology. On the other hand, the philosophy of "bahujan hitaye, bahujan sukhaye" (for the benefit of all and for happiness of all), enshrined in Rig Veda, is the one of the guiding principles prescribed for human conduct in India. The field of psychiatry is unique in its place, as cultural values, norms, and ideals have an influence in its practice more than in any other branch of medicine. The current chapter discusses how culture may influence ethical principles in the context of psychiatric practice, decision-making in ethically challenging situations involving autonomy, confidentiality, and therapeutic boundaries. Being culturally sensitive at the same time adhering to the core ethical principles can lead to providing better patient care.

INTRODUCTION

The subject of ethics deals with what is good and bad, and how best to behave in order to maximize good in a society. Medical ethics serve as guiding principles used to establish professional behavior and boundaries in clinical practice. Given the responsibility of doctors toward patients, society, others in the profession and to self, several sets of principles have been drawn to guide professional behavior; the earliest recorded being the Hippocratic oath itself. The most popular current frameworks for medical ethics are the four basic principles as given by Beauchamp and Childress[1] include: (1) respect for autonomy, (2) beneficence, (3) nonmaleficence, and (4) justice. These are not meant to be rigid rules or laws, but are guiding principles. These principles, were put forth as part of international declarations of medical associations, have gradually become legislations at various levels, national or local. They have transformed clinical and research approaches in health care, and in-turn societal attitudes toward the profession.

AN OVERVIEW OF ETHICS IN PSYCHIATRY

Psychiatric ethics is concerned with the application of moral rules to situations and relationships specific to the field of mental health practice.[2] A myriad of ethical problems pervade clinical practice and research in psychiatry, which are different from those seen in other medical specialties. This is due to several factors:
- Definition of normalcy, or what is normal versus what is deviant behavior is not absolute. It is dependent on norms defined by the society and culture from time to time.

- The nature of psychiatric diagnoses, which may add the baggage of stigma, prejudice, and discrimination to the patient.
- The need for involuntary treatments in patients whose judgment may be impaired, as a result of the mental illness.
- The nature of the therapeutic relationship, in which several intimate personal and emotional details are shared, requires a high degree of confidentiality to be maintained.

Psychiatry, as a branch of medicine, even today continues to grapple with accusations of being an inexact science. Thomas Szasz[3] vehemently indicted the field of being an "agency" of political or societal forces to act against deviant behavior, and exert social control, thus calling all of mental illness a "myth". There have been several instances in the past where psychiatry has drawn severe criticism, for practices that are known to have been evidently wrong today.

Understanding these distinct difficulties, the World Psychiatric Association drew up guidelines for professional ethics to the field of psychiatry in 1977, known as the Hawaii Declaration, which was to serve as professional ethical guidelines that are universally applicable to psychiatrists practicing all over the world. This was later revised in 1996, which is currently known as the Madrid Declaration,[4] to include certain newer dilemmas that had come up with the advances in the field of medicine. Issues as diverse as genetic research, conflict with third party players, addressing media and organ transplantation relevant to mental health have been addressed in the document.

The essence of all these recommendations is that psychiatric patients should be treated with dignity and respect, and address specific issues such as the procedure for involuntary admissions, use of physical restraints, the rights of the mentally ill, and the need for adequate resource allocation to have access to mental health care for all.

Considering the various dimensions of psychiatry, ethics plays a crucial role in safeguarding psychiatry as a profession. Ethics helps psychiatrists to be transparent and accountable in their practice. It also helps us to protect the rights of the persons with mental illness.

It is well known; that cultural differences may change the way the field of psychiatry is practiced in different societies. In view of this, the first question that comes to mind, as worded by Norman Sartorius[5] is "Is there one set of rules that should govern psychiatry as a profession, or are there as many sets of rules as there are societies?"

To answer this, we shall first try to understand the philosophy behind the framing of four basic principles. Then, by looking at the influence of culture in the practice of psychiatry, we shall look at certain situations where culture may blur the lines drawn by the ethical principles.[6]

PHILOSOPHICAL UNDERPINNINGS OF THE ETHICAL PRINCIPLES

Two main philosophical schools are considered to be the fundamental roots of contemporary ethics: (1) deontologism (Immanuel Kant) and (2) utilitarianism (Bentham and Mill).[1]

Utilitarianism, also known as consequentialism, states "the ends justify the means". This means, if the final outcome of any act, turns out to be "good", that is, whatever be the method used, leads to the betterment of the individual (or patient) or the society, then the act is considered justifiable.

The problem with utilitarianism lies in determining what can be termed as "good" in an outcome. There are differences between societies and also individuals within a society as to what "good" means. For example, the outcome of experimentation on Jews during the Nazi regime, or the indiscriminate use of psychosurgery, were all carried out under the notion that they were for the betterment of humanity. People can be treated unfairly if it will benefit the community. Acts that would be generally considered evil are acceptable under utilitarianism if they are likely to benefit the society.

Deontologism, on the other hand, also known as "rule-based ethics", posits that every act has to be done according to certain rules or laws. No matter what the outcome, these rules have to always be followed and no transgression is acceptable at any time. Immanuel Kant, an 18th century philosopher, gave the concept of the "categorical imperative", and argued that certain ways of behaving are obligatory regardless of the consequences. A simple example of a deontological stance is that it is always wrong to lie and steal, no matter what the outcome is. It also stresses the importance of respecting individuals because they are rational creatures. The principles of autonomy and informed consent have been derived from the deontological school of ethics. In short, patients are not just a "means to an end" but the end itself, and should always be taken into consideration.

Both these seemingly contrasting viewpoints on ethics have their individual merits and demerits, but can be taken together. In deciding an ethical course of action, one needs to balance the concerns of there different schools of thought. "Rule-based" utilitarianism is what forms the foundation of contemporary medical ethics.

The above basic ethical principles have been devised based of philosophies derived from Europe and Britain. They have been implemented world-over and have been incorporated in the curriculum of both undergraduate and postgraduates of every specialty curriculum. These ethical norms periodically also undergo revision, as it is understood that values can changes with time, and with advancements in medical technologies, new ethical problems keep cropping up. The Declaration of Helsinki, which is considered to be the cornerstone document of the World Medical Association regarding medical research human experimentation, underwent its latest revision 2013.

Virtue-based ethics, which is considered to be the oldest of the schools as it is based on Aristotelian concept of phronesis ("practical wisdom"), is seeing a re-emergence in medical ethics.[7] It posits that in order to safeguard against ethical problems, professionals are required to acquire certain attributes or "virtues" which are specific to their field. For example, Radden stated the virtues necessary of a psychiatrist may be as follows—compassion, humility, fidelity, respect for confidentiality, prudence, warmth, sensitivity, perseverance. Certain groups have argued that virtue ethics alone can provide or inform more prescriptive codes of ethics in psychiatry.[7]

Wig[8] explored how Indian philosophy is also in many ways virtue-based (termed "subjective"-based in his paper). The chief components of subjective ethics are austerity, self-control, renunciation, nonattachment, and concentration. In Hinduism, leading an ethical life means living simply; not being greedy; being charitable, compassionate, gentle, and pious; acting in consideration of the welfare of others; providing succor to distressed persons; being of service to all; and bearing no ill will toward others.

CULTURE AND ITS INFLUENCE IN THE PRACTICE OF PSYCHIATRY

The influence of culture in almost every aspect of the practice of psychiatry cannot be overemphasized, and this has been documented as early as by Emil Kraepelin himself.[9] Culture can be understood in many ways. Leininger[10] defined culture as *"learned, shared and transmitted values, beliefs, norms and life ways of a particular group that guides their thinking, decisions, and actions in patterned ways."* Barrett[11] defined culture as that which encompasses the symbols and conventions, human beings construct to understand and interact in the world, and cultural variety lends to extraordinary plasticity and diversity to human behavior. Culture operates at two levels: (1) at the macroscopic level it represents the social and institutional pattern of a society at large and (2) at the microscopic level it influences the individual thinking and behavior, both consciously and unconsciously.[12]

There is sufficient evidence now to say that culture may influence aspects of the occurrence, causes, manifestation, prognosis, course of various psychiatric illness. Culture affects the presentation of psychiatric illness in various ways—in the generation of symptoms, in the expression of symptoms, in the experience of symptoms and coping mechanisms, help seeking behavior, etc.

In the clinical setting, culture plays a part in the interaction patterns, expectations and even prescribing patterns of clinicians and the expectations of the patients. Cultural competence can be defined as the ability of individuals to see beyond the boundaries of their own cultural interpretations, to be able to maintain objectivity when faced with individuals from cultures different to their own, and to be able to interpret and understand behaviors and intentions of other people nonjudgmentally and without bias. Cultural competence requires cultural sensitivity, cultural knowledge, and cultural empathy.[13]

KEY DIFFERENCES IN WESTERN VERSUS EASTERN SOCIETIES

The differences given in **Table 1** represent a broad mainstream norm in comparing Western and Eastern cultures. Each of the two groups encompasses several countries, religions, ethnicities, sects, races, between which also there may be a wide variation of cultural practices. With increasing globalization, we may be heading toward a more uniform society.[14]

How these cultural differences and dynamics pattern the sociodynamics, which in turn further reflect in and determine the psychodynamics; and cultural relativism of dependence is beautifully illustrated by JS Neki in his scholarly articles published in

TABLE 1: Some of the key differences between Eastern (traditional) and Western cultures with respect to mental health care.

Western culture	Eastern (Traditional) culture
Autonomy is valued	Interdependence, affiliation, and cohesion are valued
Individualism (independence) is the ideal of development	Collectivism (Family and group orientation) is the developmental goal
Nuclear family orientation	Extended or joint family set-ups common
Locus of control internal	Locus of control external
Status achieved by own efforts	Status determined by age and position in the family, care of the elderly
Doctor-patient relationship is defined by principle of consumerism	Doctor-patient relationship is defined by respect and reverence for the physician
Guilt proneness is more	Less of guilt proneness, more prone to shame
Malpractice suing is likely	Malpractice suing is generally unlikely

British Journal of Medical Psychology (1976).[15] Analysis and understanding of patient's psychodynamics, therefore, requires a deep understanding of patient's sociocultural world on part of the psychiatrist to be therapeutically effective.

Also, when there are differences between a clinician's cultural values and belief systems with that of the patient, ethical dilemmas may arise.[16,17] They can arise in several aspects of care, including the diagnosis, types of treatment chosen, communication patterns and boundaries of the therapeutic alliance with the patient and significant others, just to name a few.

AUTONOMY AND INFORMED CONSENT

Autonomy refers to the patient's right to make decisions about his or her own health care. Clinicians recognize and respect the autonomy of patients by engaging them in decision-making discussions about their medical care through the process of informed consent. Attempts to influence a patient to accept a course of action may be limited to persuasion, after having provided patients with a rational understanding of their diagnosis and options for treatment. The importance for autonomy has gradually risen since the last few decades, and in several clinical encounters can override the principle of beneficence, unless it can be demonstrated that the patient's judgment is incapacitated and is not fit to be engaged in the decision-making process. Informed consent is now part of nearly every aspect of clinical practice.

Of the four core ethical principles elucidated by Beauchamp and Childress, respect for autonomy is be the one most closely tied to Western "individualist" societal values. In individualist society, the individual is viewed as unique, independent and in charge of his or her own destiny. However, in Eastern societies, where individual autonomy is not prized as much as interdependence and family cohesion, the emphasis on autonomy may seem out of place.

Being an interdependent society, locus of decision-making is generally the elders in the family or the head. An individual decision that is not in keeping with the collective may leave the decision-makers alone in bearing responsibility of the outcome and may deprive them of family support. When the decision is taken collectively by both patient and family members, the negative consequences of the decision are then not the patient's fault alone and the patient does not have to bear the guilt of having made a wrong decision.

Treatments against the patient's will, such as involuntary hospitalizations, use of physical restraints or somatic treatments and surreptitious medications are commonly undertaken with consent from family members, and this generally does not lead to ethical or legal problems when the family is well-informed regarding the rationale, risks of these measures.

It is also generally the case in clinical encounters especially in Indian settings that the entire onus of decision-making lies with the clinician himself. Until recent times, the "doctor" in an Indian society was likened to God, and was bestowed upon the privilege that all decisions made by the clinician were not to be questioned, no matter what the end result would be. Certain patients and their families would tend to look that the process of "informed decision-making" to be cumbersome and not by no means empowering in any sense. Taking an informed consent is generally perceived a mere signing of a piece of paper, the purpose of which no questions are generally asked. Thus, assuming a "paternalistic" attitude may be expected in a clinician in these societies. JS Neki proposed *guru-chela* relationship as the more appropriate paradigm in psychotherapy in Indian setting where the therapist is seen as embodiment of knowledge and the patient as seeker holds the therapist in higher esteem, which can be seen as antithetical to the principle of autonomy in Western setting.[18]

CONFIDENTIALITY

Disclosure of information regarding all aspects of health care including diagnosis, nature and purpose of the proposed treatment, risks, and prognosis should be limited only the patient or anyone else whom that patient wants it to be known to. Confidentiality is one of the most crucial components in a therapeutic relationship in a psychiatric setting. In Western cultures, awareness of confidentiality helps foster a sense of trust, which would enable the patient to confide in personal and intimate details, which would aid in the therapeutic process.

In Eastern settings, it is generally the family who supports the patient through his or her treatment, and tends to accompany the patient in most visits. Family members generally tend to ask questions regarding the patient's illness as a matter of right and these are generally required to be entertained by the clinician without the necessity of seeking the consent of the patient for disclosing information. Many patients feel comfortable in discussing their problems in presence of family members and do not like to maintain confidentiality. Often the patients in psychotherapy are accompanied by their family members to visit the psychiatrist's office, who would like to know all that transpires during the session and the patient may feel obliged to share.

A common ethical dilemma encountered in India is when families seek advice regarding the patient's marriage prospects, on recovery from an illness. Due to reasons of stigma, families prefer to hide facts about mental illness to other families. Certain clinicians advise family to only partially disclose information, to the other party, as full disclosure may weaken the prospects of getting married. Full disclosure regarding the illness and treatment is ideally encouraged, but is often toned down or partially shared by the family. Another situation is about disclosure of a serious diagnosis such as cancer to the patient. Many families in India prohibit the doctor from informing the patient of his/her diagnosis of cancer despite the doctor wanting to do so. This is a situation of conflict of medical ethics with social practice that is often encountered in India.

BOUNDARY VIOLATIONS

A boundary may be defined as the "edge" of appropriate professional behavior, transgression of which involves the therapist stepping out of the clinical role. Certain boundary violations may be harmless and nonexploitative, such as accepting inexpensive gifts, self-disclosure, and occasional meetings in nontherapeutic settings. Gabbard has conceptualized that there is a "slippery slope" to sexual boundary violation, which begins with seemingly benign nonsexual exchanges.[19]

There can be no doubt whatsoever, in any cultural setting, that an exploitative boundary violation, can be a serious offense. However, there can be variation in what constitutes a nonsexual boundary violation.

Refusal of nontherapeutic exchanges may hamper the fiduciary relationship between the clinician and patient. For example, patients may get offended on refusal to accept a gift as a token of appreciation, in Japanese culture.

Other nonsexual boundary violations, such self-disclosure by the therapist, physical contact such as handshake, giving blessings (purely Indian)—also may be culturally influenced by what is acceptable and what is not.

BENEFICENCE AND NONMALEFICENCE

Beneficence involves preventing harm, removing harm, and promoting good.[1] Physicians are expected to act in the best interest of their patients. Nonmaleficence is the principle of "first do no harm", and requires refraining from acts that cause harm to patients. Providing psychiatric care based on sound knowledge and using somatic treatments and psychotherapy with documented benefit are expectations of psychiatry.

These principles are generally agreed-upon, without much variation in most cultures. However, along with different explanatory models of illness that accompany various cultures, there may be different notions of what is perceived as beneficial or harmful.

The most common ethical dilemma encountered in this context is with regards to the engagement of certain spiritual or magico-religious faith healing in patients.[20] Despite significant growth in the availability and access to mental health care infrastructure, a parallel line of care for many still continues to be faith healers. Certain faith healers may simply prescribe wearing certain ornaments (e.g., a *tabeez*), or performing an elaborate *"puja"*. However, some of the rituals involve inflicting pain by branding with rods, chaining inside temples, exorcism, etc., are performed in inhumane environments. These are overtly harmful practices, but culturally accepted and are generally not questioned from an ethical or legal standpoint.

Quite often, psychiatrists in India are faced with a query from family members whether a patient can be taken to a faith healer or for religious healing practice. This may elicit feelings of negative countertransference within a clinician trained in modern medicine. However, prohibiting patients and their families to engage in the healing practices of their faith may also be violating their autonomy, and can damage the rapport to the extent that patient may be taken against medical advice or without the knowledge of the doctor. A culturally competent clinician should navigate through this being aware of the faith healing process that is planned, and discussing its risks and possible benefits. At the same time, psychoeducation to ensure their continuation and adherence to the current treatment should be undertaken, without blatantly challenging the families' belief systems. There are also circumstances when the psychiatrist uses analogies and metaphors from religion and mythology to make a point in psychotherapy with a patient who shares the same belief system. An example is that of using Shivling as a phallic symbol in psychotherapy in a patient with Shaivite belief system (Nand, 1961);[21] or using "hanuman complex" from Indian mythology in treatment of patients (Wig, 2004).[22]

CONCLUSION

It can thus be seen that in order for ethical principles to aid in the health care, especially in the field of psychiatry, cultural factors need to be taken into account. After all society and culture define the morals and ethical principles. Principles of medical ethics may need to be interpreted and applied in the cultural context for it to prove useful to patients, and the society.

REFERENCES

1. Beauchamp TL, Childress JF. Principles of Biomedical Ethics. USA: Oxford University Press; 2001.
2. Bloch S, Green S. Psychiatric ethics. In: Gelder MG, Juan JL, Nancy A (Eds). New Oxford Textbook of Psychiatry. Oxford: Oxford University Press; 2004.

3. Szasz TS. The myth of mental illness. Am Psychol. 1960;15:113-8.
4. Okasha A. The Declaration of Madrid and its implementation. An update. World Psychiatry. 2003;2:65-7.
5. Okasha A, Arboleda-Florez J, Sartorius N. Ethics, Culture, and Psychiatry: International Perspectives. Arlington, VA: American Psychiatric Publishing; 2008.
6. American Psychiatric Association. Ethics Primer of the American Psychiatric Association. Arlington, VA: American Psychiatric Publishing; 2008.
7. Radden J, Sadler JZ. The Virtuous Psychiatrist: Character Ethics in Psychiatric Practice. New York: Oxford University Press; 2010.
8. Wig NN. Mental health and spiritual values. A view from the East. Int Rev Psychiatry. 1999;11:92-6.
9. Bhugra D, Bhui K. Textbook of Cultural Psychiatry. Cambridge: Cambridge University Press; 2011.
10. Leininger MM, McFarland MR. Culture Care Diversity and Universality: A Worldwide Nursing Theory. United States: Jones and Bartlett Learning; 2006.
11. Barrett RA. Culture and Conduct: An Excursion in Anthropology. Belmont, CA: Wadsworth; 1984.
12. Chowdhury AN. Culture, psychiatry and cultural competence. In: Tseng WS, Streltzer JM (Eds). Cultural Competence in Clinical Psychiatry: Core Competencies in Psychotherapy. USA, American Psychiatric Publication; 2004. pp. 69-104.
13. Tseng WS, Streltzer JM. Introduction: culture and psychiatry. In: Tseng WS, Streltzer JM (Eds). Cultural Competence in Clinical Psychiatry. Washington, DC: American Psychiatric Publishing; 2004. pp. 1-20.
14. Sartorius N, Gaebel W, Lopez-Ibor JJ, Maj M. Psychiatry in Society. Sussex, UK: John Wiley and Sons Ltd.; 2002.
15. Neki JS. An examination of the cultural relativism of dependence as a dynamic of social and therapeutic relationships. Br J Med Psychol. 1976;49:1-22.
16. Hoop GJ, DiPasquale T, Hernandez JM, Roberts LW. Ethics and culture in mental health care. Ethics Behav. 2008;4:353-72.
17. Math SB, Viswanath B, Maroky AS. Ethical issues in psychiatry in Southeast Asia: research and practice. In: Trivedi JK, Tripathi A (Eds). Mental Health in South Asia: Ethics, Resources, Programs and Legislation. Netherlands: Springer; 2015. pp. 19-34.
18. Neki JS. Psychotherapy in India. Indian J Psychiatry. 1977;19:1-10.
19. Gabbard GO. Boundary violations. In: Bloch S, Chodoff P, Green SA (Eds). Psychiatric Ethics, 3rd edition. New York: Oxford University Press; 1999. pp. 141-160.
20. Sarkar S, Sakey S, Kattimani S. Ethical issues relating to faith healing practices in South Asia: a medical perspective. J Clinic Res Bioeth. 2014;5:190.
21. Nand S. A comparative study of scientific and religious psychotherapy with a special study of the role of the commonest Shaivite symbolic model in total psychoanalysis. Indian J Psychiatry. 1961;3:261-73.
22. Wig NN. Hanuman complex and its resolution: an illustration of psychotherapy from Indian mythology. Indian J Psychiatry. 2004;46:25-8.

CHAPTER 12

Interface with Politics

Sangha Mitra Godi, Sai Krishna Tikka

INTRODUCTION

Politics has played an important role in the origin and evolution of psychiatry. From the historical times to the modern world of global climate crisis and war, politics had a profound impact on the mental health of the society and its people through the political behavior of leaders, governing mechanisms, policies, and legislations. The interface of politics and psychiatry is a double-edged sword with both advantages and disadvantages that affect the disciplines with rising conflict and controversy. On the positive side of this interface, the international and national political partners have started emphasizing the role of mental health by celebrating World Mental Health Day, bringing reforms in existing laws, incorporating mental health indicators to be achieved in the global sustainable goals of World Health Organization (WHO) Mental Health Action Plan, and thereby paving way to the universal coverage for mental health services. However, the catastrophic effects of intrusion of political ideology into the realm of mental health has carved a strong impression in the face of history of the world politics. These include inquisition and witch hunts in the late middle ages to the extermination of thousands of incurable psychiatric patients in the Nazi "Holocaust" and incarceration of political dissidents in the psychiatry hospitals of Soviet Union.[1] The Nazi political ideology of the corrosive nature, of Jewish thought to poison the sources of idealism and feeling for race and nation has affected the Jewish psychoanalysts also. With this Nazi's notion of psychoanalysis, Freud's books had been publicly burned and all the offices of German Psychoanalytic Society had been taken over by non-Jewish members during 1933.[2] This influence of politics on psychiatry was also questioned when Julius Wagner Jauregg, a psychiatrist of Nazi era, was awarded the noble prize for unethical practices of malaria therapy on patients with mental illness.[3] Moving towards the current civilized and modern world, the world again is now bracing the fear of nuclear threat with changing political climate, leaving the fate of mental health of the world community at stake. So, this chapter provides a bird's-eye view of the different aspects, changing trends, and challenges that come into play at the interface of politics and psychiatry.

POLITICAL PSYCHOLOGY

Political psychology is an interdisciplinary branch of science that studies the influence of psychological processes on political behavior as well as the influence of political behavior on psychological process of the individual, group, and community. The political behavior, processes, and the phenomenon can be explained on the basis of various psychological theories. Many factors that influence and shape this interface of psychology and politics are existing belief systems of society, cultural beliefs and values, personality characteristics, individual and group motivations, attitudes, knowledge, cognitive processes, and learning principles. The bidirectional link between both fields is dynamic and always subjected to constant change from time to time. The psychology plays an important role in the shaping of political behavior and dynamics that are operating at the individual, group, state, national, and international level. The personality and the psychological processes of the leader affect the group behavior, societal control, regulation as well as the domestic and international foreign relations.[4] The behavioral theory of politics explains the political attitudes are learned from parents in childhood which are later reinforced and strengthened by social contingencies, individual experiences, and observation. The other psychological theories explain that certain cognitive traits result in polarized beliefs while the formation of polarized attitudes is influenced by contextual factors such as social media.[5,6] Social learning theories have elucidated the psychological basis of political authoritarianism and charismatic leadership.[7-9] Human beings are attracted to the political ideologies for the need of affiliation, power, identity, and security in the society as well as by modeling by their leaders. The Milgram experiment of social psychology also helps to understand the political obedience displayed by many loyal servants when asked by an authority.[10] Much research on personality, psychology, and political leadership has focused on leaders of authoritarian regimes. For example, Hitler's association with Holocaust can be understood based on political obedience to authority, the principles of mob psychology, and his dictatorship personality. The group dynamics of social psychology also explains about how bandwagon effect of adopting the behavior most people do influences the voting behavior and mass protests.[10] The principles of mob psychology and authority figure role of a leader can also be used for improving mental health literacy, reducing stigma, improving coordination between agencies and professionals, building public-private alliances, and training as well as for effective diffusion and delivery of mental health services.

MENTAL HEALTH OF POLITICIANS AND EFFECT OF MENTAL HEALTH ON POLITICS

The research on the interface of politics and mental health from the perspective of political mind is gaining much attention as mental health influences the mental health-participation and political participation particularly at voting ballet as well as due to the increasing pressure of global focus on mental health.[10,11] At the same time, it is important for us to understand the mental health of politicians as they can influence the future of mental health of their country's citizens and society.[12] It is always an area of interest in political psychology to understand the behavior, personality traits, and other factors that are shaping the political attitudes and behavior of the leaders that further define the political outcomes. Personality has been identified as an important factor that predisposes various political outcomes and attitudes including political participation, interest, voting, and ideologies.[4] The most common personality trait linked to politics was openness to experience that showed negative relation with conservative political attitudes and right-wing authoritarianism.[4,13,14] Historically, the personality trait of Machiavellianism is often used to describe the devious political behavior that is characterized by manipulativeness, deceitfulness, cold or callous behavior, and immoral means to gain power. Often, Machiavellianism along with personality traits of narcissism and psychopathy are labeled as the dark triad/traits that are associated with political participation and this can further shape the political ideologies.[15] The political attitudes do have an effect the stigma surrounding mental health and various studies have found that conservative political attitudes were associated with negative stereotype and stigma.[16]

The medieval to modern history has numerous examples of discussion on the mental health or personality of the political leaders. The personality of cult leaders such as Stalin, Adolf Hitler, Mao Tse Tung, Kim Jong, Donald Trump, and Vladimir Putin were often topic of discussion usually categorized and discussed as alike personalities as well as mental health of these leaders was also debated on television.[17] However, its implications on mental health professionals surfaced with Goldwater case in 1964. The mental health and fitness of the presidential candidate, Barry Goldwater, was questioned and was declared as unfit to bear the office by psychiatrists. This led to creation of American Psychiatric Association's (APA) "Goldwater Rule." The Goldwater rule refrains the psychiatrists from giving an opinion about public figures whom they did not examine directly and obtain consent to talk about their mental health.[18] This rule again came into limelight recently in the 2016 presidential campaign as the question of mental status of the presidential candidate, Donald Trump, surfaced with different opinions in the media as grandiose, maniac, narcissistic, etc.[19] However, there are few exceptions and safeguards while discussing about the psychological status of public figures in cases of deceased public figures of historical interest and when there is a duty to warn the victims or law enforcement of the possible threat mentioned in Tarasoff rule.[20] Although the Goldwater rule applies only to members of APA, mental health professionals should be careful while expressing their opinions about political figures or leaders as there has been some public discussion about the mental health of candidates in almost every decade when the leadership changes or political climate suffers persecution particularly during elections or political emergencies.

Epistemic Injustice

Epistemic injustice as a form of social injustice was conceptualized by Fricker, where the person's capacity as a knower or reasoner or questioner is dismissed by undermining their capacity to engage in testifying or making sense of one's own experiences. The existing prejudices, stigma, and sometimes for the sociopolitical or religious advantages, the credibility of the voice or expression of the patient with mental illness was often questioned and face "epistemic exclusion". This was existing in the society since ancient times as patients with mental illnesses are vulnerable group of society surrounded by negative stereotypes. This often leads to what is referred to as "Hermeneutic Marginalization" where a social group has an unequal opportunity to contribute to public discourse and expression.[21-23]

Martha Mitchell Effect

In the 1970s, accusations of corruption by the US Attorney General's wife, Martha Mitchell, on administration were dismissed as delusions which were later proved to be true. This misdiagnosis of true facts as mental illness by the psychiatrists or mental health professionals was termed as "Martha Mitchell effect."[24] The similar cases of labeling true facts as delusional is common in political milieu around the world where the conspiracy theories of persecution, paranoia, and power politics are intermingled and synonymous are sometimes used for political advantage. The true claims of persecution from the leading party or administration are often misdiagnosed as delusional and the raised voices of activists often labeled as antisocial or as grandiose delusions or the activists are labeled as bipolar patients. The book, The Protest Psychosis, explained how schizophrenia became a Black's disease and the circumstances of 1960s in Ionia State Hospital, Michigan, where the African Americans with civil rights' ideas were diagnosed with schizophrenia.[25] Often the antiauthoritarian voices are labeled as political maniacs and shifted to psychiatry hospitals to suppress the will and credibility of their movement for political advantage.

HUMAN RIGHTS

Mental health is an integral part of health and is an absolute human right of everyone irrespective of gender, race, culture, ethnicity, and nationality. Although the Mental Health Care Act 2017 of India and United Nations' Convention on the Rights of Persons with Disabilities made an initiative for the rights of person with mental illness as a legal asset to protect the people with mental illness and disability from discrimination and disadvantage, only time and political climate can decide the real fate and liberty of their rights. The Universal Declaration of Human Rights also emphasize that every person with a mental illness have the right to exercise all civil, political, economic, social, and cultural rights and this was also re-emphasized in the "WHO Resource Book on Mental Health, Human Rights, and Legislation" on paving way for the countries in drafting or revising mental health laws.[26,27] The right to access to basic mental health care through integration of mental health into primary healthcare services becomes accessible only through effective political awareness, determination, and partnership toward mental illness.[28] The lack of access, institutionalization, stigma, and discrimination were often the major challenges in achieving this goal. Sometimes patients go through a "betrayal funnel" when they perceive their civil rights and moral career are compromised in relation to their involuntary hospitalization by their caregivers and feel betrayed but not due to metal illness as explained by Erving Goffman.[29] So, these gray areas of involuntary hospitalization, treatment, covert medication, and consent when capacity is questionable are still a challenge in the face of ambiguity and instability of psychiatric diagnosis. The political empowerment of people with mental illness, acknowledging mental illness, and prioritizing mental health in economic policies can only turn the tide of this global epidemic.

ANTIPSYCHIATRY

The first of the major steps in the direction of antipsychiatry was taken by L Ron Hubbard, the founder of Church of Scientology with the goal of eradicating psychiatry from this earth. Later in 1969, the Scientology founded Citizens Commission of Human Rights to expose the dark side and evils of psychiatry. Gradually during 1960s, the antipsychiatry surfaced as an international movement with psychiatrists started opposing psychiatry with arguments against the actual existence of mental disorders, medicalization of political behavior, inhumane treatments, and illegitimate involuntary confinement in asylums. Many psychiatrists such as Thomas Szasz, David Cooper, RD Laing, Michael Foucault, and Erving Goffman have raised their voice as part of antipsychiatry movement questioning the validity of mental illness, institutionalization, labeling of mentally ill, and the abuse of psychiatry.[30,31]

Restrictive Asylum Policy and Deinstitutionalization

Asylums, which were often referred as mad houses, function by segregation of the "socially deviant" who were perceived as a burden on the society and economy. The ideology of this segregation was stated to be meant not only for a political transformation or maintaining social order but also to change the cultural image of madness into a concept of mental illness. The lunatic asylums played a prominent role in the political frames and purposes around the world that were reflected in punitive psychiatry.[30,32] However, this approach gave rise to various obligations from antipsychiatry movement such as deindividualization, stigmatization, discrimination, and wrongful confinement. The antipsychiatry movement against the institutionalization and involuntary confinement in asylums paved way for deinstitutionalization that is reflected in the current aim toward community-based treatment of mental illnesses.[30]

Labeling

Thomas Sheff's "labelling theory" states that individuals are "labelled as deviant or mentally ill because their behaviour is considered as unacceptable or deviant from social norms followed by the society."[30] In 1851, Samuel Cartwright created a mental illness "drapetomania" to describe the phenomenon of runaway of African slaves from their owners and prescribed treatment of the removal of both great toes. He also proposed a new diagnosis of dysaesthesia aethiopica to describe laziness of African slaves.[33] The labeling of behavior or mental illness carries stigma and prejudice that refrain the individual from their civil rights as well as political/community participation.[34]

The political behavior and the appropriate use of terms associated with mental illness as well as spread of awareness by political leaders in position of authority create a nonstigmatizing environment that enables the social inclusion and enhanced mental health access in the community.[35]

PSYCHOLOGICAL COSTS OF WAR AND PSYCHOLOGICAL WARFARE

One of the definite consequences of war is its catastrophic impact on the nation as well as on the mental health of its population due to the uncertainty looming around the future and life. The usual behavioral state adapted by the civilian population during war is either flight or fright reaction. The terror heightened emotional–physiological state and continuing stress levels associated with war also often lead to various physical and mental health problems ranging from depression, anxiety, insomnia to psychosomatic problems.[36] The development of "Inter-agency standing committee guidelines on mental health and psychosocial support in emergency settings" in the recent past highlights the importance of mental health during emergencies including political emergencies or war.[37] Psychological warfare denotes use of any psychological methods with the aim of effecting the emotions, motivation, attitudes, belief systems, and behaviors of the enemy or opposition group or government or organization or country.[38,39] In the modern era with advent of technology and internet, the cyberwar is used as a method of effecting the psychology and belief systems of the people through misinformation and hacking. This psychological warfare invokes a fear of impending danger, perception of threat, "fear mongering," anticipatory anxiety, and "moral panic" that break the morale of the group through false information propaganda or threat of chemical or nuclear war, etc.[39]

These instances were seen throughout the world as a part of military strategy from world war times to current ongoing Russia-Ukraine War. According to these military strategies adopted by different countries, attacking the mind of enemy is the most important element in winning the war. During World War I and World War II, the western societies and Adolf Hitler-led Germany employed these psychological tactics to influence the minds of people.[40] In 2022, the Russia and Ukraine War situation has showcased so much evidence of ongoing psychological warfare from both ends to demoralize the other countries military troops. The nuclear anxiety gained momentum since the Hiroshima Nagasaki nuclear warfare and the Hibakusha (Atom bomb survivors) were studied by various researchers. The extensive work of Robert Lifton's at that time has led to the identification of post-traumatic stress disorder (PTSD) in the survivors of nuclear war and its entry into the Diagnostic and Statistical Manual of Mental Disorders III (DSM-III).[41] Since the rise of nuclear power in the world, the fear of nuclear threat or war has constantly building the anxiety as well as effecting the mental health.[42] A recent article emphasized the significant mental health costs that the war bears on the civilian combats irrespective of the outcome of the conflict, addressing the current Russia-Ukraine War crisis.[43]

MIGRATION AND MENTAL HEALTH

Migration is a universal and complex phenomenon that is as old as the age of human existence on earth. It involves movement of people from one geographical area to another for several reasons often seeking for betterment in new place than in place of origin. Lee's "Push–pull" theory of migration elucidated various factors that push the people from their native place or pull them to the other geographical places and among those factors, political fear or persecution, lack of political freedom, poor medical care, discrimination, and war are some that not only lead to migration of people but also creating turbulence in mental health of people and social order.[44] The concept of migration is a broader one and different synonyms have been used for the people who migrate. It is based on the type of process involved in it and the reasons for such migration. These terms are emigrant, immigrant, refugee, asylum seeker, etc. A refugee is a person who migrates from his or her origin due to fear of persecution on reasons of either race, religion, nationality, or political opinion, whereas asylum seeker is a person who migrates to another country with purpose of shelter and protection in other country. The migration of refugees was observed over the past decade in different countries, i.e., from Syria to Turkey and in current Ukraine-Russia war where the civilians are fleeing from Ukraine to other neighboring European countries. The process of migration adds stress if there are barriers that lead to bullying, discrimination, lack of political and social support that further stirs various mental health issues such as anxiety, depression, PTSD, somatic symptoms, and helplessness.[44] A study on effect of migration on mental health in Norwegian emigrants to USA found that migration precipitated schizophrenia in genetically predisposed individuals and even some Indian studies found that psychiatric morbidity was higher in the migrant refugees.[44-48]

GOVERNANCE OR GOVERNMENTALITY OF MENTAL HEALTH

The constant push to democratize the decision-making process related to the health globally resulted in placing importance on the partnerships in the delivery of health care that applies aptly to mental health also, as integrated health care has become a fundamental feature in the framework or principles of almost all national or global health policies.[28] There is significant search and advocacy for shift from health governance to governmentality in the recent times but how much it would be feasible for traditional psychiatry to accept this notion is unanswered. The health governance focuses on the rules laid to govern the duties, responsibilities, and interactions between health service providers, users, and the decision makers of the ruling government that channel the healthcare system including mental health care at different levels of the society. The barriers for the mental health sector in India and failure of the mental health programs are poor mental health governance at various levels including poor political, financial support and lack of structured leadership at national, state, and district levels. Some programs related to health sector such as other tuberculosis, malaria and maternal and child health care have been successful in succeeding those barriers.[28,49] The role that power politics play in mental healthcare system establishment and penetration can be better understood through the 'Theory of power' by Thomas Hobbes. It highlights the role of power whether it is sovereign where the individual rights are transferred from one person to other people ensuring safety of their rights with the governing person or social or democratic where power is distributed and collective of all people in a society.[50] So, it is an undeniable fact that the politics determines whether government is democratic or monarchial or sovereign or republic and has a torch bearer role in taking mental health care of the society forward.

POLICYMAKING AND POLITICAL ECONOMY OF MENTAL HEALTH

Mental health systems in many countries are seriously underdeveloped, yet mental health problems not only have huge consequences upon quality of life, but also contribute to continued economic burden and reinforce poverty, particularly in low-and middle-income countries.[51] The 'social drift' theory also claims that people with mental illnesses are at increased risk of downward drift in their socioeconomic class to lower economic class due to unemployment, reduced work productivity, stigma, and high cost of healthcare expenditure spent in illness. Faris and Dunham in their ecologic study of psychosis also found an inverse relationship between social class and rates of schizophrenia. Apart from this, the unemployment, low socioeconomic class, and poverty were considered as causation or risk factor for psychiatry illnesses according to social causation theory.[52] The political decision-making, micro-and macroeconomic policies that include insurance coverage for mental health could determine the healthcare costs and accessibility of health to all, which were mostly said than done over decades. This gap in political determinism to mental health and its economic policies is seen in allocation of budget to mental health that not only affects the mental health of population but also affects its economy due to reduced work productivity. However, the recent changes brought by Government of India by incorporating insurance coverage to 17 categories of mental illness in Ayushman Bharat is a positive initiative to address the financial barriers. Although it covers the costs of inpatient management only, it includes medication, blood tests, electroconvulsive therapy (ECT), transcranial magnetic stimulation (TMS), and other neuroimaging techniques.[53] Apart from political participation in policy making, political representation of people with mental illness in making of policies related to them offers an opportunity of experiential support to overcome information and economic barriers in the development of mental healthcare services.[11] The use of prevalence, disability burden and quality of life descriptions, and antistigma campaigns may also help in attracting the politicians for devising better mental health policies as the current rising trends of mental health-related problems influenced the leaders/government globally, which is reflected in their "something must be done" approach. This message was also traced in Indian politics with the President of India's statement in 2017 warning "India might face the possible mental health epidemic."[54]

According to WHO report, the investment of 1 US Dollar in treatment of common mental illness further produces a return of 5 US Dollars due to increased work productivity which was often neglected or ignored in the budget allocation to mental health. The report also says that many low-and middle-income countries currently allocate <1-2% of the health budget to the mental health, including India. The economic loss to India on account of mental health disorders is estimated to be US $1.03 trillion, and yet the budget allocation to mental health faces constriction during budget preparation every year.[55,56] Although, the Indian government has highlighted mental health in the 2022 Union Budget by announcement of a national telemental health program, its share of budget allocation did not change much. Allocation of funds to central organizations such as NIMHANS (National Institute of Mental Health and Neurosciences) without much focus on NMHP (National Mental Health Programme) that caters mental healthcare services at the community level may not reduce the huge treatment gap of 83% treatment gap in India.[57,58]

JUDICIAL PSYCHIATRY

Psychiatrists perceive hospitalization as a means to provide and promote mental health care, whereas the legal representatives are concerned with the rights and liberty of the individual and this language as well as perspective gap between the two disciplines often create a controversy.[59] The political system can act as a bridge or a moderator between psychiatry and legal system for obtaining the collaborative approach of right-based cum evidenced-based mental health care. The national politicians and politics also play a vital role in creating and passing Acts and legislations in any country. The Government of India's judicial attitude regarding mental health reforms is clearly evident in the fact that it took 37 very long years from submission in 1950 by the Indian Psychiatric Society (IPS) for the mental health bill to be adopted by Lok Sabha in 1987. The new Mental Health Care Act 2017 placed a great emphasis on the role of patients, caregivers, nongovernmental organizations (NGOs), community, law makers, legal experts, and government by incorporating chapters on advanced directives, nominated representatives, mental health review boards, and insurance for involvement of every stakeholder of the mental healthcare services. Another welcoming aspect of the Act is decriminalization of suicide that often carries stigma and underreporting due to the laws that created gap rather than lending aid.[27] The Mental Health Care Act 2017 had a waiting period of 30 years to get passed and yet the implementation of it is still awaited and only testing times will decide how long mental health has to wait to be considered as an asset to the economy and become a political priority.

WORLD POLITICS AND PUNITIVE PSYCHIATRY

The evolution of mental health as a medical discipline since the beginning of the 19th century has been politically influenced worldwide in both the Western and non-Western world. Over the past two centuries, the political history of psychiatry has paved two roads to define and refine psychiatry. One considers psychiatry as a "social control of deviance" to protect the social order, whereas the other spreads the message of "psychiatry as advocacy with right to be different" to democratize the rights of people with mental illness.[1] These contrary political notions of repression and liberalization of psychiatry often face conflict time and again, but the notion of psychiatry as tool for controlling social deviance has been abused and misused for political reasons over the ages. This concept of political abuse of psychiatry is also termed as punitive psychiatry to describe the misuse of psychiatry to obstruct the human rights of individuals particularly for political purposes by misusing the psychiatry diagnosis or treatment methods or hospitals. This includes labeling with psychiatry diagnosis and inhumane treatments to incarceration in the psychiatry hospitals. Often the political motives include oppression of religious and political dissenters, activists, protestors, or antiauthoritarians to silence and weaken the morale of the movements.[60,61] Psychiatrists have also been involved in professional malpractice by suppression of their individual rights with politicization of mental illnesses for the political advantages either voluntarily or involuntarily based on their tendency toward the political ideologies. This political abuse of psychiatry where psychiatry is deployed as a political tool has a long history starting from the Nazi era and the Soviet rule to Ankang institutions in China and worldwide.[1,60]

Non-Western Countries

Among the non-Western countries, the Soviet Union and China faced serious allegations and pressure from World Psychiatric Association (WPA) for abusing psychiatry for political purposes. The meticulous research of Robin Munro surfaced the political abuse of psychiatry observed in China since the 1960s. The Cultural Revolution has damaged psychiatry greatly with evidence depicting abuse in various forms including labeling large numbers of people with mental illness, and involuntary confinement of political dissidents. In 1990s, as a tool against Falun Gong followers, political dissidents who complained against the republic party were incarcerated. Moreover, the diagnosis of Qigong syndrome too was created in the later years to silence the WPA claim of political incarceration in Chinese mental hospitals. The special forensic mental hospitals or the Ankang institutes were the places of political abuse of psychiatry in China with political dissidents often incarcerated with diagnosis of political maniacs or paranoid schizophrenia. There is ongoing debate on political abuse of psychiatry seems to still continue in China even after lot of criticism from psychiatry communities worldwide with mere mention in 2002 WPA world congress.[60,62,63]

The political abuse of psychiatry in the Soviet Union originated from the concept that people who opposed the Soviet regime were mentally ill and with diagnosis of sluggish schizophrenia in political dissidents. However, in the WHO Pilot Study on Schizophrenia where schizophrenia was found to be more frequently diagnosed in Moscow than other countries and later were far more frequently reassigned to nonpsychotic categories. The issue of systematic political abuse of psychiatry in the Soviet Union received condemnation from the WPA.[60,64]

In India, the system of asylums/mental hospitals which were started during British rule of India with all inherent flaws and drawbacks are powerful institutions and shelters for care of mentally ill who often received much stigma and left out by the society. At the same time, the asylums have been charged with various allegations of involuntary confinement of opposers, people feigning with mental illnesses to avoid participation in war. Later in the post independence era when Indira Gandhi government announced the state of emergency between 1975 and 1977, that period saw violations of human rights of the people which further affected the mental health of people.

Western Countries

Although the non-Western world received more outrage and condemnation for the political abuse of psychiatry, the Western countries including United Nations and most of the European nations also suffered political abuse of psychiatry in different forms. When we look at German history, it involved abuse of the "duty to care" of psychiatrists who were involved in euthanasia or killing of the socially unfit. Psychiatrists were instrumental in identifying, notifying, transporting, and killing hundreds of thousands of mentally ill and sending those deemed as socially unfit in mental hospitals to jails. The political abuse of psychiatry in Germany was blooded in the history with the Holocaust.[1,40] America's political history has numerous examples of political abuse of psychiatry such as Goldwater rule, Martha Mitchel effect, and diagnosing drapetomania in Black slaves to how schizophrenia became a Black's disease to silence the certain groups of society or for political gain of power.[20,33,65]

In order to fight against political misuse of psychiatry, International Association on the Political Use of Psychiatry (IAPUP) was formed in 1980, which was later renamed as Geneva Initiative on Psychiatry (GIP), in 1995. Over the past decades, similar scenarios were documented in other countries such as Romania, Czechoslovakia, Hungary, and Bulgaria as well and IAPUP was approached with requests to deal with political abuse of racial discriminatory policy of Apartheid in South Africa and similar abuses in other countries. In 2005, IAPUP was renamed as Global Initiative on Psychiatry (GIP) that focuses not only on political abuse of psychiatry but also human rights monitoring throughout the world with the goal of implementing humane, ethical, and effective mental health care.[60]

CONCLUSION

As we are aware that the political environment is a part of the social dimension of the bio-psychosocial model of mental health, it is important to study and understand the existing and changing dynamics of the political psychiatry interface and its bidirectional effects. Ever since the COVID pandemic has begun, different countries have been experiencing the common occurrence of arguments among family members and friends over politics and political decisions of the leaders. This trend is continuing with unexpected emergence of Russia-Ukraine War that brought uncertainty and fear associated with political decisions over war and displacement of people to other countries. This psychopolitical driven era and its decisions were strongly shaped by the media and its projection on the minds of people through journalism. Although psychiatry as a branch survived the antipsychiatry movement, the questions about its validity and legitimacy remained. This gave rise to birth of modern revolution of postpsychiatry that is advocating to democratize the mental illness with socio-cultural context based understanding and an ethical approach with minimization of medication to see through a new lens, distancing from psychiatry and antipsychiatry approach.[66] This advocacy of right to be different needs the political acceptance and commitment. Rather than just being mental health professional's duty for helping people with mental illness, it should be the common goal of proponents and opponents of psychiatry.

REFERENCES

1. Jablensky A. Politics and mental health I. Int J Soc Psychiatry. 1992;38(1):24-9.
2. Frosh S. Psychoanalysis, Nazism and "Jewish science." Int J Psychoanal. 2003;84(Pt 5):1315-32.
3. Brown EM. (2000). Why Wagner-Jauregg won the Nobel Prize for discovering malaria therapy for General Paresis of the Insane. [online] Available from: https://journals.sagepub.com/doi/10.1177/0957154X0001104403. [Last accessed April 2022].
4. Frontiers | Editorial: Political Psychology: The Role of Personality in Politics | Political Science. [online] Available from: https://www.frontiersin.org/articles/10.3389/fpos.2021.737790/full. [Last accessed April 2022].
5. van Baar JM, FeldmanHall O. (2021). The polarized mind in context: Interdisciplinary approaches to the psychology of political polarization. American Psychologist. [online] Available from: https://doi.org/10.1037/amp0000814. [Last accessed April 2022].
6. Brietzke E. Understanding and navigating the repercussions of the politically polarized climate in mental health. Trends Psychiatry Psychother. 2021.
7. Madsen D, Snow PG. The Charismatic Bond. Cambridge: Harvard University Press; 1996.
8. Altemeyer B. The Authoritarian Specter. Cambridge: Harvard University Press; 1996.
9. Bandura A. (1999). Moral disengagement in the perpetration of inhumanities. [online] Available from: https://journals.sagepub.com/doi/10.1207/s15327957pspr0303_3. [Last accessed April 2022].
10. Rosema M, Bakker BN. Social psychology and political behaviour. In: Steg L, Keizer K, Buunk AP, Rothengatter T, (Eds). Applied Social Psychology, 2nd edition. Cambridge: Cambridge University Press; 2017.
11. Frontiers | Mental Health and Political Representation: A Roadmap | Political Science. [online] Available from: https://www.frontiersin.org/articles/10.3389/fpos.2020.587588/full. [Last accessed April 2022].
12. Weinberg A. The mental health of politicians. Palgrave Commun. 2017;3(1):1-4.
13. Verhulst B, Eaves LJ, Hatemi PK. Correlation not causation: the relationship between personality traits and political ideologies. Am J Polit Sci. 2012;56(1):34-51.
14. van Hiel A, Kossowska M, Mervielde I. The relationship between openness to experience and political ideology. Personal Individ Differ. 2000;28(4):741-51.
15. Peterson RD, Palmer CL. The dark is rising: contrasting the dark triad and light triad on measures of political ambition and participation. Front Polit Sci. 2021.
16. DeLuca JS, Vaccaro J, Seda J, Yanos PT. Political attitudes as predictors of the multiple dimensions of mental health stigma. Int J Soc Psychiatry. 2018;64(5):459-69.
17. Turner T. Prophets, cults and madness. BMJ. 2001;322(7287):680.
18. Levin A. Goldwater Rule's origins based on long-ago controversy. Psychiatr News. 2016;51(17):1-1.
19. Levin A. History of Goldwater Rule recalled as media try to diagnose Trump. Psychiatr News. 2016;51(17):1-1.
20. Park S-C. The Goldwater Rule from the perspective of phenomenological psychopathology. Psychiatry Investig. 2018;15(2):102-3.
21. Crichton P, Carel H, Kidd IJ. Epistemic injustice in psychiatry. BJPsych Bull. 2017;41(2):65-70.
22. Drożdżowicz A. Epistemic injustice in psychiatric practice: epistemic duties and the phenomenological approach. J Med Ethics. 2021;47(12):e69.
23. Newbigging K, Ridley J. Epistemic struggles: the role of advocacy in promoting epistemic justice and rights in mental health. Soc Sci Med. 2018;219:36-44.
24. Verhagen P, Praag HMV, Lopez-Ibor JJ, Cox J, Moussaoui D. Religion and Psychiatry: beyond Boundaries. Hoboken: John Wiley & Sons; 2012. p. 844.
25. Luhrmann TM. The protest psychosis: how schizophrenia became a Black disease. Am J Psychiatry. 2010;167(4):479-80.
26. Kelly BD. Mental health, mental illness, and human rights in India and elsewhere: what are we

26. aiming for? Indian J Psychiatry. 2016;58(Suppl 2):S168-74.
27. Duffy RM, Kelly BD. The right to mental healthcare: India moves forward. Br J Psychiatry. 2019;214(2):59-60.
28. van Rensburg AJ, Rau A, Fourie P, Bracke P. Power and integrated health care: shifting from governance to governmentality. Int J Integr Care. 2016;16(3):17.
29. Goffman E. The moral career of the mental patient. Psychiatry J Study Interpers Process. 1959;22:123-42.
30. Desai NG. Antipsychiatry: meeting the challenge. Indian J Psychiatry. 2005;47(4):185-7.
31. Berlim MT, Fleck MPA, Shorter E. Notes on antipsychiatry. Eur Arch Psychiatry Clin Neurosci. 2003;253(2):61-7.
32. Goffman E. Asylums: Essays on the social situation of mental patients and other inmates. New York: Penguin; 1961.
33. Bynum B. Discarded diagnoses. Lancet. 2000;356(9241):1615.
34. Pasman J. The consequences of labeling mental illnesses on the self-concept: a review of the literature and future directions. 2011;2.
35. Hall T, Kakuma R, Palmer L, Minas H, Martins J, Kermode M. Social inclusion and exclusion of people with mental illness in Timor-Leste: a qualitative investigation with multiple stakeholders. BMC Public Health. 2019;19(1):702.
36. Murthy RS, Lakshminarayana R. Mental health consequences of war: a brief review of research findings. World Psychiatry. 2006;5(1):25-30.
37. Inter-Agency Standing Committee (IASC) Reference Group for Mental Health and Psychosocial Support in Emergency Settings, A Common Monitoring and Evaluation Framework for Mental Health and Psychosocial Support in Emergency Settings, IASC, Geneva, 2017.
38. Linebarger PMA. Psychological warfare. Nav War Coll Inf Serv Off. 1951;3(7):19-47.
39. Speier H. The future of psychological warfare. Public Opin Q. 1948;12(1):5-18.
40. Freis D. Psycho-politics between the World Wars: psychiatry and society in Germany, Austria, and Switzerland. 2021;39(2):314-5.
41. Zwigenberg R. Healing a sick world: psychiatric medicine and the atomic age. Med Hist. 2018;62(1):27-49.
42. Poikolainen K, Aalto-Setälä T, Tuulio-Henriksson A, Marttunen M, Lönnqvist J. Fear of nuclear war increases the risk of common mental disorders among young adults: a five-year follow-up study. BMC Public Health. 2004;4(1):42.
43. Bryant RA, Schnurr PP, Pedlar D; 5-Eyes Mental Health Research and Innovation Collaboration in military and veteran mental health. Addressing the mental health needs of civilian combatants in Ukraine. Lancet Psychiatry. 2022.
44. Virupaksha HG, Kumar A, Nirmala BP. Migration and mental health: an interface. J Nat Sci Biol Med. 2014;5(2):233-9.
45. Sethi BB, Gupta SC, Mahendru RK, Kumari P. Migration and mental health. Indian J Psychiatry. 1972;14(2):115-21.
46. Banal R, Thappa J, Shah HU, Hussain A, Chowhan A, Kaur H, et al. Psychiatric morbidity in adult Kashmiri migrants living in a migrant camp at Jammu. Indian J Psychiatry. 2010;52(2):154-8.
47. Kirmayer LJ, Narasiah L, Munoz M, Rashid M, Ryder AG, Guzder J, et al. Common mental health problems in immigrants and refugees: general approach in primary care. CMAJ Can Med Assoc J. 2011;183(12):E959-67.
48. Lavik NJ. [Mental health among Norwegian immigrants to America. Ornulv Odegård's migration research in a historical perspective]. Tidsskr Nor Laegeforen. 1993;113(17):2085-8.
49. van Ginneken N, Jain S, Patel V, Berridge V. The development of mental health services within primary care in India: learning from oral history. Int J Ment Health Syst. 2014;8(1):30.
50. Read JH. Thomas Hobbes: Power in the State of Nature, Power in Civil Society. [online] Available from: https://www.jstor.org/stable/3235060. [Last accessed April 2022].
51. Antler D. The Political Economy of Psychiatry-Power, Knowledge, and Subjectification in the State/Psychiatry Apparatus. [online] Available from: https://curve.carleton.ca/9e06b49b-031a-47e3-928b-a34cb439eef2. [Last accessed April 2022].
52. March D, Hatch SL, Morgan C, Kirkbride JB, Bresnahan M, Fearon P, et al. Psychosis and place. [online] Available from: https://academic.oup.com/epirev/article/30/1/84/623015. [Last accessed April 2022].
53. Singh OP. Insurance for mental illness: government schemes must show the way. Indian J Psychiatry. 2019;61(2):113-4.
54. Ideas For India. (2021). Understanding India's mental health crisis. [online] Available from: http://www.ideasforindia.in/topics/human-development/understanding-india-s-mental-health-crisis.html. [Last accessed April 2022].
55. Lancet T. Mental health: time to invest in quality. Lancet. 2020;396(10257):1045.
56. World Health Organization. (2013). Investing in mental health: evidence for action. [online]

Available from: https://apps.who.int/iris/handle/10665/87232. [Last accessed April 2022].
57. Business Insider. OPINION: India has taken a much-needed step towards mental health reforms, but it will be crucial how it builds on the momentum [online] Available from: https://www.businessinsider.in/india/news/opinion-india-has-taken-a-much-needed-step-towards-mental-health-reforms-but-it-will-be-crucial-how-it-builds-on-the-momentum/articleshow/89462737.cms. [Last accessed April 2022].
58. Gururaj G, Varghese M, Benegal V, Rao GN, Pathak K, Singh LK, et al. National Mental Health Survey of India, 2015–16: prevalence, patterns and outcomes. Bengaluru, National Institute of Mental Health and Neuro Sciences, NIMHANS Publication. 2016(129).
59. Zemishlany Z, Melamed Y. The impossible dialogue between psychiatry and the judicial system: a language problem. Isr J Psychiatry Relat Sci. 2006;43(3):150-4; discussion 155-8.
60. Voren R van. The abuse of psychiatry for political purposes. In: Mental Health and Human Rights Vision, praxis, and courage. Oxford, UK: Oxford University Press; 2013.
61. Heath-Kelly C. Cold War Psychiatry, Extremism, and Expertise: The "Special Committee on the Political Abuse of Psychiatry." Int Polit Sociol. 2021;olab034.
62. Birley J. Political abuse of psychiatry in the Soviet Union and China: a rough guide for bystanders. J Am Acad Psychiatry Law. 2002;30(1):145-7.
63. Kent A. Dangerous minds: Political psychiatry in China Today and its Origins in the Mao Era. By Human Rights Watch and Geneva Initiative on Psychiatry. China Q. 2003;176:1091-3.
64. Clark F. Is psychiatry being used for political repression in Russia? Lancet. 2014;383(9912):114-5.
65. ProQuest. (1979). Stigmatization and Stonewalling: The Ordeal of Martha Mitchell. [online] Available from: https://www.proquest.com/openview/a96492336bd0aff1f2dce9a2219d64ea/1?pq-origsite=gscholar&cbl=1816657. [Last accessed April 2022].
66. Bracken P, Thomas P. Postpsychiatry: a new direction for mental health. BMJ. 2001;322(7288):724-7.

CHAPTER 13

Interface with History

Ajit Avasthi, Abhishek Ghosh

INTRODUCTION

History refers to the narrative of the past events and their sequence, with an attempt to conjure up a cause-effect relationship. It looks at every object from the perspectives of space and time. Although history is supposed to inform about events, at a deeper level, it would be the insignia of the dominant beliefs, mores, and cultural practices of a particular period and people living in a specific geographic area. Psychiatry, on the other hand, is a branch of medical science, which observes and interprets human behavior, mood, cognition, and perceptions. It has an injunction to diagnose and treat disorders of mental health. In this chapter, we wish to draw your attention to the possible points of intersections between history and psychiatry, the disparate entities. This chapter would not be about the history of psychiatry but would endeavor to look into the changing philosophy and practice of psychiatry from a historical standpoint. Given the authors' limited knowledge and understanding of history, this chapter should never be perceived as an exhaustive and conclusive account of the link between history and psychiatry, rather this chapter should be viewed as a reflection of the authors' viewpoint.

To uncover the associations, we would like to concentrate on each of the four epochs: (1) the medieval age, (2) the Renaissance period, (3) the modern age (or the age of industrial revolution), and (4) the postmodern age.

MIDDLE AGE AND RENAISSANCE

In his book, Madness and Civilization: A History of Insanity in the Age of Reason, Michel Foucault provides a vivid and unbiased account of mental illness during 13th to 19th century Europe. According to Foucault, a couple of narratives dominated the social construction of mental illness (during this period): the great confinement and individual responsibility.[1] He identified the lazar houses (for confining people with leprosy) as the precursors of asylums for the people with mental illness. These establishments were built in the outskirts of the cities and mostly in places, uninhabitable and "would belong to the nonhuman". The principle of exclusion, used for patients with leprosy was extended to individuals with mental illness. Mentally ill people were grouped with the homeless, libertines, "witches", "idles", and "prostitutes" and formed an undifferentiated mass.[2] The "slightly deranged" and the "crazed lunatics" were clubbed and housed together. In today's context, it would be akin to grouping paranoid schizophrenia and anxiety disorders together. The rationale for the exclusion was their ostensible opposition to reason and progress. Readers can understand, the Renaissance was the age of reason, and "insanity" would come across as a direct contradiction to the same.

Hence, the "great confinement" was justifiable. The historical basis of the second social construction, individual responsibility, fostered and cultivated from the medieval age to the age of reason. Earlier references to mental illness labeled it as an inner devil.[2] In Christianity, reason and sanity signify "in harmony with God". In fact, Socrates focused on self-control and self-discovery for the "cure" of people with mental illness.[3] Foucault asserts, "Western culture saw madness as the weakening of disciplines and the relaxation of morals." Isolation of this "immoral" and "deviant" group did not create any conflict with the existing norms of the society. Although Foucault's Madness and Civilization was criticized for its oversimplification, premature generalizations, and presenting predominantly a French perspective, even his detractors would not argue on the horrendous conditions of the asylums. The conditions of these establishments were comparable to the animal farms in the 21st century.[2]

However, the period of enlightenment had also brought about certain positive developments. The most notable of these developments was perhaps the concept of Moral Treatment, championed by Philippe Pinel. It was proposed during the late 18th and the early part of the 19th century. Pinel, in the Salpetriere Hospital in Paris, unchained all patients with mental illness.[4] Treating a human being with dignity and avoiding all morally degrading treatment methods were the fundamental tenets of the Moral treatment. Nevertheless, he encountered a lot of resistance from the Catholic-influenced nurses. However, the split-off between the Catholic Church and the State and the belief that the Church would only rule religious matters, not the ethical and social matters must have come to Pinel's rescue. Generally, the period of Renaissance had liberalized psychiatry and persons with mental illness from the religious proscriptions and moral injunctions. It helped psychiatry to establish as a scientific and medical discipline.[3]

MODERN AGE

The late 19th and the early 20th century define the age of modernism and the epoch of industrial revolution.

Modernism: Freud, Nietzsche, and Schopenhauer

Sigmund Freud was one of the most influential psychiatrists who had shaped the 20th-century mind through his psychoanalytic theories. We would like to trace Freud's theory to the writings of other dominant thinkers of his time. One of them was Friedrich Nietzsche. In 1887, in The Genealogy of Morals, Nietzsche had talked about the "oblivion" and its description was quite similar to Freud's repression. Nietzsche's bad conscience was akin to Freud's severe superego. Nietzsche's account of man's esthetic capacity to merely curb the unconscious sexual drives was uncannily similar to Freud's sublimation. In his Birth of Tragedy, Nietzsche explained about the Dionysian and Apollonian mental processes which were primitive/instinctual and organized/logical, respectively. The readers could see its semblance with Freud's primary and secondary process thinking. There was apparent overlap in Freud's and Nietzsche's concepts of paranoia and dream as well. Despite these striking similarities, Freud had repeatedly stated that he had never read Nietzsche.[5] Although Chapman and Chapman-Santana had their reservations for Freud's claim, it is possible that both Nietzsche and Freud's thinking represented the common pattern of thinking which predominated during the early 20th century, characterized by self-consciousness, and rejection of the idea of realism. Freud's theory had a few oblique connections with another late 19th-century thinker, Schopenhauer. Freud's death instinct had a parallel with Schopenhauer's death as "true result and to that extent the purpose of life".[6] All these thinkers epitomize the philosophy of modernism.

Psychiatry and World War 1

Shell Shock: New Diagnosis in Psychiatric Lexicon

The modern age had witnessed mass destruction during the time of World War 1 (WW1). Let us look at the effect of the WW1 in psychiatry. WW1 supposedly was the trigger for the birth of military psychiatry. It was during the WW1 that a new disorder, Shell shock and a new treatment, Forward Psychiatry were introduced in the psychiatric lexicon.[7] "Forward Psychiatry" comprised of three principles: (1) proximity to battles, (2) immediacy, and (3) an expectation of recovery. These principles were used extensively during World War 2 (WW2). Although the detractors of "Forward Psychiatry" complained of the inflated claims of its followers, Jones and Wessely in their essay had talked at length about its usefulness in the Vietnam War, Korean War, and during the Israeli and Lebanon's conflicts.[8]

World War 1 and the Death Instinct

In his Beyond the Pleasure Principle, Freud had drawn direct references to the WW1 while discussing his death instinct.[9] To Freud human has the compulsion to repeat traumatic experiences either in their dreams or an awake state. The compulsion to repeat is so primitive and instinctual that it can override the pleasure principle. This realization was derived from Freud's work with the WW1 veterans who would often re-enact their traumatic war experiences.[10]

Growth of Existentialism

World War 1 could also have set off the philosophy of existentialism. As per Nietzsche, existentialism starts by denying the existing value and is an attempt to transvalue it.[11] Existentialism was also regarded as the philosophy of crises. The WW1 created an undeniable crisis and perhaps helped in sowing the seeds of existentialism. In psychiatry, phenomenology of Jasper was a derivative of existential thinking. It was a direct departure from the existing values of science, which looked at everything objectively and as quantifiable. However, the very concept of phenomenology was enshrined in the tenets of existential philosophy like, "I am what I am" or "I am because I am." Heidegger's thinking of Being in the World acknowledged being as a subject, irreplaceable and unique. When a being is confronted with the world, the psychic reality determines the so-called reality of the world.[12] This was quite analogous to the understanding of the phenomenology from the standpoint of an individual. Further growth of existentialism in psychiatry happened following the second crisis of the 20th century, the WW2.

Psychiatry in the Immediate Aftermath of the World War 2

Blatant Violation of Human Rights and the Advent of Ethics in Research

World War 2 had witnessed severe atrocities committed against patients with psychiatric disorders. Strous affirms that psychiatrists' role "was central and critical to the success of Nazi policy, plans, and principles".[13] Sterilization and euthanasia were two predominant categories of crimes against humanity, committed during the WW2, unchecked and unabated. The philosophy of racial hygiene and the idea of eugenics were the main driving force behind such crimes. Finally, at the end of the WW2, some of these doctors were tried in the International court, known as the Nuremberg's trial or the Doctors' trial (a component of the entire trial), took place in 1946. Following the trial, the code of ethics for scientific experimentation involving human subjects was laid down, also known as the Nuremberg's code. It was for the first time that the International court spelled out ethical principles, explicitly. The main components of the Nuremberg's code comprised of a need for informed consent, absence of coercion, need for a sound scientific rationale for any experimentation, and beneficence.[14] Subsequently, the Declaration of Helsinki and the Belmont report would uphold all these codes of ethics. Nazi psychiatrists contributed to the formulation of these ethical codes, of course in an ambiguous way.

World War 2 and the War Neurosis

World War 2 had brought about further growth in military psychiatry. The Shell shock equivalent of the WW2 was the psychoneurosis or the war neurosis. Both these conditions would be analogous to post-traumatic stress disorder (PTSD) of our current nosology.[15]

World War 2 and Logotherapy

Logotherapy, which was also known as the Third Viennese School of Psychotherapy was developed by Viktor Frankl, a neurologist, and a psychiatrist. Frankl spent several years in the concentration camps of Nazi Germany. In his brilliant book, "Man's Search for Meaning", Frankl gave a detailed background of the logotherapy, explaining the purpose and meaning of life and will to meaning. As opposed to Freud's psychoanalysis, which is led by the pleasure (or beyond pleasure), principle or Adler's "Individual Psychology" determined by the will of power, the primary motivational force in Frankl's logotherapy is the need to find meaning in life. Logotherapy provided a structure to practice existentialism in psychotherapy.[16]

Growth of North American Psychiatry

Authors have also tried to establish a link between WW2 and the growth of the North American psychiatry. A couple of points were put forth to explain this: migration and asylum seeking because of social and political turmoil in Europe and the hostile atmosphere of Europe, which was not conducive for study or research.[17] Following the WW2, the prolific growth of the psychoanalytic psychiatry in the United States was noteworthy. The American Psychoanalytic Society expanded its organizational efforts and critical development in the self-psychology and the ego psychology.[17] The first Diagnostic and Statistical Manual of Mental Disorders (DSM) was published in the year 1952, which would eventually come out as one of the most widely practiced diagnostic systems in psychiatry. It was heavily influenced by the US military and the navy. The classification scheme Medical 203 which was regarded as the precursor of the DSM was headed by a military psychiatrist by the name of Brigadier General William Menninger. Therefore, the effect of the War on psychiatry in general and American psychiatry, in particular, was significant and permanent.

POSTMODERN AGE

Despite some controversy, the end of the Second World War was said to usher in the beginning of the postmodern period. Postmodernity is a condition or a state of being associated with changes to institutions and creations.

Postwar Humanism and Deinstitutionalization

The context of deinstitutionalization comprised of the combined elements of idealism and pragmatism, which echoed justifiable anxiety for the well-being of persons with mental illness, a substantial majority of them, were living miserable lives inside the mental hospitals.[18] Atrocities committed during the WW2 had made the society acutely aware of the miseries of this vulnerable group. Hence, institutional care of the mentally ill came under the scanner for its potential violation of human rights and dignity. Among the several vitally essential assumptions behind deinstitutionalization, it was widely, even fervently, presumed that community-based care would be inherently more humane than hospital-based care.[19]

The arrival of person-centered therapy by Carl Rogers is another example of the influence of humanistic principles in psychotherapy. Although the seed of humanistic psychology was sown in the mid-20th century, it was after the massacre of the WW2 it had found a strong foothold in the arena of psychiatric practice. The three basic tenets of the person-centered approach, unconditional positive regard (nonjudgmental attitude), an empathic understanding, and congruence (nonauthoritative approach) are closely linked to the beliefs of humanism. Abraham Maslow's "hierarchy of needs" and "self-actualization" were also derived from the principles of humanistic psychology. In 1961, Maslow founded the first scientific journal, "Journal of Humanistic Psychology".[20] Later in the 1990s the inception and progress of positive psychology by Martin Seligman and others has come up as a follow-through of earlier humanism.[21]

History of Civil Right Movement and Psychiatry

The 1970s had observed fights for civil rights across the society—women's movement, disability rights movement, and the gay rights movement to name a few. In this background, the psychiatric survivors' movement emerged to eliminate the inhumane, coercive, and unethical treatments received by patients with mental illness. Judi Chamberlain, the intellectual leader of this movement, wrote a moving account in 1978, "On Our Own: Patient Controlled Alternatives to the Mental Health System".[22] Given the several centuries of mistreatment and decades of social welfare approach, survivors' movement was a remarkable development. In 1988, several such psychiatric survivors' group came together and formed the "Support Coalition International (SCI)". The name was changed in 2005 as "Mind Freedom International".[23] The European and World Networks of Users and Survivors of Psychiatry are other two influential groups, contributed significantly to the formulation of the United Nation's "Conventions on Rights of Persons' with Disability".

Vietnam War and Psychiatry

Vietnam War was supposedly the most protracted conflict the United States had fought so far. According to military psychiatry, the War could be classified into three stages: (1) the stage of advisory with a minimum engagement of combatants and minimum psychiatric morbidity; (2) the buildup period with a substantial number of combatants but not much psychiatric casualties; and (3) a large number of psychiatric morbidities took place during the last phase, i.e., the withdrawal phase. Wessely and Jones regarded the War as the watershed line for the understanding of the effect of unprecedented trauma on the human psyche.[24] Strikingly high mental health morbidity in Vietnam War veterans attracted several speculations. One school of thought talks about its "exceptionalism" regarding engagement of civilians as combatants. The other school blames the post-Vietnam reaction of the American public, which rendered the veterans unappreciated and rejected.[25] The diagnosis of PTSD was introduced in the

DSM-III predominantly to understand the clinical presentations of the War veterans, not amenable to the usual forms of therapy. Eye Movement Desensitization and Reprocessing (EMDR) came up as one of the unique forms of therapy for patients with PTSD.

History of the Refugee Crisis and Psychiatry

Since the WW2, the world has witnessed several refugee crises. Refugees are broadly of two types: (1) "convention refugees" are those who have been granted residency visas before the arrival to a country; and (2) "asylum seekers", the other type, are the individuals arriving without prior authorization. Studies on the refugee mental health have been conducted since the 1970s from Canada, the United States, Europe, and the Southeast Asian countries.[26] The systematic reviews, published in 2005 have summarized the existing literature. Refugees have been found to have a modestly increased risk for psychiatric disorders, depression and PTSDs are the most common ones. Several sociodemographic characteristics (being older, women, well educated, and coming from a higher socioeconomic status), and a few postdisplacement-related factors (being internally displaced, coming from countries with persistent conflict, living in institutions, having limited economic opportunities) are associated with higher risk for psychiatric disorders.[27-29] Recent refugee crisis in Europe, which has witnessed the displacement of nearly 1 million people, has rekindled the refugee issue. Recognizing the graveness of this fact, the World Psychiatric Association has issued a position statement on Migrant and refugee crisis in 2016.

Antipsychiatry Movement

The "Antipsychiatry" movement paradoxically was led by the dissenting members of psychiatry. The pioneer, Thomas Szasz, who ardently claimed about the "the myth of mental illness" was himself a psychiatrist in the New York State Hospital.[30] The other two renegade soldiers, David Cooper and Ronald Laing, were also from the psychiatric fraternity. Although they were psychiatrists, their theories were highly influenced by the social sciences.[31] All of them categorically and radically dismissed the concept of mental illness as a metaphor. The root of the antipsychiatry movement could be traced back to the post-World War sentiments, dominated by an individual's autonomy and human rights. Societal acceptance of deviant behavior had increased significantly resulting in greater freedom of expression and a compassionate and empathetic attitude toward others. These changes affected psychiatry from within, resulted in deinstitutionalization and humanistic philosophy for treating patients with mental illness. The same changes might also be held responsible for the inception and propagation of the antipsychiatry.

Although the birth and growth of biological psychiatry and psychopharmacology and the protest from the antipsychiatry quarters could be considered as parallel historical events, the former was mostly responsible for taking the shine off the later.

History of Political Dissidence and Psychiatry

The disorder which exemplifies such political abuse of psychiatry was sluggish schizophrenia, coined by a Soviet psychiatrist Andrei Snezhnevsky et al. This disorder was never recognized by the World Health Organization and in any country outside the Soviet Union. Sluggish schizophrenia was seen as a measure to contain and confine political dissidents. Even after their discharge, the "patients" were deprived of their basic rights and employability.[32] In 2002, Robert Munro wrote Dangerous Minds: Political Psychiatry in China Today and its Origins in the Mao Era and it was published by the Human Rights Watch. This book describes the human rights violations which occurred in China during the late 1960s to 1970s and during the late 1990s. According to Munro involuntary confinements of political dissidents, individuals with religious affiliations, and whistleblowers were taken place throughout these periods. In the 1990s, the Falun Gong, a certain form of spiritual practice drew the ire from the political authority, and several million were allegedly detained on the pretext of mental illness.[33] World Psychiatric Association, suspecting some foul play wanted access to the treatment records of the "patients admitted" in the Chinese mental hospitals, but the access was denied. History of political abuse of psychiatry mired the scientific image of the discipline but was contained to specific countries and times.

INTERFACE OF HISTORY AND PSYCHIATRY IN INDIA

The recorded link between history and psychiatry in the precolonial India is at best, patchy. Asoka, the great ruler of the Indian subcontinent (>200 years before the Christ), built a separate enclosure for segregating and dispensing various treatments for mentally ill.[34] However, evidence is not conclusive to say with confidence that these structures were built exclusively for people with mental illness. Direct reference to asylums was made during mid-15th century, under Mohammad Khilji's rule.[35]

Institutional care (by specialists and professionals) and the western medical model to treat psychiatric illness were brought to India by the British. The rapid expansion of asylums in India was preceded by the implementation of the first Lunacy Act (1858). However, it was after the formulation of the Indian Lunacy Act (1912), which inspired the development of mental hospitals with better medical and professional care. The European Hospital in Ranchi was established in 1918 by Col Owen AR Berkeley-Hill.[36] Nevertheless, Ernst (1987) would argue that the mental hospitals in British India were providing "less conspicuous form of social control". These establishments would act more as detention centers, rather than their purported use for treatment.[37]

The wave of deinstitutionalization would hit the shore of independent India as well. It responded with the establishment of the general hospital psychiatric units, the creation of outpatient services, and greater involvement of family members in the care of a person with mental illness.[38] Later in 1982 the National Mental Health Programme (NMHP) was launched envisioning community-based care for psychiatric illness. During the subsequent years, the government initiated the District Mental Health Programme (1996) and restrategized NMHP (2003).[39] The latter one came up on the wake of the Erwadi tragedy, where 26 people with mental illness died in a horrific fire accident in a "faith-based" mental asylum. The restrategized NMHP called for modernization and upgradation of the state-run mental hospitals and the general hospital psychiatric units. Although much later than the West the civil rights movements of patients with mental illness also started to express their concerns since early to mid-2000. Following the footsteps of the "Conventions on Rights of Persons' with Disability" the government of India rolled out its Mental Health Care Act (2017), with the individual's right and dignity at the center stage.

CONCLUSION

There have been several instances in the past when the disciplines of history and psychiatry would meet, interact, and influence each other. Sometimes these interactions would result in visible changes, which would reflect a direct and unambiguous effect of the historic events on the practice of psychiatry. Examples of such interactions are recognition of new mental health problems during or at the end of major Wars. However, many times the interaction would bring about a transformation in psychiatry through an oblique and insidious way. One such example is a growth of existentialism and humanism in psychiatry in the aftermath of World Wars. Sometime historical events would change the societal perceptions and attitudes, which through its ripple effect would affect psychiatry and the lives of patients with mental illness. Evolution of the civil rights movement and its contagion effect on the survivors' movement is an example. Finally, both historical events and psychiatric practice might be influenced by a common substrate, the prevailing cultural mores, norms, and existing philosophical underpinnings. Influence of Nietzsche and Schopenhauer on Freud's theory of ego psychology is a prototypical example. It would not be imprudent to acknowledge that all these interactions should give a better understanding of the inception, evolution, and transformation of psychiatry to its present shape.

SUMMARY

The medieval period was aptly described as the age of "great confinement" and "individual responsibility", whereas the period of Renaissance had liberalized psychiatry and persons with mental illness from the religious proscriptions and moral injunctions. The Modern and the postmodern era, with the change of the social fabric, changing mores, beliefs, and practices, with the devastating experiences of two major Wars and their aftermath, have witnessed the advent of new practices in psychiatry or have brought about significant transformations in the previous practices. We wanted to walk our readers through these developments and transformations. We also have alluded to the history of Indian psychiatry vis a vis the rest of the world.

ACKNOWLEDGMENT

None

CONFLICT OF INTEREST

None

REFERENCES

1. Foucault M. Khalfa J, Murphy J. History of Madness. New York: Routledge; 2006.
2. Porter R. Madness: A Brief History. New York: Routledge; 2002.
3. Scull A. The Insanity of Place/The Place of Insanity: Essays on the History of Psychiatry. New York: Routledge; 2006.
4. Woods EA, Carlson ET. The psychiatry of Philippe Pinel. Bull Hist Med. 1961;35:14-25.
5. Chapman AH, Chapman-Santana M. The influence of Nietzsche on Freud's ideas. Br J Psychiatry. 1995;166:251-3.
6. Grimwade R. Freud's philosophical inheritance: Schopenhauer and Nietzsche in beyond the pleasure principle. Psychoanal Rev. 2012;99: 359-95.
7. Shephard B. A War of Nerves: Soldiers and Psychiatrists in the Twentieth Century. Cambridge, Massachusetts: Harvard University Press; 2003.
8. Jones E, Wessely S. "Forward psychiatry" in the military: its origins and effectiveness. J Trauma Stress. 2003;16:411-9.
9. Freud S. Beyond the pleasure principle. Psychoanal Hist. 2015;17:151-204.
10. Freud S. Beyond the pleasure principle. In: Strachey J (Ed). The Standard Edition of the Complete Psychological Works of Sigmund Freud, Volume XVIII (1920-1922): Beyond the Pleasure Principle, Group Psychology and Other Works. London: Hogarth Press; 1955. pp. 1-64.
11. Galdston I. Existentialism and psychiatry. Bull N Y Acad Med. 1961;37:835-47.
12. Bobbio N. Old Age and Other Essays. New York: John Wiley and Sons; 2017.

13. Strous RD. Ethical considerations during times of conflict: challenges and pitfalls for the psychiatrist. Isr J Psychiatry Relat Sci. 2013;50:122-9.
14. Avasthi A, Ghosh A, Sarkar S, Grover S. Ethics in medical research: general principles with special reference to psychiatry research. Indian J Psychiatry. 2013;55:86-91.
15. Dwyer E. Psychiatry and race during World War II. J Hist Med Allied Sci. 2006;61:117-43.
16. Frankl VE. Man's Search for Meaning. Washington DC: Simon and Schuster; 1985.
17. Menninger RW, Nemiah JC. American Psychiatry After World War II (1944-1994). Washington DC: American Psychiatric Publishing; 2008.
18. Braun P, Kochansky G, Shapiro R, Greenberg S, Gudeman JE, Johnson S, et al. Overview: deinstitutionalization of psychiatric patients, a critical review of outcome studies. Am J Psychiatry. 1981;138:736-49.
19. Brown P. The Transfer of Care: Psychiatric Deinstitutionalization and its Aftermath. London: Routledge and Kegan Paul; 1985.
20. Capuzzi D, Stauffer MD. Counseling and Psychotherapy: Theories and Interventions. London: John Wiley and Sons; 2016.
21. Seligman ME, Csikszentmihalyi M. Positive psychology: an introduction. Washington DC: American Psychological Association; 2000.
22. Crossley N. Contesting Psychiatry: Social Movements in Mental Health. London: Routledge; 2006.
23. Nelson G, Ochocka J, Griffin K, Lord J. "Nothing about me, without me": participatory action research with self-help/mutual aid organizations for psychiatric consumer/survivors. Am J Community Psychol. 1998;26:881-912.
24. Wessely S, Jones E. Psychiatry and the 'lessons of Vietnam': what were they, and are they still relevant? War Soc. 2004;22:89-103.
25. Dean ET. Shook over Hell: Post-Traumatic Stress, Vietnam, and the Civil War. New York: Harvard University Press; 1997.
26. Silove D, Ventevogel P, Rees S. The contemporary refugee crisis: an overview of mental health challenges. World Psychiatry. 2017;16:130-9.
27. Porter M, Haslam N. Predisplacement and postdisplacement factors associated with mental health of refugees and internally displaced persons: a meta-analysis. JAMA. 2005;294:602-12.
28. Fazel M, Wheeler J, Danesh J. Prevalence of serious mental disorder in 7000 refugees resettled in western countries: a systematic review. Lancet. 2005;365:1309-14.
29. Steel Z, Chey T, Silove D, Marnane C, Bryant RA, van Ommeren M. Association of torture and other potentially traumatic events with mental health outcomes among populations exposed to mass conflict and displacement. JAMA. 2009;302:537-49.
30. Rissmiller DJ, Rissmiller JH. Open forum: evolution of the antipsychiatry movement into mental health consumerism. Psychiatr Serv. 2006;57:863-6.
31. Kotowicz Z. RD Laing and the Paths of Anti-Psychiatry. London: Routledge; 2005.
32. Smulevich AB. Sluggish schizophrenia in the modern classification of mental illness. Schizophr Bull. 1989;15:533-9.
33. Munro R. Dangerous Minds: Political Psychiatry in China Today and Its Origins in the Mao Era. New York: Human Rights Watch; 2002.
34. Nizamie SH, Goyal N. History of psychiatry in India. Indian J Psychiatry. 2010;52:S7-12.
35. Sharma S, Varma LP. History of mental hospitals in Indian subcontinent. Indian J Psychiatry. 1984;26:295-300.
36. Nizamie SH, Goyal N, Haq MZ, Akhtar S. Central Institute of Psychiatry: a tradition in excellence. Indian J Psychiatry. 2008;50:144-8.
37. Ernst W. The rise of the European lunatic asylum in colonial India (1750-1858). Bull Indian Inst Hist Med Hyderabad. 1987;17:94-107.
38. Wig NN. Indian concepts of mental health and their impact on care of the mentally ill. Int J Ment Health. 1990;18:71-80.
39. Murthy RS. From local to global—contributions of Indian psychiatry to international psychiatry. Indian J Psychiatry. 2010;52:S30-7.

CHAPTER 14

Interface with Sociology

Shinjini Choudhury, Abhishek Ghosh, Debasish Basu

ABSTRACT

The disciplines of psychiatry and sociology share a dynamic relationship. Before the 20th century, interaction between these fields was regarded as inconceivable. The first several decades of the last century witnessed a rise of socially oriented psychiatrists, social epidemiological studies, and significant wide scale geopolitical changes across the world, all of which contributed to the development and predominance of a sociological view to understand mental illness. 1970s onward, the introduction of an atheoretical-empirical approach, proliferation of psychopharmacology and evidence-based medicine in conjunction with opposition from the antipsychiatry camp created a rift between the two disciplines which has only grown wider with time. Leaving aside a few exceptions, the interface today is quite distinct. This essay ends with some future recommendations which might help to reconcile sociology with psychiatry.

Keywords: Social epidemiology; antipsychiatry; biopsychosocial.

INTRODUCTION

Sociology deals with the study of groups and their collective consciousness. It is the study of social behavior or society, including its origins, development, organization, networks, and institutions.[1,2] It endeavors to explain a social phenomenon, in a particular context and time. Psychiatry, as per the current biomedical model, is a disorder of an individual sans the society. Being a medical discipline, psychiatry speaks about eliciting and alleviating "symptoms" of the disorder with treatment. Apparently these two disciplines are distinct in their approach and agenda. However, a closer look makes it inevitable to be aware of the interactions between the two. An individual lives in, to, and for a society. Therefore, societal influence on the individual is undeniable. Nevertheless, the transactions between the two disciplines depend on the mutual respect, collaboration, and the basic philosophy endorsed by them. Contrasting viewpoints and intolerance to the other have ended up with a troubled relationship between sociology and psychiatry—especially when the prevailing "sociology in psychiatry" is threatened to be replaced by "sociology of psychiatry", is resulting in a turf war between the disciplines. In this essay, we shall try to understand and analyze this relationship over the years and also try to give some future directions attempting reconciliation. We have divided the last 100 years into three parts to demonstrate the topsy-turvy course of the relationship.

BEFORE 1900: PSYCHIATRY AS AN ALIEN BRANCH

Before the dawn of the 20th century, psychiatrists were considered as *Alienists* and patients with mental illnesses were treated in *Asylums* situated far away from the mainstream society.[3] There was little or no chance of interaction with other disciplines of science. The prevailing view of patients with psychiatric disorders was the eugenic view of *Victorian Psychiatry*, where patients were considered both as the victims and the etiological sources of the disease.[4,5] Stemming from this understanding of mental disorders, patients were physically and sexually segregated from the society, leaving no opportunity for further interaction. Psychiatric epidemiology was limited to counting of *Lunatics*. Therefore, sociology despite its significant practical role in medical epidemiology (*social medicine*) was unable to find its place in psychiatry.[6]

FROM 1900 TO 1970: THE ERA OF MUTUAL COLLABORATION

Emile Durkheim's "*Suicide: A Study in Sociology*" could be considered as the first major breakthrough which laid the path for a psychiatry-sociology bonhomie in the next several decades. Durkheim argued that suicide can be caused by social factors, not just individual psychological ones. Durkheim explained it on the basis of social integration. The more socially integrated a person is, i.e., connected to society and the general feeling that they belong, that their life makes sense within the social context—the less likely they are to commit suicide.[7] The appealing theoretical validity of his hypothesis attracted critical acclaim from the psychiatric community, giving rise to a new generation of socially oriented psychiatrists. Active collaboration among psychiatrists (or psychoanalysts), psychiatric social workers, and sociologists followed shortly. This collaboration resulted in several psychiatric epidemiological studies focusing on the social angle. Faris and Dunham, Chicago School researchers, published one of the first American studies to establish a link between social class and mental illness.[8] They found high rates of schizophrenia and substance abuse disorder "*in the deteriorated regions in and surrounding the center of the city, no matter what race or nationality inhabited that region*". However, the study of social class and mental illness by Hollingshead and Redlich, a sociologist and a psychiatrist respectively, may be regarded as the first creative collaborative research in the true sense. The main conclusion of this study was that there was a significant relationship between social class and mental illness, both in type and severity of mental illness suffered, as well as the nature and quality of treatment provided.[9] Alexander Leighton and Jane Murphy, in their famous longitudinal *Stirling County Study* demonstrated the universality of depression across countries, and proposed social disintegration as a causal influence contributing to psychiatric disorders.[10] Burrow, another champion of the social causes of mental illness, introduced the term "sociatry" as a name of a new discipline.[11] All these studies paved further ways to the contribution of social sciences in understanding psychiatric disorders in general and psychiatric epidemiology in particular. During the same time, George Engel, who was working on his "*Monica project*" pioneered the role of social environment in psychosomatic medicine, which finally eventuated into his widely accepted biopsychosocial model to understand medical disorders.[12] Another concept, deeply contributed by the social sciences, is the theory of abnormal illness behavior which discussed about the role of society's reaction and attitude toward those with an illness (or perceived illness).[13] Another sociological development which caught the fancy of psychiatrists was expressed emotion

(EE), which depicts the emotional aspect of relationship between the psychiatric patient and the family members.[14] The concept was floated by a psychiatrist, Julian Leff. It has five dimensions, namely (1) critical comments, (2) hostility, (3) overinvolvement, (4) warmth, and (5) positive remarks. Role of EE in relapse and recurrent hospitalizations in patients with schizophrenia has been well-validated.[15] Currently, the concept has been extended to other psychiatric disorders as well.[16]

The contribution of social sciences was not only to understanding the genesis of mental illness, but also to their management. Maxwell Jones and Thomas Main proposed the therapeutic community, which is deeply rooted in social interaction and modeling.[17,18] It was an attempt at democratization of psychiatric treatment by substituting authoritarian doctors with the clients as active participants of their own and others agent for treatment.[19] Thus, in this era, the coexistence of sociology and psychiatry, with mutual respect and support, was a rule rather than exception.

At least two major international events occurring during this time, helped shape the collaboration between psychiatry and sociology. First, the Great Depression, which began in 1929 in the United States of America and quickly spread to the rest of the world. Its strong, incisive, and pervasive impact impelled scientists to direct their attention toward social factors. The social epidemiological studies may be an indirect indication of its influence. Additionally, the world observed two major wars during this period. The war veterans with *shell shocks* and the inmates of the concentration camps with *institutional neurosis*, revealed the inevitability of the social-environmental factors in the genesis of mental illness.[20,21]

With the examination and understanding of the collaboration between the two branches, let us move on to the hypothetical next era.

1970 ONWARD: THE PHASE OF DIVERGENCE AND DISILLUSIONMENT

Several noteworthy developments in the field of psychiatry require special mention, to understand the drift. This was the era of empiricism and a theoretical approach toward mental illness. Psychiatric disorders were started to be defined upon the basis of specific diagnostic criteria or symptoms, embracing the medical model. Mental illnesses were thus dichotomized. The continuity model of illness, which supported the social factors, became nearly redundant with the advent of a new nosology, the Diagnostic and Statistical Manual of Mental Disorders, Third Edition (DSM-III). This was closely followed by the *"decade of brain"*.[22] Biological research in psychiatry overshadowed the research on social factors. Genetic epidemiological studies of schizophrenia replaced the social epidemiological studies.[23,24] Several drugs were introduced in the market for the treatment of psychosis and depression. Psychiatry began to emphasize the inherently beneficial role of treatment services, early intervention and its equitable distribution. This contrasted the sociological view where services were seen as a threat to well-being and citizenship.[25] In principle, psychiatry ruled out sociology for the latter's lack of empiricism and poor construct validity, and instead embraced *"methodologism"* and *"quantitativism"*. Empowered by the recent biological instruments, psychiatry focused to establish the construct validity of its diagnoses.[26] All these factors acting together took away the social fervor from mental illness. Psychiatry as a discipline became closer to other branches of medicine and insidiously severed its connections with its long-term collaborator, sociology. The biomedical model began to predominate the scene. However, the *"Antipsychiatry"* movement may be regarded as the factor which finally and decisively pushed psychiatry and sociology apart. This movement, paradoxically, was led by the dissident members of psychiatry and not sociology. The pioneer, Thomas Szasz, who emphatically claimed about the "the myth of mental illness" was himself a psychiatrist in the New York State Hospital.[27] David Cooper, Ronald Laing, the other two renegade soldiers were also from the psychiatric fraternity. Although, they were psychiatrists, their theories were highly influenced by the social sciences.[28] All of them categorically and radically dismissed the concept of mental illness as a metaphor! The categorical diagnostic approach of DSM received stern criticism from sociological commentators. For Carpenter, DSM-IV represents "the psychiatric equivalent of the World Trade Organization promoting the principles of *American Universalism* as objective standard beyond reproach".[29] The drug development and trials to concur with the evidence-based medicine also met with harsh comments from the other quarter, and an unholy nexus with the pharmaceutical companies were portrayed as an ulterior motive. These defiant and intolerant discourses made the coexistence of sociology and psychiatry almost impossible.[30] Eventually by late 1980s, most of the sociologists had neither the theoretical orientation, nor the practical competence, to support social psychiatry research.[31,32] They became deskilled as social psychiatric collaborators.

The geopolitical state might help us understand the disillusionment. The post-World War sentiments were dominated by individual's autonomy and human rights. Societal acceptance to deviant behavior increased significantly resulting in greater freedom of expression and a compassionate and empathetic attitude toward others. These changes affected psychiatry from within, resulted in deinstitutionalization and humanistic philosophy for treating patients with mental illness.[33,34] The same changes might also be held responsible for the attacks imposed on psychiatry from outside, namely from the sociologists or the *antipsychiatrists*. **Table 1** represents the rise and fall of relationship between psychiatry and sociology.

A FEW NOTABLE EXCEPTIONS

George Engel proposed a holistic alternative to the reductionistic biomedical model to understand and respond adequately to patients' suffering. He named it as the biopsychosocial model. This model is both a philosophy of clinical care and a practical clinical guide. Philosophically, it is a way of understanding how suffering, disease, and illness are affected

TABLE 1: Rise and fall of relationship between psychiatry and sociology.

Before 1900 (No link between sociology and psychiatry)	1900–1970 (Era of convergence)	1970 onward (Era of dichotomy)
• No contact of psychiatry and sociology • Psychiatry was confined to the asylums	• Durkheim's contribution • Social epidemiological studies in psychiatry • Role of social factors in psychiatric disorders • *Evolution of important concepts:* Therapeutic community, expressed emotion	• Predominance of nosology • Antipsychiatry movement • Advent of biological psychiatry • Divergence of sociology and psychiatry

by multiple levels of organization, from the molecular to the societal. At the practical level, it is a way of understanding the patient's subjective experience as an essential contributor to accurate diagnosis, health outcomes, and humane care.[35] The overt emphasis on the role of the social domain, the macroenvironment could have mandated the re-entry of social sciences into the arena of psychiatry. Despite its appeal, it had received its fair share of criticism.[36] As Ghaemi thinks, "biopsychosocial model is the conceptual *status quo* of contemporary psychiatry. Although it has played an important role in combating psychiatric dogmatism, it has devolved into mere eclecticism".[37]

Pat Bracken and Phil Thomas have brought about a new concept in psychiatry, the postpsychiatry, which implies that a person with mental illness is part of a complex, interacting matrix of social influences in which the mind cannot be abstracted or studied as an independent phenomenon. They reasoned that government policies are beginning to change the ethos of mental health care.[38] The new commitment to tackling the links between poverty, unemployment, and mental illness has led to policies that focus on disadvantage and social exclusion.[39] These emphasize the importance of contexts, values, and partnerships and are made explicit in the national service framework for mental health.[40] The service framework raises an agenda that is potentially in conflict with biomedical psychiatry. In a nutshell, the government (and the society it represents) is asking for a very different kind of psychiatry and a new deal between health professionals and service users. Critics of postpsychiatry declare, "True, as Bracken and Thomas assert, community care is failing. It is failing because of government underfunding, not because of a failed model of science. We ask for bread, and you offer us postmodernism".[41] Thus, the relationship remains status quo.

The two social factors which may have found a comfortable place in psychiatry are: (1) culture and (2) migration. It is well-recognized that culture plays a profound role in the way a person experiences and expresses his/her symptoms in the process of symptom formation. Culturally mediated *idioms of distress* and *culture bound psychiatric syndrome* are frequently discussed and studied empirically.[42,43] Cultural formulation to understand the interaction of culture with mental illness, cultural competency, and culture sensitive care to factor in the role of culture for optimal management of patients with mental illness, are now commonplace in the practice of psychiatry.[44] Migration is known to cause an unprecedented change in the lifestyle, goals, and coping among individuals and families.[45] This concept is one that is central to social psychiatry, as it depicts the conflicts between man's hopes and aspirations for a better prospect in a new socioeconomic-cultural matrix (the "pull" factor), pressures and obligations forcing a person to migrate to a socioculturally alien land, outside the country or inside (the "push" factor), and the resilience of human beings and their families in the face of new challenges of change.[46,47]

Even in this era of adversity, a couple of interdisciplinary journals are still in place. *International Journal of Social Psychiatry* is a peer reviewed journal published since 1954, which provides a forum for the dissemination of findings related to social psychiatry. *Social Psychiatry and Psychiatric Epidemiology* is another journal which intended to publish research papers of psychiatric epidemiology, with social aspects (in addition to biologic and genetic). The *Indian Journal of Social Psychiatry* is dedicated to the cause of social psychiatry since 1984. 2015 onward, it is being published by the Wolters Kluwer/MedKnow Publications, an internationally acclaimed publishing house that handles and publishes more than 300 scientific journals from India and abroad. The World Association of Social Psychiatry (WASP) founded in 1964, laid down its emphasis on the role of culture and national-international collaboration across various disciplines related to social psychiatry. All these are encouraging developments for psychiatry in general and social psychiatry in particular.

FUTURE: BREAKING THE BARRIER

Breaking the apparently insurmountable barrier needs special and combined efforts from both the fraternities. Multidisciplinary journals, conferences, and professional bodies are required to take the lead in the much awaited reconciliation. Socially informed psychiatrists must come together and assert, not for the benefit of sociology, but for the sake of psychiatry. The biological and social psychiatry should not be viewed as divergent and incompatible, but must be used judiciously to complement each other.

Among other possibilities, social capital might be seen as a bridge between sociology and psychiatry. Social capital is a multidimensional construct which has risen to prominence in the last few decades. It cuts across the fields of sociology, economics, politics, administration, health and behavior among others. It is defined as, "Features of social organization, such as trust, norms and networks that can improve the efficacy of society by facilitating coordinated actions".[48] This concept has been in vogue in medical epidemiology for quite some time now, since its potential role in mortality has been probed.[49] However, application of social capital in psychiatry is a relatively recent phenomenon. The evidence of its role in a wide spectrum of mental illness

BOX 1: The way forward.
- More interdisciplinary journals and conferences
- *Change of viewpoint and attitude:* Flexibility to accept the view of one another
- Adoption of the biopsychosocial model to understand and treat behavioral disorders
- Application of the social capital in psychiatry

starting with common mental disorders to schizophrenia has been investigated successfully.[50-53] Social capital has also found its place in recovery of mental illness.[54] More research on the association between mental health and social capital is warranted in future.

The human race in general, and science in particular has made such rapid progress not through noncooperation and cold wars, but through mutual respect, collaboration, debate, discussion, and pragmatism. We hope that psychiatry will break the current proverbial barrier and reach out to sociology, thus bestowing a fair chance upon the revival of the prestige of social psychiatry **(Box 1)**.

ACKNOWLEDGMENT

None

CONFLICT OF INTEREST

None

REFERENCES

1. Siddiqui JA, Kumari M. American sociological review (2010-2014): a bibliometric study. Indian J Lib Inf Sci. 2015;9(3):197-203.
2. Ashley D, Orenstein DM. Sociological Theory: Classical Statements. Allyn and Bacon; 2005.
3. Forsythe B. Mental and social diagnosis and the English Prison Commission 1914-1939. Soc Policy Admin. 1990;24:237-53.
4. Bentall R. Reconstructing Schizophrenia. London: Routledge; 1992.
5. Kleinman A. Some Uses and misuses of the social sciences in medicine. In: Fiske DW, Shweder RA (Eds). Metatheory in Social Science: Pluralisms

and Subjectivities. Chicago: Chicago University Press; 1986
6. Rosen G. Madness in Society. New York: Harper; 1979.
7. Symonds RL. Emile Durkheim's Suicide: A Study in Sociology. London: Routledge; 1994.
8. Faris RE, Dunham HW. Mental disorders in urban areas: an ecological study of schizophrenia and other psychoses. Chicago: University of Chicago Press; 1939.
9. Hollingshead AB, Redlich FC. Social class and mental illness: a community study. New York: John Wiley; 1958.
10. Murphy JM, Laird NM, Monson RR, Sobol AM, Leighton AH. A 40-year perspective on the prevalence of depression: the Stirling County Study. Arch Gen Psychiatry. 2000;57:209-15.
11. Burrow JW. Evolution and Society. Oxford: CUP Archive; 1966.
12. Engel GL. The clinical application of the biopsychosocial model. Am J Psychiatry. 1980;137:535-44.
13. Pilowsky I. Abnormal illness behaviour. Br J Med Psychol. 1969;42:347-51.
14. Kavanagh DJ. Recent developments in expressed emotion and schizophrenia. Br J Psychiatry. 1992;160:601-20.
15. Leff J, Kuipers L, Berkowitz R, Vaughn C, Sturgeon D. Life events, relatives' expressed emotion and maintenance neuroleptics in schizophrenic relapse. Psychol Med. 1983;13(4):799-806.
16. Hooley JM, Gotlib IH. A diathesis-stress conceptualization of expressed emotion and clinical outcome. Appl Prev Psychol. 2000;9:135-51.
17. Jones M, Bonn EM. From therapeutic community to self-sufficient community. Psychiatr Serv. 1973;24:675-80.
18. Jones M. The concept of a therapeutic community. Am J Psychiatry. 1956;112:647-50.
19. Clark DH. The therapeutic community: concept, practice and future. Br J Psychiatry. 1965;111:947-54.
20. Stone M. Shellshock and the psychologists. In: Bynum WF, Porter R, Shepherd M (Eds). The Anatomy of Madness. London: Tavistock; 1985.
21. Barton WR. Institutional Neurosis. Bristol: Wright and Sons; 1958.
22. Shorter E. A History of Psychiatry: From the Era of the Asylum to the Age of Prozac. Chichester: Wiley;1997.
23. Guze SB. Biological psychiatry: is there any other kind? Psychol Med. 1989;19:315-23.
24. Moncrieff J, Crawford MJ. British psychiatry in the 20th century: observations from a psychiatric journal. Soc Sci Med. 2001;53:349-56.
25. Pilgrim D, Rogers A. The troubled relationship between psychiatry and sociology. Int J Soc Psychiatry. 2005;51:228-41.
26. Fryers T, Melzer D, Jenkins R. Mental Health Inequalities Report 1: A Systematic Literature Review. London: Department of Health; 2000.
27. Rissmiller DJ, Rissmiller JH. Open forum: evolution of the antipsychiatry movement into mental health consumerism. Psychiatr Serv. 2006;57(6):863-6.
28. Kotowicz Z. RD Laing and the Paths of Anti-psychiatry. London: Routledge; 2005.
29. Carpenter M. 'It's a small world': mental health policy under welfare capitalism since 1945. Sociol Health Illn. 2000;22:602-20.
30. Berrios G, Porter R (Eds). A History of Clinical Psychiatry. London: Athlone Press; 1995.
31. Miller P, Rose N. The Tavistock programme: The government of subjectivity and social life. Sociology. 1988;22:171-92.
32. Parker I, Georgaca E, Harper D, Mclaughlin T, Stowell-Smith M. Deconstructing Psycho-pathology. London: Sage; 1997.
33. Shaffer J. Humanistic Psychology. Englewood Cliffs, NJ: Prentice-Hall; 1978.
34. Davidsson L. Deinstitutionalization and community based psychiatry: some aspects from literature. Med Arh. 1998;53:135-8.
35. Engel GL. The biopsychosocial model and medical education. Who are to be the teachers? N Engl J Med. 1982;306:802-5.
36. McLaren N. A critical review of the biopsycho-social model. Aust NZJ Psychiatry. 1998;32:86-92.
37. Ghaemi SN. The rise and fall of the biopsychosocial model. Br J Psychiatry. 2009;195:3-4.
38. Bracken P, Thomas P. Postpsychiatry: a new direction for mental health. BMJ. 2001;322:724-7.
39. Gray JA. Postmodern medicine. Lancet. 1999;354:1550-3.
40. Bracken P, Thomas P. A new debate on mental health. Open Mind. 1998;89:17.
41. Keen TM. Post-psychiatry: paradigm shift or wishful thinking? A speculative review of future possibles for psychiatry. J Psychiatr Ment Health Nurs. 2003;10:29-37.
42. Nichter M. Idioms of distress revisited. Cult Med Psychiatry. 2010;34:401-16.
43. Griffith L. Culture-bound syndrome. The Wiley Blackwell Encyclopedia of Health, Illness, Behavior, and Society. 2014.

44. Kleinman A. Anthropology and psychiatry. The role of culture in cross-cultural research on illness. Br J Psychiatry. 1987;151:447-54.
45. Kleiner RJ, Parker S. Migration and mental illness: a new look. Am Sociological Rev. 1959;24:687-90.
46. Bhugra D, Jones P. Migration and mental illness. Adv Psychiatr Treat. 2001;7(3):216-22.
47. Bhugra D. Migration and mental health. Acta Psychiat Scand. 2004;109(4):243-58.
48. Paldam M. Social capital: one or many? Definition and measurement. J Econ Surv. 2000;14(5):629-53.
49. Kawachi I, Kennedy BP, Lochner K, Prothrow-Stith D. Social capital, income inequality, and mortality. Am J Public Health. 1997;87:1491-8.
50. De Silva MJ, McKenzie K, Harpham T, Huttly SR. Social capital and mental illness: a systematic review. J Epidemiol Community Health. 2005;59:619-27.
51. McKenzie K, Whitley R, Weich S. Social capital and mental health. Br J Psychiatry. 2002;181:280-3.
52. Kawachi I, Berkman LF. Social ties and mental health. J Urban Health. 2001;78:458-67.
53. De Silva MJ, Huttly SR, Harpham T, Kenward MG. Social capital and mental health: a comparative analysis of four low income countries. Soc Sci Med. 2007;64:5-20.
54. Tew J, Ramon S, Slade M, Bird V, Melton J, Le Boutillier C. Social factors and recovery from mental health difficulties: a review of the evidence. Br J Soc Work. 2011;42(3):443-60.

CHAPTER 15

Interface with Mythology

Ajit V Bhide

MYTH, LEGEND AND HISTORY

The word "myth" conjures up tales of imaginary persons, Gods, Goddesses, demigods and demigoddesses, ogres, monsters, and also of happenings that mix the plausible with the fantastic. Blessings, curses, adventures, and misadventures abound, to tell stories, often of fantastic imagination. Somehow, the word myth is too quickly associated with untruths. This in itself is a fallacy, or at the least, an overvalued notion.

Actually, much of mythological compendia is traceable to real happenings recorded, granting that the recording often is distorted by the archivist. In the Japanese tradition, the history of the country is so interwoven with a charming mythology, adhered to as the truth by many of that nation to this day.

It has been argued that when real happenings of great import are recorded and retold, they are not myths but legends. Important dramatis personae of these stories then become "legendary" and remembered for some act or personal quality, as we shall see.

The author finds the fine distinction between legend and myth a confounding one, and in the present essay the two are used practically interchangeably. Historicity, which is the authenticity of a told history, is not a concern in mythology per se, though it does give rise to passionate polemics on the actuality of some tales, arguments abounding for and against. A case in point is the recent proclamation by a noteworthy leader of the country at an international science congress, that plastic surgery existed in this country eons ago, as exemplified by the implant of an animal head on a human torso, to restore a slain divine child to life. This led to an uproarious outrage from the vast majority of the scientific community, and a spirited defense by believers in the story of Ganesha.

This chapter focuses on mythology in the context of its relevance to the discipline of psychiatry and I plead the readers' indulgence for the slightly skewed emphasis on the mythology of India, particularly the puranas and the two great epics of the subcontinent.

CULTURES AND MYTHS

Myths exist wherever language does and these tales are passed on in oral or written fashion with great scope for embellishment, alteration, deletion and other forms of corruption or modification. There are certain parallels between mythical tales that are fascinating in the absence of any actual or known forms of transmission of the core content.

Thus, two legendary heroes, early in their life are set afloat in rivers, seas as neonates, fated to great futures as leaders: Karna the premarital offspring of Kunti, is a blemish on her virginity, and from a mixture of shame and compassion she disposes of her baby by safely setting him afloat in a basket, to later be rescued by strangers. He is to emerge as one of the principal warrior heroes of the Mahabharata. Moses, in the Judeo-Christian tradition, is rescued by a sleight of hand, from a campaign of infanticide of Hebrews by drowning them ordered by the Pharaoh of Egypt. He will later emerge as the rescuer of his race.

Another analogous occurrence is the story of matricide in two unrelated cultures. In the Greek tradition, Orestes murders his mother, Clytemnestra. This is on account of her having murdered his father Agamemnon with the help of her illicit lover. This avenging act of the son is after all the expected honorable path. In turn, this leads to some torturous consequences for the lad which will be resolved after a convoluted series of happenings. Similarly, in Indian puranas, there is the tale of Parashurama, son of sage Jamadagni and an avatar of Vishnu, who at his father's command slays his beloved mother Renuka, again for an act of infidelity. The pleased father offers his son a boon, and the son now asks that the mother be restored to life.

There are probably innumerable such parallels between mythologies of vastly distant cultures. Jung, who arguably was the most serious compiler, student and analyst of myths, certainly so among psychiatrists, gave us the concept of the collective unconscious of humans to understand the recurrence of such themes in different civilizations. He believed that ancient frameworks that were common across vastly separated populations existed in the minds of men and these he called archetypes.

Some recent researchers in the field of mythology have drawn parallels between phylogenetic evolution and the morphosis of myths over periods. Based on the study of myths from folklore across the world, a phylogenetic tree has been suggested to show the relatedness of myths. In India, most myths are related to the range of emotions, called the *Ashtarasa*, later modified into the *Navarasas*.

It is interesting also how narratives change in proximal cultures. In Persia, where *Zoroastrianism* was the universal religion, the supreme deity was the Ahura Mazda. Linguists believe *ahura* and *asura* are linked and good spirits in that country were the *Asuras*. In India, not geographically far from Persia, asuras are regarded as the evil ones, while suras are the virtuous and godly ones.

MYTHOLOGY AND THE MIND

Myths come about from observation as well as imagination. There can also be an admixture of the two, and quite possibly that is the most common root. In any case, characters and events from the narrative impress upon the thinking mind the presence or lack of differing qualities: virtue and vice. This serves as a template for the mind to work on especially in the vulnerable developing states but adults are not immune from such influences and can change the courses of their lives when converted by convincing tales of salvation or doom. The mind seems to need vindication of its motives, whether positive negative or mixed, and this is very often to be found in the text of various myths.

VIRTUE AND MYTHOLOGY

Western tradition speaks of four cardinal virtues: (1) prudence, (2) justice, (3) temperance, and (4) courage. After the arrival of the New Testament, the three additional Christian virtues became adjuncts: (1) faith, (2) hope, and (3) charity (love). Exemplars of each of these are many.

Prudence has itself been derived from the Goddess Prudentia, traditionally shown holding a mirror and a snake. The mirror signifies a proper perspective, the snake the need to tackle difficulties. Implicit in prudence are the subvirtues, so to say of wisdom, insight, and knowledge. Prudence is closely related to the next virtue, justice.

Justice, represented by Justitia, is the sense of fairness. The icon of the Goddess being blindfolded in order to avoid any chance of bias in arbitrating an issue brought before her, also holds a balance to weigh fairly what is presented, and a sword to signify punishment for the guilty.

Temperance (Temperantia) upholds modesty and humility, while strongly avoiding excesses of all kinds, particularly of sensual pleasures.

Fortitude or Courage is exemplified by most heroes who are fearless and unshaken in their resolve, unmitigated by threats and dangers. From the various Greek myths Jason, Samson, and Orestes are examples of such bravery, each faced with differing daunting tasks and moral dilemmas.

In Indian systems too, there are virtues listed. There are many scattered references to these. In the Manusamhita, uprighteous living calls for ten virtues: (1) dhriti (courage), (2) kshama (forgiveness), (3) dama (temperance), (4) asteya (noncovetousness), (5) shucha (purity), (6) indriyanigraha (overpowering the sensuous), (7) dhi (prudence), (8) vidya (wisdom), (9) satyam (truthfulness), and (10) akrodha (angerlessness). To this one may add vinaya (humility) and ahimsa (nonviolence). Myriad examples are to be found of these virtues in heroic figures of Indian mythology. It would suffice to give here the instance of Shri Rama, the eponymous hero of the Ramayana, who largely embodied all these good qualities and has therefore been called the *Maryada Purushottam* or ideal man.

VICE AND MYTHOLOGY

In Indian systems, there are six cardinal human failings. These are called the shadripu: (1) kama (lust), (2) krodha (anger), (3) lobha (greed), (4) mada (arrogance), (5) moha (attachment), and (6) matsarya (jealousy).

Kama and moha are well exemplified by King Shantanu, the grandsire of the principal families in the Mahabharata, who in his blind desire for the fisher princess Satyavati, makes his son Devavrata forego his rights as an heir. The Mahabharata is replete with examples of krodha that I cited in an article several years ago in the Indian Journal of Psychiatry. Mada is the undoing of King Hiranyakashipu in the Prahlada tale. Lobha and matsarya are the failings (among many other faults) of the Kaurava prince, Suyodhana (later called Duryodhana). He is morbidly jealous of his Pandava cousins for their skills, their wisdom, and also their wife Draupadi. He covets their kingdom and craftily plots to usurp it. Lobha is also evinced by the eternally hungry rakshasa, Bakasura, also in a story within the Mahabharata.

The vices in this Indian list correspond in some measure to the Western notion of the seven deadly sins: (1) lust, (2) gluttony, (3) greed, (4) sloth, (5) wrath, (6) envy, and (7) pride. Lust is the near fatal flaw in the English Arthurian legend, of Sir Lancelot for his King, Arthur's, wife. Gluttony and greed both speak of an excess of wanting, the former for consumables, the latter for covetable objects such as land and power. Wrath is the burning rage of the spirit Lyssa in Greek myths. Envy, in the Biblical story, is what caused the downfall of Cain who could not tolerate God's choosing the offering of his brother Abel, leading eventually to the former killing the latter in a cowardly manner. Extreme pride, also called hubris, is displayed by Lucifer, at one time a much favored angel of the Creator, and causes him to be condemned to hell.

Aergia, in Greek mythology is the demi-goddess guarding the entrance to the court of Hypnos, God of sleep. She is the model for sloth. The last one does not figure in the Indian list.

Most of these characters mentioned in relation to virtues and vices, in both the Indian and western systems are proverbial for embodying those qualities.

BLESSINGS AND BENEVOLENCE AND CURSES AND DAMNATION

Many mythological figures go through austerities and penance or some other acts of devotion to be blessed with unusual gifts. Thus, the egoistic asura, Hiranyakashipu, gains from Brahma the boon to never be killed by man or animal. He is eventually killed by Vishnu in the avatar of half-man half-lion (Narasimha).

In the Ramayana, Dasharatha unwittingly kills Shravana the devoted son of his parents, who upon his confession curse him to die lamenting for his own son. Forlorn at this fate, Dasharatha at least temporarily has respite for he has till now been dejected, having had no offspring from any of his three wives. The curse does mean that he will have a son. Thus is Shri Rama born with three other brothers, to the joy of the King, his queens and the populace; later by a turn of fate, Dasharatha has to face the fulfillment of the curse when his beloved son and heir apparent willfully goes into exile in the interest of his father's honor. The tale of Dasharatha with a curse that is a temporary blessing is most poignant as a paradigm for many life situations.

In a tale of within the Bhagavata, is the story of Shakuntala, the beautiful and clever daughter of sage Vishwamitra and the nymph Menaka, abandoned by the parents and brought up as a foundling by Kanva, a gentle sage himself. Shakuntala meets in the forest, where her foster father's ashram is, the handsome King Dushyant, who is besotted with her. But he has to return to his kingdom and by the time he does, she is carrying his child. Still lost in romantic mooning, Shakuntala fails to notice and answer a visiting sage. The latter, enraged curses her that the object of her preoccupation, i.e., the person on whom she was daydreaming would forget her. Twists and turns befall the girl, effectively retold by poet Kalidasa. It is interesting that many of the curses are followed by remorse of the cursed and the latter's pleas are usually met with some remedial measure.

In the Mahabharata, there are two tales of students gaining martial skills from teachers, unbeknown to the masters. Thus, Ekalavya, a skillful tribal archer seeks to refine his mastery at the feet of the guru, Dronacharya. The latter refuses as he would only impart his knowledge to princes. Ekalavya, builds an effigy of the master and starts practicing after paying obeisance to the figurine. Dronacharya chances upon this young man's superior abilities, and is impressed. Upon learning of the stratagem of the Ekalavya, he demands his fee; it is to be the archer's thumb, thus disabling him forever from archery. In another story, the Brahman warrior Parashurama, avowed foe of the Kshatriyas, is tricked into teaching his battle axe techniques to Karna who pretends to be a Brahman. On the discovery of the deceit, Karna is cursed by Parashurama to be rendered helpless when he most needs his divine armor. The curse plays out in the eventual battle between the Kauravas and Pandavas.

CONDITIONS AND SYNDROMES FROM MYTHOLOGY

A number of clinical conditions exist that in varying measure mimic the states or characters of mythology, across cultures.

Panic disorder came to be identified as a distinct variation, once subsumed in the anxiety neurosis, relatively recently. It is worth recalling that panic comes from the mischievous demigod Pan, of Greek lore, notorious for scaring away shepherdesses by startling them with the sound of his musical pipes.

Freud, fascinated and fixated by sexuality, coined the term *Oedipus complex*. He believed it to be a normal phase in the development of a boy (with of course the Electra equivalent for the female child), where there is erotic love for the parent of the opposite sex. The core was apparently derived from the story of monarch Oedipus, who ended up marrying his mother Jocasta. Most nonpsychoanalytically oriented psychiatrists do not agree with the claimed ubiquity of this phenomenon. But Freud also erred in naming it; the legendary Oedipus fell in love with a woman whom *he did not know* to be his mother.

The term *Electra complex* was actually first suggested by Freud's then acolyte, Carl Jung, as a daughter's competing with the mother for the father's attention and indulgence. Freud seems to have rejected this idea and called the condition in girls the female Oedipal attitude. He continued to believe that in normal development the boy resolved the complex through castration anxiety and the girl through penis envy. To this day most of the orthodox psychoanalysts feel these are valid concepts and claim to have found even the neuroanatomic substrates of these states.

Priapism is named for the Greek God Priapus, famed for his disproportionately large phallus on a short ugly body. In reality, priapism is a state of sustained erectile state that can be quite painful.

Narcissistic personality disorder is named after another Greek male, Narcissus, who had never seen how handsome he actually was. On seeing his reflection for the first time, he fell madly in love with that image, so much so, he could not bear to be away from it; he finally fell into the water body where he had seen his appearance, and died. Excessive self-love that interferes with normal functioning is the hallmark of this personality disorder.

Hermaphroditism is a name for a broad title for states where an individual has features, physically and/or psychologically, of both genders. It takes its name from the Greek figures of Hermes, a handsome God and Aphrodite, the Goddess of paramount beauty. In clinical practice, hermaphroditism is a complex set of conditions with very different causations.

Closer home, an eminent though self-effacing Indian psychiatrist, HS Narayanan, noted the similarities between the *Kleine–Levin syndrome* and the mythological figure of Kumbhakarna. Hypersomnolence and hyperphagia do occur in this condition and were said to be attributes of this brother of Ravana. Hypersexuality, however, has not been mentioned as a character of Kumbhakarna.

Pathological gambling could find an eponym in being called the *Yudhishthir syndrome*. This person, the eldest of the five Pandava brothers, in his preoccupation to win a game of dice gambled away all his belongings one by one, even losing their kingdom and the clothes on his back. Ultimately, he even put at stake their wife Draupadi who was humiliated publicly in the court of the wily Kauravas. In fact, Yudhishthir was trapped into this situation by Shakuni, the maternal uncle of the Kauravas, who knew the former's weakness for gambling and was working to aid his nephew Suyodhana who coveted the righteous Pandavas' kingdom and envied them (see above).

Trishanku avastha is a condition where an individual is in limbo between his goals and desires and his actual position in life, often for no fault of his. It is named after Satyavrata (later called Trishanku—three times sinner) son of King Prithu, an ancestor of Shri Rama, who could neither enter Heaven nor was allowed to return. One version has it that he was refused entry by the Devas because he had slaughtered a cow and eaten beef, another says that he had insisted on going in with his physical body. One way or the other, the sage who thought Heaven befitted Satyavrata for all his good deeds, (Vishwamitra or Kaushik in the differing versions) would not let him descend to Bhu Loka (the Earth), and so he remained, suspended between Heaven and Earth. One other version has it, that a separate Heaven was eventually constructed for Trishanku!

MYTHOLOGY AND THERAPY

There are stories in mythology that can have therapeutic value. One redoubtable doyen of Indian Psychiatry JS Neki has expanded at large on the *guru-chela paradigm* in psychotherapy in this country. NN Wig, another eminent psychiatrist has given an actual mythological example that he found useful in therapy. He christened it the *Hanuman complex.*

The anthropoid demigod Hanuman, unflinching devotee of Shri Rama had for some reason been cursed that he at crucial moments when he most needed his legendary physical strength, he would forget that he possessed it. In the Ramayana on such an occasion, he sat dejected over his inability that called for his prowess as he had become unaware of it. He had to be reminded of his power, and then stunningly rose to the occasion. This is a practical point in the therapeutic situations when a patient needs to be reminded to recall his/her own inner resources that diffidence has caused to have faded in memory.

Literature on cognitive therapy emphasizes Socratic thinking an important component of which is perseverance in questioning. In the Kathopanishad, we have the example of Nachiketa, driven to the death God Yama by his father in a fit of rage. Determined to understand the mystery of life death and the hereafter, Nachiketa asks these of Yama who has been pleased with Nachiketa. He offers him many other boons but Nachiketa will not be deterred from his quest and after dogged firmness he does get his answer.

Indian folklore is replete with other instances of therapeutic value. Thus, we have the swallowing of poison by the God Shiva in order that the Gods and good people be saved by the treasures that emerge from the churning of the ocean, for the poison precedes those treasures and must be done away with. A metaphor for taking, I believe the rough to have the smooth. We also have the unending series questions that Vetal, the vampire asks of the King Vikram.

MODERN MYTHOLOGY

Mythical stories, it is sometimes conjectured, have been over and done with. This is far from the truth. Every age has had its own fantasy stories and these abound even in this day and age. The immense popularity of the Harry Potter series is a case in point of the hold that fantastical tales, spells and potions, curses and eternal plotting have on the human mind. To name just one other example is the cult following that the recently deceased Terry Pratchett has among adolescents and mostly young adults.

There could be one important distinction between this mythology and that of the past: the new variety is almost purely fiction with little or no mixing of factual happenings. The importance of religious and spiritual content is also practically absent in modern mythology.

THE NEED FOR MYTHS: ETERNAL INDEED

The need to have mythology is probably an inbuilt one on man. Myths according to

Pattanaik, condition thoughts and feelings. "Mythology influences behavior and communication", he avers. "People outgrow myth and mythology when myth and mythology fail to respond to their cultural need."

In a lighter vein, the Anglo American poet, WH Auden asked:

> *By what myths would your priests account*
> *for the hurricanes that come*
> *twice every twenty-four hours,*
> *each time I dress or undress,*
> *when, clinging to keratin rafts,*
> *whole cities are swept away*
> *to perish in space, or the Flood*
> *that scalds to death when I bathe?*
>
> *Then, sooner or later, will dawn*
> *a Day of Apocalypse,*
> *when my mantle suddenly turns*
> *too cold, too rancid, for you,*
> *appetising to predators*
> *of a fiercer sort, and I*
> *am stripped of excuse and nimbus,*
> *a Past, subject to Judgement.*

Auden wrote this after being fascinated by an article in a popular science journal, which talked about the microbes inhabiting the human skin. Would microbes, or indeed higher life forms, ever have a mythology series of their own? One does not see the possibility of the complete disappearance of myth and mythology in the foreseeable future of the human race.

SUGGESTED READING

1. Jung CG. Selected Writings. Suffolk: Fontana; 1983.
2. Pattanaik D. Myth = Mithya: A Handbook of Hindu Mythology. New Delhi: Penguin; 2006.
3. Peck MS. Further Along the Road Less Traveled and Beyond: Mythology and Human Nature. New York: Touchstone; 1993.

CHAPTER 16

Interface with Philosophy

Pratap Sharan

INTRODUCTION

The Encyclopaedia Britannica defines philosophy (from Greek word, philosophia: love of wisdom) as the rational, abstract, and methodical consideration of reality as a whole or of fundamental dimensions of human existence and experience.[1]

Psychiatry has a close link with philosophy for long, however, philosophy of psychiatry has developed as a field of inquiry, with its specific set of questions and themes, only over the past few decades.

WHY PHILOSOPHY OF PSYCHIATRY?

There are several unresolved questions regarding psychiatry: To what extent does the practice of psychiatry fit within the medical paradigm? And how does psychiatry differentiate itself from other fields concerned with mental health, such as psychology and social work?

A major issue with mental disorders is that they cannot be defined in reference to an underlying pathology. The illness experience itself is the "disorder." The need for a biopsychosocial approach puts psychiatry at odds with the biomedical approach of medicine.

Another reason why psychiatry needs philosophy is that the discipline is faced with several tough ethical questions such as involuntary treatment, reduced criminal responsibility, and disability benefits.

PHILOSOPHY OF PSYCHIATRY

Philosophy of psychiatry is a branch of philosophy that helps make sense of issues related to the experience of mental disorder, its scientific research and clinical treatment, and associated social and political questions.[2] Some key domains of philosophy of psychiatry are:

- *Philosophy of mind and psychiatry* is concerned with questions related to the connection between the mind and the body, the self, and the experience of mental phenomena/disorders (phenomenology).
- *Philosophy of science and psychiatry* is concerned with questions about the nature of science, the nature of things like scientific theories and explanations as they pertain to the mental field, and how best to use the results of scientific investigation to effect changes in the world.
- *Ethics and psychiatry* deals with ethical issues related to how we should perceive and treat people who have been diagnosed with a mental disorder (e.g., disability benefits, stigma, and capacity).
- *Social and political philosophy and psychiatry* deals with issues related to the influence of medical, social, and political systems on the emergence and treatment of mental disorders; connections between oppression and mental health; the relationships among sexism, racism, and

other forms of bigotry and how they are supported by the institutional structures.

Social and political philosophy of psychiatry is also concerned about the nature of mental disorders (e.g., whether the experiences and problems associated with mental disorders should be seen as expressions of illness or reactions to personal problems/intolerable circumstances) and about how we should understand and support people who experience these differences (e.g., the antipsychiatry and neurodiversity movements).[2]

Philosophy of Mind and Psychiatry

It is crucial for psychiatry to have a viable understanding of the nature of mental states. Unlike physical states, mental states are meaningful (i.e., they refer to things and events outside of themselves) and they are associated with subjective consciousness.[3]

According to Cartesian dualism, a mind is a nonphysical substance that is distinct from a physical body (and may exist without it). Advances in biology, evolution, and psychiatry led to a rejection of mind–body dualism; however, the relationship between mind and body continues to be a matter of significant debate.[4]

The most prevalent viewpoint today is that mental states are brain states. One variant of this viewpoint is the "identity theory," which suggests that mental states are identical to brain states. Accordingly mental disorders are seen as brain disorders and assumed to be best understood through neuroscience and treated through biomedical procedures applied to the brain. However, this raises a question regarding exactly how does the brain form thoughts and experiences.[4]

The advocates of "functionalism" propose that mental states are best understood in terms of the informational functions (software) they perform, rather than the underlying mechanisms (hardware) that embody those functions in the brain.[5] This would suggest that mental disorders can be understood as problems with the cognitive processes embodied in the brain and could be treated through cognitive therapies (software patches) without necessarily changing the underlying mechanism (hardware). However, functionalism does not explain important features of mental states such as consciousness.[4]

Proponents of "property dualism" treat conscious mental states as nonphysical properties that may emerge from the brain but are not reducible to functional or physical processes in the brain.[6] Property dualism allows for dependency of conscious mental states upon the brain.

The biopsychosocial model suggests that the human mind is a complex phenomenon, amenable to a variety of explanatory frameworks.[4] Conscious thoughts and experiences provide a level of organization and analysis, situating the first-person perspective within the broader matrix of biological mechanisms, psychological functions, and social behaviors. It sees these levels of analysis not as competing accounts of mentality, but rather as integrated facets of a person as viewed by higher and lower levels of analysis.

Relevance of the Brain/Chemical Question to the Philosophy of Psychiatry

As science advances, we may be able to consistently associate psychiatric conditions with certain chemical and/or brain differences; however, crucial questions about what such associations "mean" would remain. The association of psychiatric conditions with chemical and brain differences does not necessarily mean that psychiatric conditions are bona fide illnesses or disorders, e.g., they could be nonpathological forms of neurodiversity. Such questions have important personal and political ramifications, e.g., conceptualization as ill versus divergent can alter a person's self-conception, impact social processes such as stigma, and state policies such as disability benefits. Almost all mental phenomena (including nonpathological) have some brain differences underlying them. Hence, brain differences should not be equated with pathology.

Phenomenology

Phenomenology concerns itself with the world as it presents itself to us.[7] Husserl suggested that it is possible to transcend presuppositions (common-sense notions, scientific explanations, other interpretations, or abstractions) and biases and to experience a state of prereflective consciousness, which allows us to describe phenomena as they present themselves to us. The phenomenological method involves three phases of contemplation: Epoché, phenomenological reduction, and imaginative variation. Epoché requires the suspension of presuppositions and interpretations to allow the perceiver to become fully aware of what is before it. Phenomenological reduction consists of describing the phenomenon that presents itself to us in its totality (physical as well as experiential features), i.e., the constituents of the experience of the phenomenon. Phenomenological reduction aims to set aside, or *bracket*, preconceived notions. Imaginative variation involves an attempt to access the structural (dimensions of time, space, or social relationships) components of the phenomenon. Imaginative variation attempts to identify the conditions associated with the phenomenon without which it would not be what it is. Finally, constituent and structural descriptions are integrated to arrive at an understanding of the essence of the phenomenon.

Intersubjectivity is an important question for phenomenology—the question if, and to what extent, we can experience the other and have epistemic access to their mind and mental states. There are two predominant approaches to intersubjectivity: Mentalistic (e.g., "theory of mind") and phenomenological.[8] Mentalist approaches assume that the other's mind is unreachable, so they emphasize the need to infer the other's mental states by observing their external behavior. Phenomenological approaches do not consider mental states as closed off but as prereflectively connected to other people and the environment. They emphasize the affective, embodied, and situated nature of interpersonal understanding.

Philosophy of Science and Psychiatry

Classification: Natural Kinds

A fundamental philosophical issue concerning psychiatric classification is the question of whether classificatory systems can classify "natural kinds."

In philosophy of science, natural kinds (e.g., NaCl, birds) are understood as classes or groupings that accurately correspond to the natural structure of the world, whereas artificial kinds (e.g., furniture, apps) are classes that reflect the interests and actions of humans. Natural kinds are thought to be naturally occurring (or real) classes that are the appropriate objects of scientific study, while artificial kinds are arbitrary classes that serve social functions, but do not have a natural basis. In science related to humans, some classifications (e.g., Hodgkin lymphoma, Down syndrome, and introversion) refer to natural kinds as these classes/dimensions can be defined with reference to a set of natural properties; other classifications (e.g., conservatives, homophilic/homophobic) are considered as artificial kinds as these classes/dimensions are defined exclusively by conventions (social properties).

Official classification systems before Diagnostic and Statistical Manual 3rd edition (DSM-III) classified mental disorders in a theoretical and etiological manner, e.g., they followed a fundamental classificatory distinction between biological and psychological causes. DSM-III and its successors purportedly took an atheoretical and descriptive approach with a focus on reliability. However, an underlying assumption of these classification systems is that mental illnesses are discrete biological diseases with clear boundaries between the normal and the sick. However, as illustrated in the need to develop the Research Domain Criteria (RDoC), there are serious doubts regarding whether officially recognized diagnostic categories map onto discrete mental disorders.

Murphy argues that purely descriptive systems of classification are incommensurate with the medical model.[9] While such models implicitly assume that mental disorders are distinct (disease) entities that reflect underlying causal differences, they prohibit reference to the causal processes and dysfunctions that distinguish them. Symptom-based approaches to classification fail to distinguish heterogeneous conditions since such categories group together different profiles as manifestations of the same disorder. He suggests that descriptive categories should be supplemented with causal information concerning the determinants of various symptoms to be consistent with the medical model.

Ian Hacking on the other hand feels that psychiatric categories cannot classify natural kinds because the objects of classification in psychiatry (and in human sciences) are inherently unstable because of the "looping effects" in contrast to the stable objects of classification in the natural sciences.[10] Looping effects are social feedback effects of classifications, wherein individuals who are classified change in response to how they are classified, e.g., individuals diagnosed with social anxiety disorder would act in accordance with the stereotypes associated with the label. Rachel Cooper argues that Hacking fails to establish that the objects classified in the human sciences are sufficiently different from the objects of classification in the natural sciences.[11] She accepts the existence of looping effects; however, she feels that the changes that looping effects produce for objects of human science classification are not of greater metaphysical significance than changes produced by other kinds of feedback effects on some objects of natural science classifications, e.g., bacterial mutations in response to antibiotics. Similarly, Tsou argues that the presence of looping effects does not render the objects of classification unstable. He feels that if psychiatric phenotypes can be associated with specific markers, the entity can be considered a natural kind that remains stable despite the looping effects of its classification.[12]

Moral Responsibilities of Psychiatric Researchers

A major question concerning philosophers of psychiatry is related to the extent to which psychiatric researchers have a moral responsibility to consider the nonepistemic (nonknowledge) consequences (e.g., harms) of their research.

Epistemic values aim to promote the attainment of truth. Intrinsic epistemic values directly promote the attainment of truth, e.g., empirical adequacy, predictive accuracy, and internal consistency. Extrinsic epistemic values promote the attainment of truth indirectly by enabling the realization of intrinsic epistemic values, e.g., generality and external consistency.[13] Nonepistemic values aim at the attainment of specific practical, moral, or social good, e.g., the minimization of harms, justice and equity, respect for autonomy, social utility, economic goods such as job creation or profit, and personal goods such as prestige or recognition. It is widely accepted that such values can play a legitimate role in pursuing the nonepistemic goals of psychiatry, such as deciding which research programs to fund, which research designs are ethically permissible, and how to apply research results to develop more efficacious treatments.[13] These goals are usually considered to be external to psychiatric research. However, there is disagreement as to whether and to what extent these sorts of values should play a role in decisions internal to psychiatric research, e.g., how to interpret research results or whether to accept or reject a hypothesis.

Research inevitably involves the possibility of error when accepting or rejecting hypotheses. Philosophers of science refer to this possibility of error as "inductive risk." Inductive risks can have nonepistemic consequences, e.g., classificatory revisions based on psychiatric research can lead to increase in false-positive or false-negative diagnoses. An increase in false-positive diagnoses risks "medicalizing" normal problems of living, while false-negative diagnoses can prolong individuals' suffering.

A (nonepistemic) value-free ideal of psychiatric research advocates for insulating psychiatric research from the influence of nonepistemic values (i.e., knowledge as a good in itself). A (nonepistemic) value-laden ideal of psychiatric research advocates for the inclusion of such values (e.g., potential harms should be factored in) while drawing inferences arising from research.

Allowing nonepistemic values to play a role in these internal stages of psychiatric research raises several concerns. The most notable of these concerns is the problem of "wishful thinking." If psychiatric researchers are expected to appeal to nonepistemic values when interpreting the results of their research, their conclusions would be more a reflection of their value judgments than the actual underlying structure of psychiatric conditions.[14] Philosophers also worry that allowing nonepistemic values during the internal stages of psychiatric research would impose the values of researchers on other stakeholders, even though researchers are not specifically trained in values. Supporters of the value-free ideal in research suggest that if one cannot make error-free decisions based solely upon epistemic values, then one should just wait for further evidence to accumulate.

Critics of value-free conception of psychiatry research argue that excluding nonepistemic values is either unattainable or undesirable. Those who adopt the former position either challenge the distinction between epistemic and nonepistemic values upon which the conception rests or contend that individuals are simply incapable of excluding nonepistemic values from their assessments of the adequacy of evidence.[15] Proponents of inclusion of nonepistemic values appeal to some version of the "underdetermination thesis" to justify their position. They state that researchers rarely have sufficient evidence to determine conclusively whether to accept or reject a hypothesis, so they can rarely rely solely upon epistemic values to minimize the risks associated with these possible errors. They contend that at least when the risks are significant, nonepistemic values should influence the standards of evidence required for accepting or rejecting hypotheses. They try to avoid the problem of "wishful thinking" by restricting the application of nonepistemic values. Steel suggests that nonepistemic values should not take precedence over epistemic values or directly determine whether scientists accept or reject a hypothesis, rather, nonepistemic values should only function to determine how much evidence is required before accepting or rejecting a hypothesis or the appropriate level of statistical significance.[13]

Critics of value-free conception of psychiatry research suggest that it is a moral responsibility of scientists to foresee and avoid the potential harms associated with psychiatric research. Adherents of the value-free ideal, on the other hand, suggest a minimalist approach to researchers' moral responsibilities. They insist on a sharp division between scientific research and public policy contexts, with nonepistemic values being reserved for the latter context.

Finally, it should be mentioned that if scientists were to disagree on research inferences based on espousal of different epistemic values, then it would be difficult to eliminate nonepistemic values from influencing research conclusions. Transparency on use of nonepistemic values during the decision-making process would be key to minimize its inappropriate use.

Causation

In general, there are two broad classes of philosophical views on causation. One set of accounts stresses the idea that causation is a matter of interdependence of events or variables (probabilistic account). The other set stresses the idea that causation is a matter of physical process or production.[16]

Although the idea that genuine causal relations are concrete local interactions seem intuitively appealing, a broad range of clear cases of causal interaction do not trade on such ideas, e.g., farmers' suicide. Also, omissions and absences can typically function as causes, but such things are "nowhere," as per definition, and hence conceptually ill-suited to figure in physical interactions.

Hence, the probabilistic account reflects better the causal reasoning employed in a variety of scientific disciplines. Currently, interventionist account (variant of probabilistic account) is gaining traction as a causal account in philosophy of psychiatry. According to interventionism, causal claims are claims about results of hypothetical interventions in specific scenarios ("If X had not occurred, Y would not have occurred," e.g., "If I hadn't taken a sip of this hot milk, I wouldn't have burned my tongue." Event Y is that I burned my tongue; cause X is that I had a hot coffee). However, interventionism leaves several objective causal processes outside of the analysis.[16]

There is a subtle connection between the two views (probabilistic vs. mechanistic)—scientists attempt to supplement the probabilistic causal account with a more mechanistic causal understanding. As discussed earlier, nonreductive physicalism is the dominant view in current philosophy of mind. The mental is perceived to be fully dependent on, yet distinct from the physical. "Nonreductive physicalism" posits that the mental is always physically realized (the physical basis of a particular mental state determines its occurrence entirely), but it can be multiply realized physically (each mental state could have had alternative physical mechanisms). In computing terms, it is akin to implementing the same software on different hardware.

Ethics and Psychiatry

Informed Consent

Informed consent is the autonomous, voluntary act of authorizing one's own medical treatment with awareness of one's illness, need for treatment, treatment options, and the risks and potential benefits of each, considering one's unique situation and personal values. It is an ongoing collaborative procedure between care providers and patients that maximizes patient self-determination and minimizes professional coercion and overreach.

Self-determination presupposes moral and epistemic agency. Agency is the ability to act on one's own behalf. Moral agency is the ability to act volitionally and deliberately as a member of a moral community (shared ethical values and principles). A moral community may be any group that tacitly or explicitly (e.g., code of ethics of professional organizations) creates rules to govern interpersonal behavior in a society. The ethics of informed consent establishes a moral community comprised of doctors and patients. Epistemic agency is the ability to be a full cognitive and intellectual participant in a community of knowers. A community of knowers has tacitly shared views on knowledge generation, what is considered knowledge, what constitutes expertise, and how to utilize knowledge in the decision-making.[17]

Informed consent requires treating patients as full moral agents capable of making their own life choices according to their own aims and values; and as full epistemic agents capable of acquiring, utilizing, and applying pertinent medical knowledge to serve their own aims. Toward the realization of these, doctors are expected to enable patients to participate in shared epistemic and moral communities by providing medical knowledge (in understandable form) necessary for patients to make their treatment decisions based on their overall interests and values.[17]

Coercion and Influence

The issue of constraint and coercion occurs in other areas of health (e.g., quarantine) but are more pressing in mental health, where involuntary treatment (hospitalization, restraint, medication) as well as more subtle forms of pressure and influence occur more frequently.

Some philosophers define coercion in terms of threat or pressure (intentional use of a credible threat to influence or control the actions of another person—by restricting choices), others in terms of enforcement. The latter emphasize the coercer's position of power or possession of the means for following through on threats.[18] While involuntary commitment is paradigmatic of coercion, there are ethical debates over what distinguishes coercion from other influences such as familial pressure.

Manipulation and persuasion are less controlling forms of influence that are often employed in mental health.[19] Manipulation covers deception, offers and inducements, the management of information, use of social and cultural norms, and interpersonal leverage. Rational persuasion is noncontrolling. Examples of manipulative influences include framing information (e.g., using clinical language rather than lay terms), incentives (e.g., making certain privileges contingent on specific behaviors), concrete threats (e.g., threatening hospitalization unless directives are followed), and deception (e.g., failing to inform patients of available options to ensure uptake of clinician's favored option). Examples of persuasion include *recommendations* (e.g., advising admission to start a new medication), and appeals to patients' *values and goals* (e.g., emphasizing compliance to take care of children).

The standard justification for use of controlling influences is that they are sometimes unavoidable in the best interest of the individual patient and/or the general public, e.g., treatment of psychiatric symptoms, may directly impact reasoning capacities and decrease the need for use of controlling influence. However, use of influence should be ethical and based on evaluation of capacity for autonomous choice, confidence in the efficacy of treatment, and the anticipated benefit to harm ratio.[18] The need to justify use of influence increases with the degree of restrictiveness (persuasion, manipulation, and coercion).

The use of psychiatric advanced directives could help in more consensual management. Efforts can also be made to reduce the use of restrictive measures by giving patients better information about their hospitalization/treatment (including its justification and duration); an increased focus on protecting patient rights; more family involvement; clearer lines of communication between the hospital and community; more meetings with service users; and better training of staff about interventions for aggressive behavior.[18]

Recently, the construct of perceived coercion (client's experience of treatment pressure) is gaining traction. More than three-fourth of patients hospitalized involuntarily and about one-fourth of those hospitalized voluntarily report the experience of perceived coercion. Importantly, perceived coercion is associated with avoidance of mental health services, lower patient satisfaction, and negative attitudes toward treatment.[18] Those reporting perceived coercion are often concerned about "procedural justice" (e.g., lack of participation in admission decision, implicit threat of involuntary admission).

Social and Political Philosophy

Neurodiversity Theory

In contrast to the earlier antipsychiatry movement, which challenged the validity of psychiatric diagnoses, neurodiversity advocates accept that diagnoses such as autism, learning disorders, attention deficit hyperactivity disorder, and schizophrenia can be useful ways of grouping underlying neurocognitive differences (psychiatric kinds); however, they feel that these kinds are not necessarily "disordered." They feel that these psychiatric kinds are minority modes of neurocognitive functioning that are disabled by a hegemonic "neuro-typical" society, which is averse to recognizing diversity.

Walker distinguishes between the neurodiversity paradigm and the pathology paradigm (current psychiatric and biomedical theory).[20] The latter seems to suggest that there is one "right," "normal," or "healthy" way for human brains and minds to be configured and to function. Individuals and groups who fall outside this dominant concept of normality (at a clinically significant level) are considered to have an "internal pathology." The neurodiversity paradigm posits neurodiversity to be a natural and valuable form of humanity. It suggests that there are more than one "right," "normal," or "healthy" type of brain or mind configuration and functioning. It is just that some will be more/less adaptive in different contexts, i.e., the context can make minority modes of being seem like they are inherently disabled. They suggest that dominant ideals of selfhood exclude (marginalize) and harm (pathologize) large numbers of people who fall outside them.[20]

The neurodiversity paradigm has challenged standard psychiatric thinking and practice, by showing how intertwined psychiatric theory is with broader normative and ideologically laden judgments.

Disciplinary Power and Biopower

Disciplinary power aims to create, disseminate, and reinforce social norms to control individuals, making them docile in relation to the extant power structure. Biopower aims to create the context for the exercise of social hygiene (controlling birth, life, and death of groups) through the classification of individuals into groups, of desirable and undesirable populations (e.g., forced sterilization of women with intellectual disabilities and mental disorders; the eugenic program of Nazi Germany). Psychiatry can aid the state in the exercise of both kinds of power through the creation of norms for behavior, correcting abnormal behavior, and reinforcing the boundaries of the normal.

In many ways, psychiatry is a social institution, not merely an academic/medical discipline. It is a social institution in the sense that it is embedded and intertwined with other social institutions (e.g., the legal system), and therefore contains and reinforces social assumptions and unavoidably carries bias (e.g., immigrants are more likely to be diagnosed with psychosis, or gender-based minorities are considered to have mental disorders).

Psychiatry has also been employed to identify and manage populations which are characterized as potential dangers to society by virtue of committing crime without apparent motive (psychiatrization of criminal danger—criminality indicating a derangement with no other symptom than the crime itself). Such crimes prompted the need for a criminal psychology that could treat social danger, characterized as danger for oneself, others, and one's descendants through heredity.[21] This has led to the growth of predictive policing with criminologists and criminal psychologists developing criteria used to predict danger.

CONCLUSION

In essence, philosophy is an effort to think clearly. The need for clear thinking in psychiatry arises because the subject deals with problems of meaning alongside empirical difficulties. Philosophy can help provide a more complete picture of the full meanings of the complex concepts by which we make sense of mental phenomena and the world around us. As an open and collegial discipline, it also supports methodological pluralism, and intellectual and cultural diversity.

At a more practical level, philosophy, by linking values with evidence (values-based practice) can help us in using science in a more patient-centered way.[22] Philosophical explication can also assist with multidisciplinary teamwork as different professional disciplines often work with very different implicit models of mental health and disorders.

REFERENCES

1. Encyclopaedia Britannica. Philosophy. [online] Available from https://www.britannica.com/topic/philosophy. [Last accessed June, 2022].
2. Tekin S, Bluhm R. Introduction to philosophy of psychiatry. In: Tekin S, Bluhm R (Eds). The Bloomsbury Companion to Philosophy of Psychiatry. London: Bloomsbury Academic; 2019. pp. 3-17.
3. Pernu TK. The five marks of the mental. Frontiers Psychol. 2017;8:1084.
4. Butler J. Understanding the nature of mental states: psychiatry, the mind-body problem, and the biopsychosocial model of medicine. In: Tekin S, Bluhm R (Eds). The Bloomsbury Companion to Philosophy of Psychiatry. London: Bloomsbury Academic; 2019. pp. 41-58.
5. Levin J. Functionalism. In: Zalta EN (Ed). The Stanford Encyclopaedia of Philosophy; 2016. [online] Available from https://plato.stanford.edu/archives/win2016/entries/functionalism. [Last accessed June, 2022].
6. Chalmers DJ. The Conscious Mind: In Search of a Fundamental Theory. New York: Oxford University Press; 1996.
7. Willig C. Introducing Qualitative Research in Psychology, 3rd edition. Berkshire (UK): Open University Press; 2019. pp. 250-97.
8. Hutto DD. Interpersonal relating. In: Fulford KWM, Davies M, Gipps R, Graham G, Sadler J, Stanghellini G, Thornton T (Eds). The Oxford Handbook of Philosophy and Psychiatry. Oxford: Oxford University Press; 2013. pp. 240-57.

9. Murphy D. Psychiatry in the Scientific Image. Cambridge, MA: MIT Press; 2006.
10. Hacking I. Kinds of people: moving targets. Proc Brit Acad. 2007;151:285-318.
11. Cooper R. Why Hacking is wrong about human kinds. Brit J Philos Sci. 2004;55:73-85.
12. Tsou JY. DSM-5 and psychiatry's second revolution: descriptive vs. theoretical approaches to psychiatric classification. In: Demazeux S, Singy P (Eds). The DSM-5 in Perspective: Philosophical Reflections on the Psychiatric Babel. Dordrecht: Springer; 2015. pp. 43-62.
13. Steel D. Epistemic values and the argument from inductive risk. Philos Sci. 2010;77:14-34.
14. Ghaemi N. Taking disease seriously: beyond "pragmatic" nosology. In: Kendler K, Parnas J (Eds). Philosophical Issues in Psychiatry II: Nosology. Oxford: Oxford University Press; 2013. p. 42.
15. Colombo M, Bucher L, Inbar Y. Explanatory judgment, moral offense and value-free science. Rev Philos Psychol. 2016;7:743-63.
16. Pernu TK. Causal explanation in psychiatry. In: Tekin S, Bluhm R (Eds). The Bloomsbury Companion to Philosophy of Psychiatry. London: Bloomsbury Academic; 2019. pp. 217-36.
17. Pouncey C, Merz JF. Informed consent in psychiatry: philosophical and legal issues. In: Tekin S, Bluhm R (Eds). The Bloomsbury Companion to Philosophy of Psychiatry. London: Bloomsbury Academic; 2019. pp. 257-82.
18. Cratsley K. The ethics of coercion and other forms of influence. In: Tekin S, Bluhm R (Eds). The Bloomsbury Companion to Philosophy of Psychiatry. London: Bloomsbury Academic; 2019. pp. 283-304.
19. Faden RR, Beauchamp TL. A History and Theory of Informed Consent. Oxford: Oxford University Press; 1986.
20. Walker N. Throw Away the Master's Tools: Liberating Ourselves from the Pathology Paradigm, Neurocosmopolitanism 2013. [online] Available from http://neurocosmopolitanism.com/throw-away-the-masters-tools-liberating-ourselves-from-the-pathologyparadigm/. [Last accessed June, 2022].
21. Foucault M. The dangerous individual. In: Politics, Philosophy, Culture: Interviews and Other Writings, 1977-1984. New York: Routledge; 2013.
22. Fulford KWM, Stanghellini G, Broome M. What can philosophy to for psychiatry? World Psychiatry. 2004;3:130-5.

CHAPTER 17

Interface with Religion

Sandeep Grover, Devakshi Dua

INTRODUCTION

Religion is part and parcel of the life of most human beings. Many people, including those with mental problems, find religion to be very important in their lives. Across the world, the majority of the people follow one or another religion, with some people following more than one religion. According to one estimate, about 4,000 religions are being observed across the globe.[1] A study that evaluated the religious affiliation of people by self-identification across the 230 countries and territories estimated that about 84% of the human beings on the earth identify themselves with a religion, with Christianity (33%) being the most commonly followed religion, followed by Islam (24%) and Hinduism (15%), Buddhism (7%), and Judaism.[2] Because a majority of the people across the globe identify themselves with one or more religions, it can be said that religion plays an essential role in the life of many human beings.

Since ancient times, there has been a link between religion and mental disease. Most mental diseases were considered to be caused by witchcraft or demonic possession in medieval times. These thoughts were not based on any systematic research. However, these beliefs have dominated until now and influence various aspects of mental illnesses. In the more contemporary research, the association of mental illnesses with religion/religiosity has been understood as the influence of religion/religiosity on symptoms of mental illness (i.e., symptoms with religious content, suicidality, substance use, etc.), help-seeking, pathways to care, medication adherence, treatment adherence, treatment response, psychosocial adaptation, relapse rates, recovery, social integration, and quality of life, etc. This chapter discusses the basic understanding of religion/religiosity and its association with mental illnesses [especially schizophrenia, bipolar disorder (BD), depression, obsessive-compulsive disorder (OCD), and suicidal behavior].

DEFINITION

According to one of the definitions, religion is defined as *"an organized system of beliefs, practices, rituals, and symbols designed to facilitate closeness to the sacred or transcendent."*[3] It is understood as an expression that involves affiliations, beliefs, practices, and rituals.[3,4] Religions usually have specific thoughts about life after death and rules about conduct that guide life within a social group.[3] It is frequently practiced in a group setting, but it can also be done alone and privately. Religiousness, orthodoxy, faith, belief, piousness, dedication, and holiness are all synonyms for religiosity.[5] These synonyms reflect what religious studies would call characteristics of religiosity rather than concepts that are synonymous with religiosity.[3]

DIMENSIONS OF RELIGION/ RELIGIOSITY

Various authors have tried to understand multiple dimensions and constructs of religion/religiosity. The most commonly described concepts of dimensions of religion/religiosity include those by Glock,[6] Allport and Ross,[7] and Huber.[8]

Glock (1965)[6] identified five fundamental elements of religion: Intellectual, ideological, public, private, and experiential. The intellectual dimension is related to the social expectation that religious people have some knowledge of religion and views on transcendence, religion, and religiosity. It is a general indicator of the frequency of thinking about religious issues. Religious ideology is the social expectation that religious people believe in the presence and substance of a transcendent reality, as well as the relationship between transcendence and humanity.[6] It is about the fundamental views of religions. Public practice means the frequency of public participation in religious rituals and communal activities such as going to a temple for Hindus, Church attendance, and Friday prayer for Muslims.[3,7] Private practices mean devoting oneself to the transcendent in personal space's individualized activities and rituals. It includes meditation and prayer and the dialogical and participative pattern of spirituality. Religious experiences are the experiences in which the religious individuals have "some kind of direct contact with an ultimate reality," which affects them emotionally.

In summary, the intellectual and ideological dimensions refer to thoughts, public and private practice measurements refer to the action, and the experiential dimension relates to experience, emotion, and perception. These dimensions can represent a person's religiosity from the sociological and psychological perspectives. All the five dimensions are considered autonomous.[7]

Extrinsic and intrinsic elements of religiosity were established by Allport and Michael.[8] *They defined extrinsic religiosity as a self-serving and pragmatic approach to religion that gives believers assurance of salvation. These people are prone to using religion for prestige, sociability, and self-justification, and they frequently tailor a religion to suit their needs. A person with intrinsic religiosity internalizes their faith's entire ideology and goes beyond just going to church, temple, or mosque.* Religion serves as a primary motivator for some people.

Their other needs are brought into harmony with their religious beliefs: *"The extrinsically motivated person uses thier religion, whereas the intrinsically motivated person lives thier religion."*[8] Huber and Huber (2012) gave the concept of personal religious construct system that suggests the blending of psychological entity with the core dimensions. This is described as the personality superstructure, which includes all personal structures relating to the personally defined world of religion and religiosity. When a person anticipates something having religious significance, a distinctive religious construct is activated.[7]

RELIGIOSITY VERSUS SPIRITUALITY

Spirituality is a multifaceted notion that resists easy categorization.[9-11] Various definitions have been used, such as *"subjective experience of the sacred."*[12] The essential element of spirituality is connectedness. Accordingly, spirituality is defined as the pursuit of an experience of self-connection, connection with others, connection with nature, and connection with the transcendent. Connectedness with the transcendence refers to something or someone that exists beyond the human realm, such as the universe, transcendent reality, a higher power, or God.[13]

There are specific fundamental differences between religiosity and spirituality. Individualistic, open-ended, liberating, and subjective quests are frequently referred to as spirituality. On the other hand, religion is described as gradually narrowing in scope, embodying the doctrinal, institutional, liturgical, and authoritarian characteristics of a particular beliefs.[14]

RELIGIOUS PRACTICES IN PATIENTS WITH MENTAL ILLNESSES

Schizophrenia

Available evidence suggests that having a mental illness does not stop people from practicing their religion. It has been shown that a majority of schizophrenia patients participate in private (91%) and public (68%) religious services or activities.[15] Some data suggest that compared to the general population, patients with schizophrenia have higher religious involvement[16] but lower religious attendance.[17]

Religion and Psychopathology

This has been one of the significant areas of research in patients with various mental disorders. An important focus has been schizophrenia. Available data suggest that many patients with schizophrenia present with delusions and hallucinations of religious nature, which can be further understood as those with religious and supernatural themes.[18,19] However, both of these are loosely understood as psychopathology with religious themes. Religious hallucinations and delusions allude to organized religious themes (e.g., prayer, sin, and possession) or religious personalities (e.g., God, Jesus, devil, and prophet). The supernatural psychopathological manifestations, on the other hand, have more universal mystic connotations (e.g., black magic, spirits, demons, being bewitched, mythical forces, ghosts, sorcery, and voodoo).[20] The prevalence of religious psychopathology in patients with schizophrenia has a wide variation, with prevalence rates of 6–63.3%,[20-24] influenced mainly by the study of methodology and the country. Comparative studies suggest that the prevalence of religious psychopathology varies from one country to another. One study suggests that religious delusions are more common in Germany than in Japan.[20] In terms of themes of delusions with religious content, the common themes include that persecution (by malevolent spiritual entities), influence (being controlled by spiritual entities), and self-significance (delusions of sin/guilt or grandiose delusions).[25,26] Religious delusions are linked to higher levels of grandiosity, passive experiences, internal evidence for their delusions (anomalous experiences or emotional states), and readiness to accept alternatives to their delusions, according to the data.[26,27]

In terms of various parameters of delusion, there is data to suggest that compared to delusions without religious content, delusions with religious content are held with more conviction and pervasiveness.[18] In terms of the association of religious delusions with the religion and religious support of the patient, available data suggest that there is no significant difference between those with and without religious delusions in terms of value given to the religion between the two groups, but patients with religious delusions report receiving lower support from their religious communities.[24,25]

Limited research has focused on the association of type of religion and religious delusions. This evidence suggests that patients who believe in Christianity have more religious delusions, especially delusions of guilt and sin, than those belonging to Islam.[22]

On the other hand, compared to patients of a Buddhism background, patients who believe in Christianity have been shown to have a lower frequency of religious-themed delusions.[28] In terms of different subgroups in the same religion, some studies suggest that Catholics experience lower religious delusions when compared to the Protestants and those without religious affiliations.[29] Other studies indicate that patients with schizophrenia with Roman Catholic affiliations have a higher prevalence of delusions of guilt with religious content than Protestants and Muslims.[26,27] Studies focused on patients with schizophrenia belonging to different cultural backgrounds suggest that the persecutors are more often supernatural beings among Christians than Muslims and Buddhists.[26,27] Studies from Asia that have compared patients belonging to different ethnic groups suggest that delusions with religious and supernatural themes are more prevalent in patients of Korean origin when compared to patients who are of Korean–Chinese or Chinese origin.[28]

According to studies examining the relationship between hallucinations and various religions and religious practices, patients who observe Judaism report having more hallucinations at night, which is linked to the idea that they are more sensitive to bad spirits and demons at night.[29] According to cross-cultural research, religion-based auditory hallucinations are more common in patients from the United Kingdom than in Saudi Arabia.[30]

In terms of the association between religiosity and the incidence of religious delusions and hallucinations, the evidence is mixed, with some research suggesting that persons with higher religiosity had a higher prevalence of religious delusions and hallucinations.[31] Others claimed there was no connection between the two.[23]

Relationship of Religion and Other Clinical Aspects in Patients of Schizophrenia

In patients with schizophrenia, religion/religiousness is associated with enhanced social integration and a lower incidence of suicide attempts,[32,33] a lower risk of substance abuse,[32,33] a lower rate of smoking,[34] and a better quality of life,[17,35,36] lower level of functioning,[31] and better prognoses.[37] Findings on the association between religion and psychosocial adaptation are mixed. Some research indicates more excellent psychosocial adaptation,[38] and others indicate poor social and psychological status in most schizophrenia patients.[16] Spirituality and religious support have also been linked to improved recovery[39-41] and a lower relapse rate.[42,43] However, in some studies, stronger religiosity has been associated with a higher risk of suicide attempts in some patients.[32]

Religious Coping

Religious coping is operationally defined as *"the use of religious beliefs or behaviors to facilitate problem-solving to prevent or alleviate the negative emotional consequences of stressful life circumstances."*[44] Available data suggest that higher use of religious coping in patients with schizophrenia is associated with better psychological and existential well-being.[45] It has also been shown that benevolent religious reappraisal is associated with better well-being, better adjustment, and less personal loss from mental illness, whereas punishing God reappraisal and reappraisal of God's powers are associated with lower well-being and adjustment, as well as more significant personal loss from mental illness.[46] The use of positive religious coping has also been shown to influence the psychological health domain of quality of life.[15] In contrast, higher use of negative religious coping has also been associated with poorer quality of life[15] and a higher level of distress.[47]

Longitudinal studies of schizophrenia patients have found that increased religious salience and good religious coping predict fewer negative symptoms, a better quality of life, and a better clinical global impression score.[41] Spiritual activity is linked to improved social functioning and the management of negative symptoms.[48]

Few studies have looked at the frequency of use of various types of religious coping that individuals with persistent mental diseases such as schizophrenia use and how they help them cope with stressful situations.[25,49,50] According to studies, up to 80% of patients use religious coping to cope with their illness.[51] Others have claimed that spirituality and religion helped 45% of patients manage with the condition.[25] Studies comparing patients with different diagnosis suggest that patients with schizophrenia, BD, and schizoaffective disorder use religious coping for a significantly longer period of time than those diagnosed with depressive disorders, and they perceive religious coping to be significantly more helpful than those diagnosed with depression.[52]

Religion and Explanatory Models of Patients with Schizophrenia

It is well known that a significant proportion of schizophrenia patients hold nonmedical explanations for their illness, with supernatural causes being the most common etiological models.[53-57] These supernatural causations include possession by witches or demons, esoteric, spiritual and mystical factors, supernatural forces, sorcery, ghosts/evil spirit, spirit intrusion, divine wrath, planetary/astrological influences, dissatisfied or evil spirits, and bad deeds of the past.[53-57] The supernatural causations are held by 66–70% of the patients from India.[55] In contrast, studies from other parts of the world have reported the presence of supernatural explanatory models in about 10% of schizophrenia patients.[57] According to a cross-cultural study involving Arab-Islamic, Jordanian, and German patients, Jordanian patients believe in esoteric elements behind their sickness and view it as more dangerous.[58]

Nonmedical explanatory frameworks, according to studies, influence insight,[59] help-seeking,[57,59] and are linked to poor outcomes.[54]

Religion and Quality of Life

A few studies suggest that spirituality and religiosity have an important influence on the overall quality of life and coping of schizophrenia patients.[60,61]

Religion and Help-seeking

Religious delusions influence help-seeking, treatment, and outcome. Patients with religious delusions take longer to establish service contact,[62,63] receive more medication, have more severe illness, and have poorer functioning.[62] Those with religious delusion/hallucination are more likely to receive magico-religious healing, are not satisfied with the psychiatric treatment,[31] and are more likely not to adhere to psychiatric treatment.[63] Evidence suggests that those with religious delusions have a poor outcome.[64-66] According to studies from India, many patients seek the help of religious healers to alleviate sickness symptoms,[67] and indigenous healing approaches are regarded supplementary to medical care of mental illness.[59] According to a survey of psychiatric patients at a hospital in Tamil Nadu, South India, 58% of psychotic patients saw a religious healer before seeking psychiatric help.[68] Due to cultural explanations for the condition, several research suggest that seeking religious care for mental disorders is often a first step in managing mental disorders.[68] Spiritual suffering has been reported in patients with schizophrenia hospitalized for long periods of time in other countries.[69] Studies that have specifically evaluated religiosity suggest that higher religiosity is associated with a lower preference for psychiatric treatment.[31]

Relationship of Religion and Treatment Adherence

Different studies have mixed findings concerning the association of various aspects of religion with treatment adherence. Some research imply that religion/religiousness is related with greater treatment adherence in patients with schizophrenia,[32,43,70] whereas others suggest that religion is associated with poor treatment adherence.[31,34]

Acceptance of Religious Assistance during Treatment

Available data suggest that the majority (85%) of the patients with mental illnesses request religious assistance.[19]

Bipolar Disorder

Religion and Psychopathology

As in patients with schizophrenia, patients with BDs also have religious delusions and hallucinations, and these may include believing one to be God, hearing messages from God, or having a divine mission.[71,72] Studies that have evaluated the prevalence of delusions with a religious content within manic episodes have estimated these at 15–33% in the USA[18,73] and 38% in India.[74] Some studies suggest that compared to patients with schizophrenia and complex-partial seizures, patients with BD have a higher frequency of hyper-religiosity. The most common theme of delusions was possession.[75] Other studies have also supported the lack of difference in the prevalence of religious delusions between patients with BD and schizophrenia.[76]

Religious Beliefs and Practices

A study from the USA evaluated the beliefs of patients with BD and reported that all patients with BD reported having faith in God. Additionally, about two-thirds of the patients endorsed views related to the devil (64%), Bible miracles (91%), afterlife (73%), and that Bible referred to daily events (82%).[77] Available data also suggest that a significant proportion of patients with BD have strong religious beliefs (78%) and frequently engage in religious practices.[78] Occasional studies that have evaluated the association of religious involvement (public, private, or subjective) and the clinical state (euthymia, mania, mixed, or depression) suggest that patients in a mixed state more often indulge in prayer/meditation. In contrast, those who are euthymic less often indulge in prayer/meditation.[79] A study from India compared patients with severe mental illnesses (SMIs) (i.e., schizophrenia, BD, and depression) and healthy controls and reported significantly lower participation in organized religious activities among persons with SMI when compared to healthy controls.[80] However, patients with SMI did not differ from healthy controls regarding nonorganized religious activities and intrinsic religiosity.[80] In terms of coping, this study also revealed that compared to healthy controls, patients with SMIs more often use negative religious coping, with no significant difference between the patients of various SMIs.[80] A study from India reported that >90% of patients with BD reported belief in God, and about 70% report that their treating psychiatrist did not pose questions to understand their religiosity.[74]

Etiological model: One of the studies from India reported that about half (45.4%) of the patients with BD attribute their illness to a supernatural/religious cause. In terms of specific reasons, the most common supernatural and religious causes included planetary influences (13.5%) and God's will (30.8%).[74] Studies from other parts of the world suggest that majority of the patients endorse mixed medical and religious explanatory models for their illness.[81]

Religious Coping

A significant proportion (79%) of the patients with BD also report using religious coping in dealing with the illness. This profile of patients with BD does not differ from other disorders such as schizophrenia.[52] Some studies suggest that religious coping mechanisms are the most common adaptive problem-solving methods used by patients with BD.[82] A study from India showed that compared to healthy controls patients with SMIs (i.e., schizophrenia, BD, and depression) more often use negative religious coping, with no significant difference between the patients of various SMIs.[80] Some data from longitudinal studies suggest that higher use of positive religious coping in the baseline is associated with better quality of life after 2 years of follow-up.

In contrast, higher use of negative religious coping at the baseline is associated with the worst quality of life in the environmental domain at a 2-year follow-up. On the other hand, higher intrinsic religiosity at the baseline is associated with better quality of life in the environmental domain at the follow-up. In contrast, higher use of negative religious coping at the baseline is associated with a higher chance of developing manic symptoms at the follow-up assessment.[83] Higher use of positive religious coping has also been shown to be positively associated with the opinion about the experiences during the episodes to be religious and pathological.[84,85]

Pathways to Care

Some studies that have evaluated help-seeking suggest that most (86.7%) of the patients with BD seek faith-healing treatment in their lifetime.[86] In another study, authors reported that about half (44.3%) of the BD patients had first treatment contact with religious/supernatural treatment providers.[74] Another study from Delhi reported that about one-third (32.8%) were the first treatment contact.[87]

Medication Adherence

In terms of the impact of religious belief on medication adherence, some data suggest that higher medication adherence is associated with weaker religious beliefs.[78] Some data indicate that a small proportion (19%) of patients report conflicting information received from the healthcare professionals and the spiritual advisors, especially regarding the intake of medications.[78]

Suicidality

A qualitative study assessed the association of suicide attempts with religiosity and reported that higher nonorganized religious activity and intrinsic religiosity were associated with a lack of history of suicide attempt(s).[88] Other studies have also reported the protective effect of moral objection to suicide.[89]

Religious Practices and Their Impact on Treatment

Some studies have evaluated the effects of fasting during Ramadan among patients with BD. One of the studies reported a lack of the impact of fasting on serum lithium levels and relapse rates.[90] Another study suggested that compared to those who did not fast, patients who fasted had nearly twice the relapse rate even after controlling for lithium level, sleep, and coffee consumption.[91]

Depression

Some of the studies have evaluated the relationship of depression with religiosity.

Compared to BD, a large amount of data is available to understand the various aspects of religiosity and depression. A systematic review of prospective studies suggests that there has been an increase in the interest in this area, with nearly half of the published studies appearing after 2010.[92]

Impact of Religiosity on the Incidence of Depression

The systematic review of prospective studies suggests that about 60% of the studies report a lack of effects of religious attendance on the incidence of depression, whereas 40% of the follow-up studies indicate that higher religious attendance is associated with lower incidence of depression.[93] Other religious parameters such as positive religious coping, private religious practices, and religious denomination are less likely to predict a lower incidence of depression over time. However, the "Composite" religious variables (combining measures of religious attendance, motivation, and contents of beliefs) are more likely to predict a lower incidence of depression over time. On the other hand, a significant number of studies (59%) suggest that religious struggle is associated with an increased incidence of depression.[93] Another review of the literature suggests that religious beliefs and practices may help people cope better with stressful life circumstances, give meaning and hope, and provide social support. At the same time, it is also suggested that religious beliefs can increase guilt.[92]

Religiosity and Clinical Characteristics

A meta-analysis of the data suggests that higher religiousness is associated with 1% lower depressive symptoms.[94] A study involving adolescents showed that many of the characteristics of religion are related to the severity of depression.[95] Even after controlling for characteristics including social support and substance misuse, forgiveness, negative religious support, and loss of faith, poor religious coping were found to have a significant relationship with depression severity.[95] Even after controlling for severity of depression at baseline, longitudinal studies reveal that loss of faith in God predicts a poorer improvement in depression scores over 6 months.[95]

Explanatory models: A study from India evaluated the explanatory models of patients with depression and reported that the Karma-deed-heredity category (77.4%) was the most common explanatory model, followed by psychological explanations (62.2%), weakness (50%), and social causes (40.2%). In terms of specific models, the most commonly reported explanations included the will of God (51.2%), followed by fate/chance (40.9%), weakness of nerves (37.8%), general weakness (34.7%), bad deeds (26.2%), the evil eye (24.4%) and family problems (21.9%).[96]

Religious coping: Data also suggest that the frequency of religious coping in patients with recurrent depressive disorders does not differ from that of patients with schizophrenia and BD.[80]

Impact of Religiosity on Treatment Outcome

A literature review suggests that higher religiosity is associated with faster remission from depression. Data also suggest that religious and spiritual interventions are associated with reducing depressive symptoms.[93]

Suicidal Behavior

Studies in patients of depression that have evaluated religiosity and spirituality about depression have done so in the form of religious affiliations,[97,98] religious participation[99] in the form of attending religious places, spiritual practices in the form of beliefs, mediation, and religious coping.[97,100] Available data suggest that suicide and suicidal behavior are negatively associated with higher religious attendance, religious worship, and having religious affiliation.[101,102] Studies that have compared suicide attempters and nonattempts suggest that nonattempters have a greater fear of social disapproval and more significant moral objections to suicide.[89,99,100,103]

Suicidal ideation severity is also found to be adversely correlated with moral objections to suicide and religious beliefs.[104] Moral objections were a significant reason for patients attempting low-lethality suicide to live, according to studies focusing on the lethality of the attempt. In terms of religious coping, data suggests that religious coping and a relationship with God helped to prevent suicide in both the general and clinical populations (including those with depression).[105] Religion, on the other hand, may have negative consequences by instilling shame and anxiety, which can lower life satisfaction.[106] Religious patients had a higher rate of psychiatric problems and suicide attempts, contradicting the popular belief that religion is always protective.[102] Studies from India suggest that suicidal ideations are more common in Hindus (compared with Christian or Muslim religions).[107] Further, studies from India involving patients with depression suggest that high religiosity is associated with lower suicidal intent and fewer attempts than those with low religiosity.[108]

Obsessive-Compulsive Disorder

The role of religiosity and other religious parameters have also been studied in patients with OCD. The original meaning of the word obsession is "actuation by the devil or an evil spirit from without," suggesting that it was initially believed to originate from one's religious life.[109] The importance of religion in the manifestation of OCD can be understood from the term "religious OCD" used to describe religious obsessions. This is also understood as scrupulosity, in which the clinical picture is dominated by religious or moral fears and includes fears that God is unreasonable and punitive.[110]

Impact on Prevalence and Occurrence of OCD

There is some data to suggest that a higher frequency of religious service attendance is associated with a lower prevalence of OCD, and in terms of specific religious affiliations, Catholic (compared to Baptists) association is associated with higher prevalence of OCD.[111] Available data also suggest that scrupulosity is moderately associated with religiosity, with highly religious persons scoring high for fear of sin and fear of God.[112] In terms of orthodoxy, studies suggest that ultra-orthodox persons have three times more religious OC symptoms than nonreligious symptoms.[113,114] Religiosity has also been linked with higher rates of obsessive personality traits.[115,116] However, some studies contradict the association of occurrence with religiosity,[117] especially the religious attitude.[118,119]

Clinical Manifestations

Available data suggest that religious matters are more common in the obsessive content in people from Egypt, India, Israel, and Turkey, which is in contrast to the higher prevalence of obsessions with aggressive themes in persons from the USA and Brazil.[109] The prevalence of religious obsessions across different studies varies from 5 to 60%, with figures in the lower range from countries such as England (5%), Singapore (7%), India (11%), and those from countries such as Egypt (60%), Saudi Arabia and Israel (50%) and Bahrain (40%) reporting toward higher range.[120] Some literature suggests that higher religiosity is associated with higher severity of obsessions and checking behavior and indicates that religiosity also significantly influences the thought-action fusion in the morality domain.[119] However, other studies do not support these findings.[120]

Explanatory Models

A study from India suggests that about half of the patients (57.3%) with OCD attribute their illness to supernatural causes.[121]

First Treatment Contact

A study from India reported that about 18% have faith healers as their first treatment contact for OCD, and those who believed in supernatural causations more often did so.[122]

Interventions

The importance of religion in the management of OCD can be understood from the perspective that many authors have incorporated religious principles in the management of OCD, and some have described the role of religious cognitive-behavior therapy (RCBT) in the management of OCD.[122] A literature review explicitly focusing on the Islamic population concluded that OCD patients who are religious and receive religious psychotherapy show more rapid improvement in symptoms and require a lower dosage of medications for a lesser duration.[123]

Suicidal Behavior

Religiosity is believed to have some protective role in suicide.[106] Contemporary research shows that suicide rates are lower in religious countries than secular ones.[124] Suicidal gestures/suicidal attempts/suicidal ideations are inversely connected to religious commitment, religious affiliations,[3,125] and strong moral objections.[3,125] It is also believed that religious commitment/ participation is linked to less aggressive behavior,[3] impulsivity,[102,103,126] better social ties,[3,125] reduced alienation,[3,125] and better social support.[3,127] All these factors possibly contribute to lower suicidal behaviors.

Some of the studies have compared subjects of different religions regarding the prevalence of suicidal ideations and suicide attempts. These studies suggest that Hindus have higher rates of suicidal ideations compared to those belonging to other (Muslims, Christians, Jains, and Sikhs) religious affiliations.[128,129] Another study suggested that compared to Buddhists, rates of suicidal ideation are higher among Christians.[130] However, this finding contradicts other studies that report higher suicidal ideations among those who are non-Christians.[131] On the other hand, some of the studies which have compared people of different religious affiliations have not found any difference in the prevalence of suicidal ideations.[132]

Studies that have evaluated the relationship of suicide attempts with religious affiliations suggest that the rate of suicide attempts is higher among Hindus when compared to those belonging to other (Muslims, Christians, Jains, and Sikhs) religious affiliations.[128] However, Catholics and Taoists do not differ significantly from Christians.[130] Studies that have evaluated people of the Muslim religion have reported higher rates of suicide attempts among Jews than that Muslims.[132]

Higher religious attendance appears to serve a protective effect in the development of suicidal ideations[133-140] and suicide attempts,[135-143] according to studies. Recurrence of suicide attempts is linked to "purpose of life," according to a longitudinal study.[144] However, some studies have found negative results, such as a lack of link between religious attendance and suicidal ideation and attempt.[145-147] Occasionally, studies have found a greater rate of history of suicide attempts among people with religious affiliation, as well as a higher rate of suicidal ideation among depressive patients who value religion more and attend religious services more frequently.[106]

Private religious activities have also been linked to lower incidence of suicide ideation.[148] According to a recent systematic analysis of the relationship between religion and suicidal behavior, religious affiliation may not always protect against suicidal ideation among the many components of religion. Suicide attempts are protected by religious affiliation.[106] After controlling for social support as a covariate, another aspect of religion, religious service attendance, did not appear to be protective against suicidal ideation; however, religious service attendance did emerge as a protective factor against suicide attempts.[106]

CONCLUSION AND FUTURE DIRECTIONS

This chapter provides ample evidence that religiosity and its various dimensions influence many mental illnesses. The influence of religiosity and its dimensions has been understood concerning the development of the disorder (especially depression), with some evidence to suggest that religiosity plays a protective role in the development of depression. Contemporary research also sheds light on the association of religiosity/religious beliefs on symptoms of mental illness (i.e., symptoms with religious content, suicidality, etc.), help-seeking, pathways to care, medication adherence, treatment response, psychosocial adaptation, relapse rates, social integration, and quality of life, etc. Hence, it is vital to assess religiosity and its various dimensions among patients with mental illnesses. Further, the management of mental illnesses should consider the explanatory models held by the patients, and efforts much be made to address the contradictory explanatory models owned by the patients/caregivers from that by clinicians. Religious principles should be taken into account while planning treatment, and clinicians should encourage their patients to use positive religious coping to deal with their illness.

However, it is essential to remember that, at present, there is limited research in this area. Future research in this area is required to address many unresolved issues.

REFERENCES

1. World Population Review. Religion by Country 2022. [online] Available from https://worldpopulationreview.com/country-rankings/religion-by-country. [Last accessed June, 2022].
2. Pew Research Center. The Global Religious Landscape. [online] Available from https://www.pewforum.org/2012/12/18/global-religious-landscape-exec/. [Last accessed June, 2022].
3. Koenig H, King D, Carson VB. Handbook of Religion and Health. USA: Oxford University Press; 2012.
4. Moreira-Almeida A, Lotufo Neto F, Koenig HG. Religiousness and mental health: a review. Rev Bras Psiquiatr. 2006;28:242-50.
5. Holdcroft B. What is religiosity? Cathol Educ J Inq Pract. 2006;10:89-103.
6. Glock CY, Stark R. Religion and Society in Tension. Chicago: Rand McNally; 1965.
7. Huber S, Huber OW. The Centrality of Religiosity Scale (CRS). Religions. 2012;3:710-24.
8. Allport GW, Michael J. Personal religious orientation and prejudice. J Pers Soc Psychol. 1967;5:432-43.
9. Hill PC, Pargament KI, Hood RW, McCullough J Michael E, Swyers JP, et al. Conceptualizing religion and spirituality: points of commonality, points of departure. J Theory Soc Behav. 2000;30:51-77.
10. George LK, Larson DB, Koenig HG, McCullough ME. Spirituality and health: what we know, what we need to know. J Soc Clin Psychol. 2000;19:102-16.
11. Moberg DO. Assessing and measuring spirituality: confronting dilemmas of universal and particular evaluative criteria. J Adult Dev. 2002;9:47-60.

12. Vaughan F. Spiritual issues in psychotherapy. J Transpersl Psychol. 1991;23:105-8.
13. de Jager Meezenbroek E, Garssen B, van den Berg M, van Dierendonck D, Visser A, Schaufeli WB. Measuring spirituality as a universal human experience: a review of spirituality questionnaires. J Relig Health. 2012;51:336-54.
14. Yonker JE, Schnabelrauch CA, DeHaan LG. The relationship between spirituality and religiosity on psychological outcomes in adolescents and emerging adults: a meta-analytic review. J Adolesc. 2012;35:299-314.
15. Nolan JA, McEvoy JP, Koenig HG, Hooten EG, Whetten K, Pieper CF. Religious coping and quality of life among individuals living with schizophrenia. Psychiatr Serv. 2012;63:1051-4.
16. Mohr S, Borras L, Nolan J, Gillieron C, Brandt PY, Eytan A, et al. Spirituality and religion in outpatients with schizophrenia: a multi-site comparative study of Switzerland, Canada, and the United States. Int J Psychiatry Med. 2012;44:29-52.
17. Cohen CI, Jimenez C, Mittal S. The role of religion in the well-being of older adults with schizophrenia. Psychiatr Serv. 2010;61:917-22.
18. Appelbaum PS, Robbins PC, Roth LH. Dimensional approach to delusions: comparisons across types and diagnoses. Am J Psychiatry. 1999;156:1938-43.
19. Gearing RE, Alonzo D, Smolak A, McHugh K, Harmon S, Baldwin S. Association of religion with delusions and hallucinations in the context of schizophrenia: Implications for engagement and adherence. Schizophr Res. 2011;126:150-63.
20. Tateyama M, Asai M, Kamisada M, Hashimoto M, Bartels M, Heimann H. Comparison of schizophrenic delusions between Japan and Germany. Psychopathology. 1993;26:151-8.
21. Krzystanek M, Krysta K, Klasik A, Krupka-Matuszczyk I. Religious content of hallucinations in paranoid schizophrenia. Psychiatr Danub. 2012;24 (Suppl 1):S65-9.
22. Stompe T, Friedman A, Ortwein G, Strobl R, Chaudhry HR, Najam N, et al. Comparison of delusions among schizophrenics in Austria and in Pakistan. Psychopathology. 1999;32(5):225-34.
23. Rudaleviciene P, Stompe T, Narbekovas A, Raskauskiene N, Bunevicius R. Are religious delusions related to religiosity in schizophrenia? Medicine. 2008;44:529-35.
24. Wilson W. Religion and psychosis. In: Koenig H, (Ed). Handbook of Religion and Mental Health. San Diego: Academic Press; 1998. pp. 161-73.
25. Mohr S, Borras L, Betrisey C, Pierre-Yves B, Gilliéron C, Huguelet P. Delusions with religious content in patients with psychosis: how they interact with spiritual coping. Psychiatry. 2010;73:158-72.
26. Tateyama M, Asai M, Hashimoto M, Bartels M, Kasper S. Transcultural study of schizophrenic delusions: Tokyo versus Vienna versus Tubingen (Germany). Psychopathology. 1998;31:59-68.
27. Getz GE, Fleck DE, Strakowski SM. Frequency and severity of religious delusions in Christian patients with psychosis. Psychiatry Res. 2001;103:87-91.
28. Kim K, Li D, Jiang Z, Cui X, Lin L, Kang JJ, et al. Schizophrenia delusions among Koreans, Korean-Chinese and Chinese: a transcultural study. Int J Soc Psychiatry. 1993;39:190-9.
29. Greenberg D, Brom D. Nocturnal hallucinations in ultra-orthodox Jewish Israeli men. Psychiatry. 2001;64:81-9.
30. Kent G, Wahass S. The content and characteristics of auditory hallucinations in Saudi Arabia and the UK: a cross-cultural comparison. Acta Psychiatr Scand. 1996;94:433-7.
31. Huang CL, Shang CY, Shieh MS, Lin HN, Su JC. The interactions between religion, religiosity, religious delusion/hallucination, and treatment-seeking behavior among schizophrenic patients in Taiwan. Psychiatry Res. 2011;187:347-53.
32. Mohr S, Brandt PY, Borras L, Gilliéron C, Huguelet P. Toward an integration of spirituality and religiousness into the psychosocial dimension of schizophrenia. Am J Psychiatry. 2006;163:1952-9.
33. Huguelet P, Mohr S, Jung V, Gillieron C, Brandt PY, Borras L. Effect of religion on suicide attempts in outpatients with schizophrenia or schizoaffective disorders compared with inpatients with non-psychotic disorders. Eur Psychiatry. 2007;22:188-94.
34. Borras L, Khazaal Y, Khan R, Mohr S, Kaufmann YA, Zullino D, et al. The relationship between addiction and religion and its possible implication for care. Subst Use Misuse. 2010;45:2357-410.
35. Gaite L, Vázquez-Barquero JL, Borra C, Ballesteros J, Schene A, Welcher B, et al. A quality of life in patients with schizophrenia in five European countries: the EPSILON study. Acta Psychiatr Scand. 2002;105:283-92.
36. Murray-Swank A, Goldberg R, Dickerson F, Medoff D, Wohlheiter K, Dixon L. Correlates of religious service attendance and contact with religious leaders among persons with co-occurring serious mental illness and type 2 diabetes. J Nerv Ment Dis. 2007;195:382-8.

37. Flics DH, Herron WG. Activity-withdrawal, diagnosis, and demographics as predictors of premorbid adjustment. J Clin Psychol. 1991; 47:189-98.
38. Huguelet P, Mohr S, Borras L, Gillieron C, Brandt PY. Spirituality and religious practices among outpatients with schizophrenia and their clinicians. Psychiatr Serv. 2006;57:366-72.
39. Huguelet P, Borras L, Gillieron C, Brandt PY, Mohr S. Influence of spirituality and religiousness on substance misuse in patients with schizophrenia or schizoaffective disorder. Subst Use Misuse. 2009;44:502-13.
40. Webb M, Charbonneau AM, McCann RA, Gayle KR. Struggling and enduring with God, religious support, and recovery from severe mental illness. J Clin Psychol. 2011;67:1161-76.
41. Mohr S, Perroud N, Gillieron C, Brandt PY, Rieben I, Borras L, et al. Spirituality and religiousness as predictive factors of outcome in schizophrenia and schizoaffective disorders. Psychiatry Res. 2011;186:177-82.
42. Rund BR. Fully recovered schizophrenics: a retrospective study of some premorbid and treatment factors. Psychiatry. 1990;53:127-39.
43. Huguelet P, Binyet-Vogel S, Gonzalez C, Favre S, McQuillan A. Follow-up study of 67 first-episode schizophrenic patients and their involvement in religious activities. Eur Psychiatry. 1997;12:279-83.
44. Koenig H. Handbook of Religion and Mental Health. San Diego: Academic Press; 1998.
45. Pieper JZT. Religious coping is highly religious psychiatric inpatients. Ment Heal Religion Culture. 2004;7:349-63.
46. Phillips R, Stein C. God's will, God's punishment, or God's limitations? Religious coping strategies reported by young adults living with serious mental illness. J Clin Psychol. 2007;63:529-40.
47. Nurasikin MS, Khatijah LA, Aini A, Ramli M, Aida SA, Zainal NZ, et al. Religiousness, religious coping methods and distress level among psychiatric patients in Malaysia. Int J Soc Psychiatry. 2013;59:332-8.
48. Revheim N, Greenberg WM, Citrome L. Spirituality, schizophrenia, and state hospitals: program description and characteristics of self-selected attendees of a spirituality therapeutic group. Psychiatr Q. 2010;81:285-92.
49. Smith S, Suto MJ. Religious and/or spiritual practices: extending spiritual freedom to people with schizophrenia. Can J Occup Ther. 2012; 79:77-85.
50. Smolak A, Gearing RE, Alonzo D, Baldwin S, Harmon S, McHugh K. Social support and religion: mental health service use and treatment of schizophrenia. Comm Ment Health J. 2013;49:444-50.
51. Tepper L, Rogers SA, Coleman EM, Malony HN. The prevalence of religious coping among persons with persistent mental illness. Psychiatr Serv. 2001;52:660-5.
52. Reger GM, Rogers SA. Diagnostic differences in religious coping among individuals with persistent mental illness. J Psychol Christianity. 2002;21:341-8.
53. Napo F, Heinz A, Auckenthaler A. Explanatory models and concepts of West African Malian patients with psychotic symptoms. Eur Psychiatry. 2012;27(Suppl 2):S44-9.
54. Johnson S, Sathyaseelan M, Charles H, Jeyaseelan V, Jacob KS. Insight, psychopathology, explanatory models and outcome of schizophrenia in India: a prospective 5-year cohort study. BMC Psychiatry. 2012;12:159.
55. Kate N, Grover S, Kulhara P, Nehra R. Supernatural beliefs, aetiological models and help-seeking behavior in patients with schizophrenia. Ind Psychiatry J. 2012;21:49-54.
56. Saravanan B, Jacob KS, Johnson S, Prince M, Bhugra D, David AS. Belief models in first-episode schizophrenia in South India. Soc Psychiatry Psychiatr Epidemiol. 2007;42:446-51.
57. Unal S, Kaya B, Yalvaç HD. Patients' explanation models for their illness and help-seeking behavior. Turk Psikiyatri Derg. 2007;18:38-47.
58. McCabe R, Priebe S. Explanatory models of illness in schizophrenia: comparison of four ethnic groups. Br J Psychiatry. 2004;185:25-30.
59. Saravanan B, Jacob KS, Deepak MG, Prince M, David AS, Bhugra D. Perceptions about psychosis and psychiatric services: a qualitative study from Vellore, India. Soc Psychiatry Psychiatr Epidemiol. 2008;43:231-8.
60. Shah R, Kulhara P, Grover S, Kumar S, Malhotra R, Tyagi S. Contribution of spirituality to quality of life in patients with residual schizophrenia. Psychiatry Res. 2011;190:200-5.
61. Shah R, Kulhara P, Grover S, Kumar S, Malhotra R, Tyagi S. Relationship between spirituality/religiousness and coping in patients with residual schizophrenia. Qual Life Res. 2011;20:1053-60.
62. Siddle R, Haddock G, Tarrier N, Faragher EB. Religious delusions in patients admitted to hospital with schizophrenia. Soc Psychiatry Psychiatr Epidemiol. 2002;37:130-8.

63. Moss Q, Fleck DE, Strakowski SM. The influence of religious affiliation on time to first treatment and hospitalization. Schizophr Res. 2006;84: 421-6.
64. Rocca P, Castagna F, Marchiaro L, Rasetti R, Rivoira EF. Neuropsychological correlates of reality distortion in schizophrenic patients. Psychiatry Res. 2006;145:49-60.
65. Doering S, Muller E, Kopcke W, Pietzcker A, Gaebel W, Linden M, et al. Predictors of relapse and rehospitalization in schizophrenia and schizoaffective disorder. Schizophr Bull. 1998;24:87-98.
66. Thara R, Eaton WW. Outcome of schizophrenia: The Madras longitudinal study. Aust N Z J Psychiatry. 1996;30:516-22.
67. Compton J, Bhugra D. Experiences of religious healing in psychiatric patients in South India. Soc Psychiatry Psychiatr Epidemiol. 1997;32: 215-21.
68. Padmavati R, Thara R, Corin E. A qualitative study of religious practices by chronic mentally ill and their caregivers in South India. Int J Soc Psychiatry. 2005;51:139-49.
69. Yang CT, Narayanasamy A, Chang SL. Transcultural spirituality: the spiritual journey of hospitalized patients with schizophrenia in Taiwan. J Adv Nurs. 2012;68:358-67.
70. Kirov G, Kemp R, Kirov K, David AS. Religious faith after psychotic illness. Psychopathology. 1998;31:234-45.
71. Menezes A, Moreira-Almeida A. Religion, spirituality and psychosis. Cur Psychiatry Rep. 2010;12:174-9.
72. Raab K. Manic depression and religious experience: the use of religion in therapy. Ment Health, Relig Cult. 2007;10(5):473-87.
73. Koenig HG. Religion, spirituality, and psychotic disorders. Arch Clin Psychiatry. 2007;34(Suppl 1): 95-104.
74. Grover S, Hazari N, Aneja J, Chakrabarti S, Avasthi A. Influence of religion and supernatural beliefs on clinical manifestation and treatment practices in patients with bipolar disorder. Nord J Psychiatry. 2016;70:442-9.
75. Brewerton TD. Hyperreligiosity in psychotic disorders. J Nerv Ment Dis. 1994;182:302-4.
76. Cothran MM, Harvey PD. Delusional thinking in psychotics: correlates of religious content. Psychol Rep. 1986;58:191-9.
77. Kroll J, Sheehan W. Religious beliefs and practices among 52 psychiatric inpatients in Minnesota. Am J Psychiatry. 1989;146:67-72.
78. Mitchell L, Romans S. Spiritual beliefs in bipolar affective disorder: their relevance for illness management. J Affect Disord. 2003;75:247-57.
79. Cruz M, Pincus HA, Welsh DE, Greenwald D, Lasky E, Kilbourne AM. The relationship between religious involvement and clinical status of patients with bipolar disorder. Bipolar Disord. 2010;12:68-76.
80. Grover S, Dua D, Chakrabarti S, Avasthi A. Religiosity and spirituality of patients with severe mental disorders. Indian J Psychiatry. 2021;63:162-70.
81. Ouwehand E, Zock H, Muthert JKH, Boeije H, Braam AW. 'The Awful Rowing toward God': interpretation of religious experiences by individuals with bipolar disorder. Pastor Psychol. 2019;68:437-62.
82. Çuhadar D, Savaş HA, Ünal A, Gökpınar F. Family functionality and coping attitudes of patients with bipolar disorder. J Relig Health. 2015;54:1731-46.
83. Stroppa A, Colugnati FA, Koenig HG, Moreira-Almeida A. Religiosity, depression, and quality of life in bipolar disorder: a two-year prospective study. Revista Brasileira de Psiquiatria. 2018;40:238-43.
84. Ouwehand E, Braam AW, Renes JW, Muthert HJK, Zock HT. Holy apparition or hyper-religiosity: prevalence of explanatory models for religious and spiritual experiences in patients with bipolar disorder and their associations with religiousness. Pastoral Psychol. 2020a;69:29-45.
85. Ouwehand E, Zock H, Muthert H. Religious or spiritual experiences and bipolar disorder: a case study from the perspective of dialogical self-theory. Religions. 2020b;11:1-21.
86. Grover S, Avasthi A, Chakravarty R, Dan A, Chakraborty K, Neogi R, et al. Bipolar disorder course and outcome study from India (BiD-CoIN study): sample description and methods. J Affect Dis. 2021;280:16-23.
87. Sahu A, Patil V, Purkayastha S, Pattanayak RD, Sagar R. Pathways to care for patients with Bipolar-I disorder: an exploratory study from a tertiary care centre of North India. Indian J Psychol Med. 2019;41:68-74.
88. Caribé AC, Studart P, Bezerra-Filho S, Brietzke E, Nunes Noto M, Vianna-Sulzbach M, et al. Is religiosity a protective factor against suicidal behavior in bipolar I outpatients? J Affect Disord. 2015;186:156-61.
89. Dervic K, Oquendo MA, Grunebaum MF, Ellis S, Burke AK, Mann JJ. Religious affiliation and

suicide attempt. Am J Psychiatry. 2004;161: 2303-8.
90. Farooq S, Nazar Z, Akhtar J, Akhter J, Irfan M, Irafn M, et al. effect of fasting during Ramadan on serum lithium level and mental state in bipolar affective disorder. Int Clin Psychopharmacol. 2010;25:323-7.
91. Eddahby S, Kadri N, Moussaoui D. Fasting during Ramadan is associated with a higher recurrence rate in patients with bipolar disorder. World Psychiatry. 2014;13(1):97.
92. Bonelli R, Dew RE, Koenig HG, Rosmarin DH, Vasegh S. Religious and spiritual factors in depression: review and integration of the research. Depress Res Treat. 2012:962860.
93. Braam AW, Koenig HG. Religion, spirituality, and depression in prospective studies: a systematic review. J Affect Disord. 2019;257:428-38.
94. Smith TB, McCullough ME, Poll J. Religiousness and depression: evidence for a main effect and the moderating influence of stressful life events. Psychol Bull. 2003;129:614-36.
95. Dew RE, Daniel SS, Goldston DB, McCall WV, Kuchibhatla M, Schleifer C, et al. A prospective study of religion/spirituality and depressive symptoms among adolescent psychiatric patients. J Affect Disord. 2010;120:149-57.
96. Grover S, Kumar V, Chakrabarti S, Hollikatti P, Singh P, Tyagi S, et al. Explanatory models in patients with first-episode depression: a study from North India. Asian J Psychiatry. 2012;5:251-57.
97. Sun F, Park NS, Roff LL, Klemmack DL, Parker M, Koenig HG, et al. Predicting the trajectories of depressive symptoms among southern community-dwelling older adults: the role of religiosity. Aging Ment Health. 2012;16:189-98.
98. Koenig HG, George LK, Peterson BL. Religiosity and remission of depression in medically ill older patients. Am J Psychiatry. 1998;155:536-42.
99. Kleiman EM, Liu RT. Prospective prediction of suicide in a nationally representative sample: religious service attendance as a protective factor. Br J Psychiatry. 2014;204:262-6.
100. Rasic DT, Belik S-L, Elias B, Katz LY, Enns M, Sareen J. Spirituality, religion and suicidal behavior in a nationally representative sample. J Affect Disord. 2009;114:32-40.
101. Lawrence RE, Oquendo MA, Stanley B. Religion and suicide risk: a systematic review. Arch Suicide Res Off J Int Acad Suicide Res. 2016;20:1-21.
102. Colucci E, Martin G. Religion and spirituality along the suicidal path. Suicide Life Threat Behav. 2008;38:229-44.
103. Nkansah-Amankra S, Diedhiou A, Agbanu SK, Agbanu HLK, Opoku-Adomako NS, Twumasi-Ankrah P. A longitudinal evaluation of religiosity and psychosocial determinants of suicidal behaviors among a population-based sample in the United States. J Affect Disord. 2012;139:40-51.
104. Dervic K, Grunebaum MF, Burke AK, Mann JJ, Oquendo MA. Protective factors against suicidal behavior in depressed adults reporting childhood abuse. J Nerv Ment Dis. 2006;194:971-4.
105. Wang M-C, Lightsey OR, Tran KK, Bonaparte TS. Examining suicide protective factors among black college students. Death Stud. 2013;37:228-47.
106. Lawrence RE, Brent D, Mann JJ, Burke AK, Grunebaum MF, Galfalvy HC, et al. Religion as a risk factor for suicide attempt and suicide ideation among depressed patients. J Nerv Ment Dis. 2016;204:845-50.
107. Patel V, Ramasundarahettige C, Vijayakumar L, Thakur J, Gajalakshmi V, Gururaj G, et al. Suicide mortality in India: a nationally representative survey. Lancet. 2012;379:2343-51.
108. Gupta S, Avasthi A, Kumar S. Relationship between religiosity and psychopathology in patients with depression. Indian J Psychiatry. 2011;53(4):330-5.
109. Yorulmaz O, Gencoz T, Woody S. OCD cognitions and symptoms in different religious contexts. J Anxiety Dis. 2009;23:401-6.
110. Pirutinsky S, Siev J, Rosmarin DH. Scrupulosity and implicit and explicit beliefs about God. J Obsessive Compuls Relat Dis. 2015;6:33-8.
111. Himle JA, Taylor RJ, Chatters LM. Religious involvement and obsessive-compulsive disorder among African Americans and Black Caribbeans. J Anxiety Dis. 2012;26:502-10.
112. Abramowitz JS, Huppert JD, Cohen AB, Tolin DF, Cahill SP. Religious obsessions and compulsions in a non-clinical sample: The Penn Inventory of Scrupulosity (PIOS). Behav Res Ther. 2002;40:825-38.
113. Greenberg D, Shefler G. Obsessive-compulsive disorder in ultra-orthodox Jewish patients: A comparison of religious and non-religious symptoms. Psychol Psychother. 2002;75(Pt 2): 123-30.
114. Greenberg D, Witztum E. The influence of cultural factors on obsessive-compulsive disorder: Religious symptoms in a religious society. Isr J Psychiatry Relat Sci. 1994;31: 211-20.
115. Lewis CA, Maltby J. Religious attitude and practice: the relationship with obsessionality. Pers Individ Differ. 1995;19:105-8.

116. Lewis CA. Religiosity and obsessionality: the relationship between Freud's "religious practices." J Psychol. 1994;128:189-96.
117. Hermesh H, Masser-Kavitzky R, Gross-Isseroff R. Obsessive-compulsive disorder and Jewish religiosity. J Nerv Ment Dis. 2003;191:201-3.
118. Assarian F, Biqam H, Asqarnejad A. An epidemiological study of obsessive-compulsive disorder among high school students and its relationship with religious attitudes. Arch Iran Med. 2006;9(2):104-7.
119. Cinar T, Tan O, Keskin R, Sayar GH. The relationship between obsessive-compulsive symptoms and religious attitudes. J Neurobehav Sci. 2021;8:36-41.
120. Tek C, Ulug B. Religiosity and religious obsessions in obsessive-compulsive disorder. Psychiatry Res. 2001;104:99-108.
121. Grover S, Patra BN, Aggarwal M, Avasthi A, Chakrabarti S, Malhotra S. Relationship of supernatural beliefs and first treatment contact in patients with obsessive-compulsive disorder: an exploratory study from India. Int J Soc Psychiatry. 2014;60:818-27.
122. Almasi A, Akuchekian SH, Maracy MR. Religious Cognitive Behavior Therapy (RCBT) on Marital Satisfaction OCD patients. Procedia Soc Behav Sci. 2013;84:504-8.
123. Mohamed NR, Elsweedy MS, Elsayed SM, Rajab AZ, Elzahar ST. Obsessive-compulsive disorder, an Islamic view. Menoufia Med J. 2015;28:289-94.
124. Stack S. The effect of religious commitment on suicide: a cross-national analysis. J Health Soc Behav. 1983;24(4):362-74.
125. Nock MK, Borges G, Bromet EJ, Cha CB, Kessler RC, Lee S. Suicide and suicidal behavior. Epidemiol Rev. 2008;30:133-54.
126. Perroud N, Baud P, Mouthon D, Courtet P, Malafosse A. Impulsivity, aggression and suicidal behavior in unipolar and bipolar disorders. J Affect Disord. 2011;134(1-3):112-8.
127. Parker M, Lee Roff L, Klemmack DL, Koenig HG, Baker P, Allman RM. Religiosity and mental health in southern, community-dwelling older adults. Aging Ment Health. 2003;7(5):390-7.
128. Sidhartha T, Jena S. Suicidal behaviors in adolescents. Indian J Pediatr. 2006;73:783-8.
129. Maniam T, Mariani M, Firdaus M, Kadir AB, Mazzini MJ, Azizul A, et al. Risk factors for suicidal ideation, plans and attempts in Malaysia--results of an epidemiological survey. Compr Psychiatry. 2014;55 (Suppl 1):S121-5.
130. Fang C-K, Lu H-C, Liu S, Sun Y-W. Religious beliefs along the suicidal path in northern Taiwan. Omega. 2011;63:255-69.
131. Snarr JD, Heyman RE, Slep AMS. Recent suicidal ideation and suicide attempts in a large-scale survey of the US Air Force. Suicide Life Threat Behav. 2010;40:544-52.
132. Gal G, Goldberger N, Kabaha A, Haklai Z, Geraisy N, Gross R, et al. Suicidal behavior among Muslim Arabs in Israel. Soc Psychiatry Psychiatr Epidemiol. 2012;47:11-7.
133. Langille DB, Asbridge M, Kisely S, Rasic D. Suicidal behaviors in adolescents in Nova Scotia, Canada: protective associations with measures of social capital. Soc Psychiatry Psychiatr Epidemiol. 2012;47:1549-55.
134. Taliaferro LA, Rienzo BA, Pigg RM, Miller MD, Dodd VJ. Spiritual well-being and suicidal ideation among college students. J Am Coll Health J ACH. 2009;58:83-90.
135. Taylor PJ, Gooding P, Wood AM, Tarrier N. The role of defeat and entrapment in depression, anxiety, and suicide. Psychol Bull. 2011;137:391-420.
136. Robinson J, Yuen HP, Gook S, Hughes A, Cosgrave E, Killackey E, et al. Can receipt of a regular postcard reduce suicide-related behavior in young help seekers? A randomized controlled trial. Early Interv Psychiatry. 2012;6:145-52.
137. Hoffman S, Marsiglia FF. The impact of religiosity on suicidal ideation among youth in Central Mexico. J Relig Health. 2014;53:255-66.
138. Rushing NC, Corsentino E, Hames JL, Sachs-Ericsson N, Steffens DC. The relationship of religious involvement indicators and social support to current and past suicidality among depressed older adults. Aging Ment Health. 2013;17:366-74.
139. Robins A, Fiske A. Explaining the relation between religiousness and reduced suicidal behavior: social support rather than specific beliefs. Suicide Life Threat Behav. 2009;39:386-95.
140. Rasic D, Kisely S, Langille DB. Protective associations of importance of religion and frequency of service attendance with depression risk, suicidal behaviors, and substance use in adolescents in Nova Scotia, Canada. J Affect Disord. 2011;132:389-95.
141. Blackmore ER, Munce S, Weller I, Zagorski B, Stansfeld SA, Stewart DE, et al. Psychosocial and clinical correlates of suicidal acts: results from a national population survey. Br J Psychiatry. 2008;192:279-84.
142. Kaslow NJ, Price AW, Wyckoff S, Bender Grall M, Sherry A, Young S, et al. Person factors associated

with suicidal behavior among African American women and men. Culture Divers Ethnic Minor Psychol. 2004;10:5-22.
143. Sisask M, Varnik A, Kolves K, Bertolote JM, Bokhari J, Botega NJ, et al. Is religiosity a protective factor against attempted suicide: a cross-cultural case-control study. Arch Suicide Res Off J Int Acad Suicide Res. 2010;14:44-55.
144. Mandhouj O, Perroud N, Hasler R, Younes N, Huguelet P. Characteristics of spirituality and religion among suicide attempters. J Nerv Ment Dis. 2016;204:861-7.
145. Blum RW, Halcón L, Beuhring T, Pate E, Campell-Forrester S, Venema A. Adolescent health in the Caribbean: risk and protective factors. Am J Public Health. 2003;93:456-60.
146. Chatters LM, Taylor RJ, Lincoln KD, Nguyen A, Joe S. Church-based social support and suicidality among African Americans and Black Caribbeans. Arch Suicide Res. 2011;15(4):337-53.
147. Stroppa A, Moreira-Almeida A. Religiosity, mood symptoms, and quality of life in bipolar disorder. Bipolar Disord. 2013;15(4):385-93.
148. Cole-Lewis YC, Gipson PY, Opperman KJ, Arango A, King CA. Protective role of religious involvement against depression and suicidal ideation among youth with interpersonal problems. J Relig Health. 2016;55:1172-88.

CHAPTER 18

Interface with Art Therapy

Debasis Bhattacharya, Rahul Bhattacharya

INTRODUCTION: INTERFACE BETWEEN ART AND PSYCHOLOGY

It is difficult to have clear boundaries in art therapy. One of the challenges lies in defining "art". In this chapter, we have focused on visual or nonverbal art. Art therapy is a dynamic encounter between the two entities: (1) art and (2) mind. It exploits new potentials through a range of diverse activities and it is not restricted to either *form* or *content*.[1,2] Therefore, the field of art therapy is essentially interdisciplinary. While conventional therapy or psychotherapy involves verbal communication, "art therapy" offers the opportunity to delve into the *nonverbal* and transcend verbal and linguistic barriers. Therefore, art therapy is therapy distinct from what is commonly referred to in the west as "talking therapy". It is recognized that nonverbal communication plays a key role in human interactions. Art therapy offers an opportunity to tap into these powerful and sometimes raw and unprocessed emotions or urges which may be otherwise difficult to articulate verbally.[3-5]

"Art" has evolved and has been redefined over human history. What constitutes art is sometimes all encompassing and esoteric? The domain of "art" refers to the diverse range of activities with the use of imagination to express ideas of feeling. This broad conceptual frame also includes music, theater, film, installation, crafts, drama in addition to painting and sculpture. Within visual arts, creative processes include drawing, painting, sculpture, and other related works of visual media. All these modalities emphasize on a nonverbal mode of communication and encourage creative expression. In this chapter, however, we would be referring to art synonymously to "visual art" particularly in relation to drawing and painting.

There is a shifting of paradigm from "art as a recreational activity" to "art as a transformative process" in art therapy.[6-8] The emphasis is on "collaboration" rather than "transaction". The client (receiving art therapy) defines their goal through the collaborative and interactive process of art-making in art therapy. This is different from a didactic plan of treatment. The process of art therapy is not manualized in detail. It is fluid and keeps faith in the process of shared exploration by the therapist and the client (or patient). The therapist does not play the role of an expert. The therapist participates as a learner and if needed takes on a role of a guide or a facilitator. The whole process maintains a balance between rationality, imagination and sensitivity.

Exploring nonverbal communication with the therapist is also a creative venture. The art therapist helps to access and thereby potentially awaken their client's personal and latent creativity. Through the use of a chosen art-medium a path of guided creativity is pursued. The focus of this process is not on attaining artistic skills or focusing on the "theories of art"; instead, the therapist provides scaffolding and a safe environment for the client to create. It also provides an opportunity to connect with the clients' urges and feelings through the artwork and then allow further exploration of their psyche. The creative processes of this venture aim to find patterns and to make connections between the creative phenomena and linking these to the clients' world. By avoiding a verbal "dialogue" or didactic communication, art therapy provides an opportunity to explore subtleties which are often difficult to access or too painful to articulate in verbal therapy sessions.[6,7]

VERBAL AND NONVERBAL LANGUAGE: EVOLUTIONARY AND HUMAN DEVELOPMENTAL PERSPECTIVE

Though language is an innate faculty in human beings, it develops through complex sociocultural interaction.[1,4,5] Human communication systems use sounds and words for verbal language. Similarly, in visual language, there is a plethora of signs and symbols which include abstract visuospatial forms. Visual art can be seen as an expression of visual language. The expression of cave paintings of early human beings as early as 30,000 BC was the imprint of early human communication.[9-11] With evolution, we find the "pictographs" representing images evolving to depict more crystallized ideas, i.e., "ideographs". In such symbolic transformation of communication lies the predecessor of an alphabetic "one-sound, one-sign" communication system.

Similarly, if we examine the general principles of human development, we find the expression begins with preverbal communication. Infants look and recognize before they speak. Gradually, they become attentive to sounds and images and finally get tuned to categorical perceptions of verbal and visual language.[12]

Alphabets, words and grammar offer structure to communication. Such communication is regulated by sophisticated rules and is highly manualized. We can apply these rules in our mind better once we have processed our thoughts and feelings. Verbal language often involves a degree of cognitive processing as it does not offer a direct avenue for our sensory experiences. It serves only to share labels or names what we have seen or heard or thought.

Perceptual experience may be far more subtle, subjective and contextual.[5] Our memory retains this sensory component and before memory is stored away. Perceptions pass through a transient "sensory memory" phase followed by processing through "working memory" before being coded in "long-term memory". It is hypothesized this process is disrupted, causing flashback and nightmare leading to "reliving" symptoms in post-traumatic stress disorder (PTSD).[7] Visual language offers an opportunity to tap into such sensory experiences and allow suitable expression. One may hypothesize such an avenue allows "processing" or shaping of fears and trauma, through agreed goals in art therapy.[4]

When someone has not managed to distill their feelings or thoughts either due to cognitive or emotional challenges, verbal communication may not be easy and may lack clarity. In such situations, visual language offers an alternative avenue which is not restricted by vocabulary or verbal syntax or semantics. Visual art therapy can on such situations rely on visual idioms to mediate our psychological pain, anxieties, cognitive dissonance and confusion.

VISUAL LANGUAGE

The characteristics of visual communication may be categorized under two dimensions: (1) *mimetic* or representational and (2) *non-mimetic* or abstract quality.[4,5,12] The power of mimesis facilitates discharge of our basic instinctual urges. Mimesis may also reflect symbolic meaning of the content.

On the other hand, "nonmimetic" aspect constitutes the abstract components and their psychic organization which can be approached as the whole or the "Gestalt" (as proposed by Gestalt psychology). Our mind seeks pattern and simple "whole" or "Gestalt" through our eyes. This is an innate ability of our human mind. The perceiving eye tends to bring together elements to complete a form and appreciate the "Figure" as well as the "Ground". Gestalt psychology has examined some basic perceptual laws.[4,5] It has been found that tensions between perception and balance of human mind may be expressed by the abstract pattern of "dots" **(Figs. 1 to 3)**.

The grouping of "dots" or "shapes" follows the innate perceptual laws—grouping by: *proximity*, *continuity*, and *similarity* has also been demonstrated in **Figures 4 to 6**.

Every visual stimulus is a dynamic affair. Perceptual qualities of wedge shape, oblique, direction or expanding pattern give the experience, which can be explored as a metaphor. We do not have the appropriate terminology to describe how we perceive visual forces. However, all the illusionary experience of depth and distance are appreciated by the laws of perception. The perception of "movement" is an illusion. Perhaps the viewer generates within his body an appropriate kinesthetic reaction **(Figs. 7A and B)**.

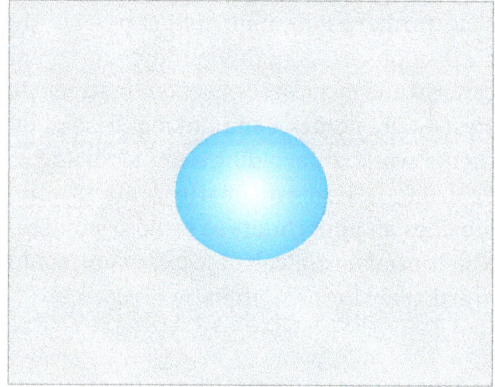

Fig. 2: Stable.

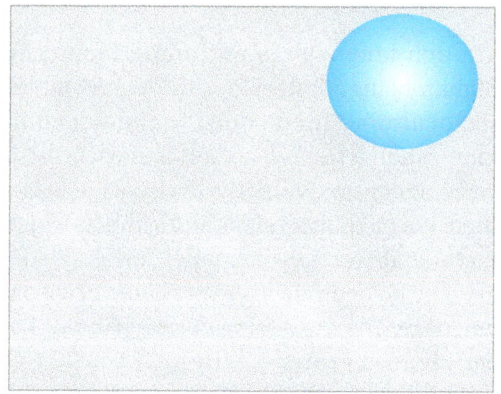

Fig. 3: Needs some breathing space.

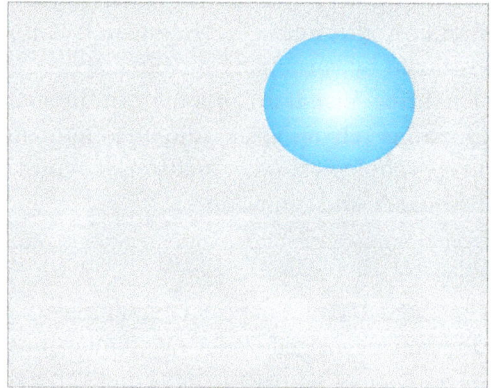

Fig. 1: Restless and tension.

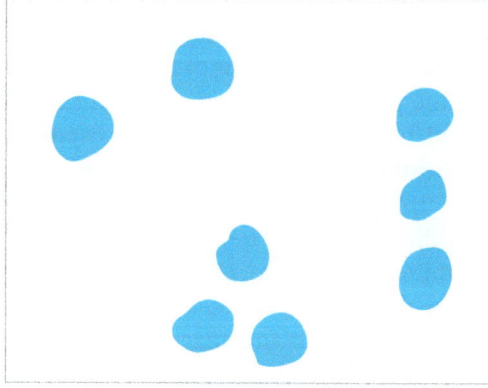

Fig. 4: Proximity.

Color is one of the most essential components of visual language. Naming colors is problematic. The world of colors is an assortment of potentially innumerable hues derived from the range of electromagnetic waves within the visible spectrum creating vision-sensory neuronal stimuli. Colors might have a particular connotation for the individual client. Psychologists have studied some of the generic nonmimetic qualities of colors, e.g., red looks stable, yellow tends to expand, and blue suggests introversion or retraction. Colors may also have a representational meaning, e.g., blue sky, yellow sunflower, or red rose. However, colors may also bear some personal association evolving personal or cultural idiom and may bear symbolic meaning. So, the therapist needs to be mindful of these individual meaning(s), a color might hold for a client. So, when the client starts splashing colors, he or she opens avenues to explore a potentially layered narrative. In fact, there is a complementary relation between mimetic and nonmimetic elements. The combination and application of these various elements are abundant in wide range of folk art, craft, design as well as highly acclaimed "abstract art". As such visual language is relatively universal and transcends linguistic and cultural nuances; later in this chapter, we discuss its potential in a multilingual country like India.

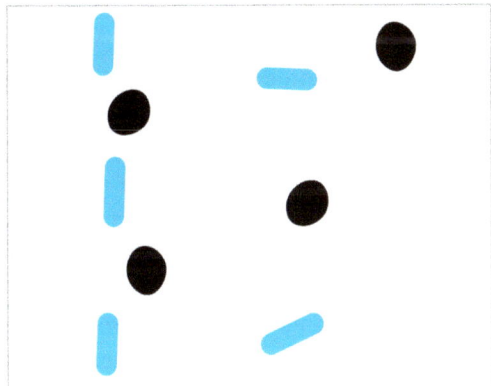

Fig. 5: Continuity.

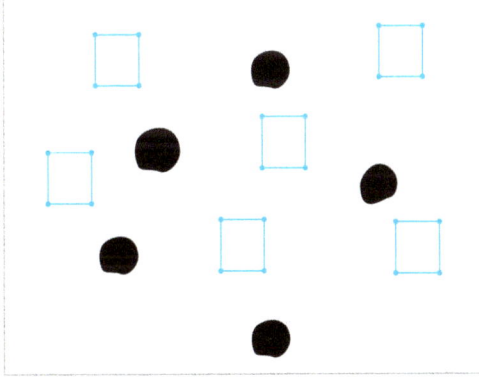

Fig. 6: Similarity.

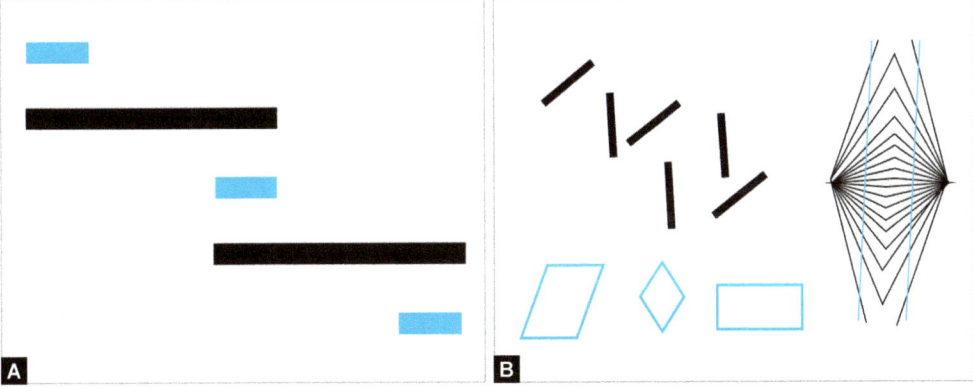

Figs. 7A and B: Movement.

THERAPEUTIC APPROACHES

The structured attempt of art therapy began around the mid-20th century arising independently in Europe and the United States. In 1940s, the artist Adrian Hill did pioneering work in the field of art therapy. He had an analytic approach where he believed that the client builds up a "defense" against his miseries and misfortunes by involving himself in art-making. Subsequently, Edward Adamson started an art-studio in an asylum in the United Kingdom. Adamson also emphasized on the importance of the exhibiting those artworks or the "products". He used such shows as an instrument to interpersonal interaction as well as a sociocultural intervention. In the United States around the same period, Margaret Naumburg and Dr E Kramer introduced psychodynamic art therapy.[7,8] The ideas of Sigmund Freud largely influenced this classical phase of art therapy. The therapists focused on searching for meaning (or mimesis) in the created images. There was a tendency to explore projection of unconscious urges of sex and aggression through the facilitated *catharsis* of art therapy.[8,13]

Jung's concept of analytical and archetypal psychology also crossed over to art therapy. Jung believed, human beings not only share a similar anatomy they also share a common tendency to enshrine their deepest experiences in some overarching universal motifs or symbols (*archetypes*) like the "mandala". The Sanskrit word "mandala" means "sacred circle". Creation of circular design had been part of spiritual practices of different traditional cultures. It broadly signifies "wheel of time" or life cycle. In contemporary practice, it often represents unit of life or a cell or outerworld or the universe. In Jungian concept, it is described as symbol of "unconscious self".[14] More recently "mandala" has become a multicultural idea of "art therapy" with it being associated with the "primordial circle".

Gestalt therapist encouraged active participation and enactment of sensorimotor activation. The therapist looked beyond the "meaning" of the content of artwork. He appreciates the expression of the abstract pattern and the dynamic wholeness or the "gestalt" of the creation. This is a shift from the mimetic to the nonmimetic form of visual expression.[15]

Contemporary art therapists usually tend to subscribe to an eclectic approach and assume that there is a continuity of expression of both the mimetic and nonmimetic components of visual language. The task of interpretation of artwork or search of meaning is the task of psychometrician. Many such interpretive psychological tests (e.g., Thematic apperception test, Rorschach's inkblot test, Bender Gestalt test, Draw-a-Man test, etc.) have developed but these no longer belong to the domain of art therapy.

In contrast to this attitude of "detecting" psychopathology, the therapist in art therapy primarily encourages the client to build resilience by releasing their pent-up emotions. Hence, the "process" not the "product" is considered to be of prime importance.[16] The therapist stimulates the creative drive (or an urge to produce new ideas) and a creative skill (an ability to reach a creative outcome from the idea). Creative process is the act of grasping and nurturing of the inspiration through stimulation or through brainstorming. The focus is not on memory or recall.[7,14]

The medium of art also offers an avenue to the sensory experience and may provide cues that open avenues of discourse. Hence, the emotional release possible through rubbing a pastel on a sheet may offer special opportunities which watercolor may not offer. Similarly, scribbling with pen or splashing

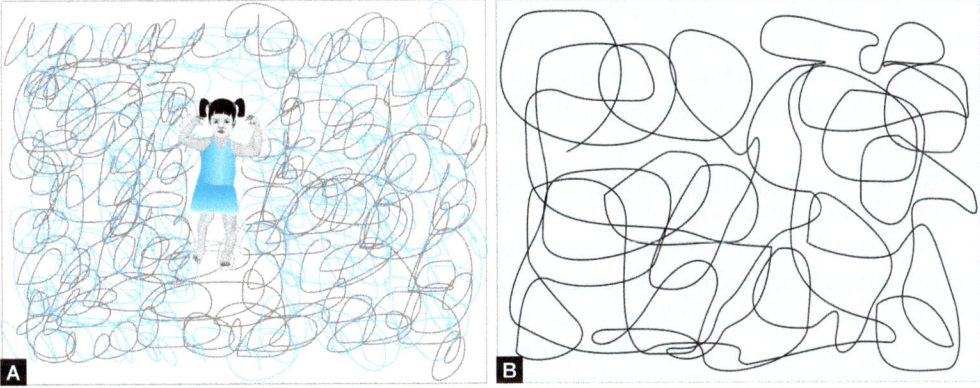

Figs. 8A and B: Scribbling.

colors on canvas might be relevant in certain situations.[15,17,18]

The usual starting phase often is the process of scribbling. Scribbling is an immensely powerful way to spur new ideas and explore inner self.[19] When you are scribbling, you are telling your brain to hold off on evaluating the value of the idea. This facilitates maximal generation of ideas in absence of conscious inhibitory control. The process of doodling allows relaxation and familiarity with the process of art therapy **(Figs. 8A and B)**.

Alternative starting rituals may involve splashing of colors or arranging different shapes to make a pattern **(Fig. 9)**.

Here art is considered as a "tool". When the client starts composing, he wants to remember or exhibit what really matters and thus he or she tries to make the relevant choices about what to communicate. So, therapeutically "good" artwork is one of significance to oneself.[19]

The therapeutic process of art therapy fosters self-awareness, encourages emotional growth, and enhances relationships with the *other* through access to imagination. The creative process of art therapy generally has the ability to pick up on allegorical expressions and use of metaphors. Allegory often reveals conflict while metaphors break barriers in

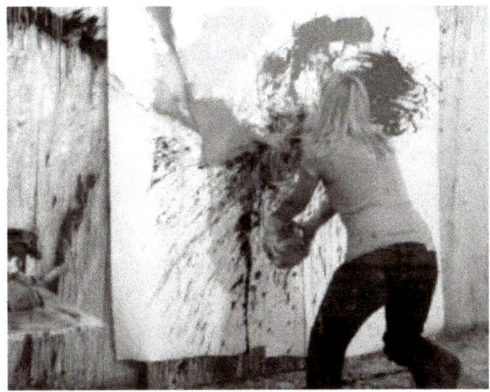

Fig. 9: Splash of color.

communication, e.g., help overcome taboos and inhibitions.[16,19,20]

EVIDENCE BASE OF ART THERAPY

Does art therapy work? The evidence base so far has not been robust, though it is stronger for nonpsychotic mental illnesses compared to psychotic conditions. In 2015, in a major meta-analysis and quantitative review was carried out in the United Kingdom which found, 15 randomized controlled trials (RCTs) exploring the efficacy of art therapy in nonpsychotic conditions. The studies looked into different conditions and used different comparators (or control groups) while measuring efficacy. As the studies were varied (what statisticians would call "heterogeneous"), statistical meta-analysis combining or pooling the data was not feasible. There was clinical heterogeneity and insufficient comparable data on outcome measures across studies. The meta-analysis concluded that art therapy was associated with significant positive changes relative to the control group in mental health symptoms in 10 out of the 15 studies. The control groups varied between studies but included waitlist/no treatment, attention placebo controls and psychological therapy comparators. Themes relating to benefits of art therapy for patients or service users included the relationship with the therapist, personal achievement and distraction. Areas of potential harms were noted as activation of unresolved or traumatic emotions, lack of skill of the art therapist and sudden termination of art therapy. Eleven of the studies were conducted in adults while four were conducted in children.[21] A clinical trial (RCT) aiming to measure efficacy of art therapy in personality disorder (CREATE trial) was abandoned due to poor recruitment. Evidence base in the field of personality disorder and art therapy remains poorly explored.

In the United Kingdom, the NICE (National Institute for Health and Clinical Excellence) guidelines for schizophrenia recommend that art therapies are considered for all people with schizophrenia, particularly for the alleviation of negative symptoms.[22] However, this recommendation has been challenged. A review of qualitative evidence of art therapy for people with psychosis in the Lancet Psychiatry, Angelica Attard and Michael Larkin[23] found little quantitative evidence for its effectiveness with only a few qualitative studies suggesting that it could be beneficial. A large pragmatic trial of group art therapy (MATISSE) found little evidence to suggest benefit of art therapy in schizophrenia.[24] The Royal Australian and New Zealand College of Psychiatry 2016 guidelines for schizophrenia note that art therapy is included in the NICE guidelines, but conclude that the evidence from RCTs is inconclusive.[25]

A recent Cochrane review of evidence base of art therapy in dementia only found two trials of suitable quality. These two studies found no clear changes in memory or most other outcomes looked at when comparing art therapy to other activities. It also noted high drop out in therapy as a potential challenge in this population.[26]

Questions are raised in planning of psychotherapy (and art therapy in particular) with respect of sample-characteristics, research-design, procedures, data-evaluation and assessment.[27-29] However, in spite of the rather equivocal evidence base for art therapy when researched as a condition-specific RCT, there are several positive stories. It is possible art therapy as a modality does not lend itself well to RCT. Moreover art therapy cannot be 'blinded' in RCTs. Art may facilitate communication which might be rewarding to the patient but may not offer associated symptom relief. Unfortunately, most studies set out to measure symptom reduction rather than personal well-being. Subjective well-being is difficult to measure. We believe art therapy may need to be offered to patients where a need for this that has been identified. Client or patient factors such as an interest in art and a difficulty in verbal communication may also need to be considered. Though we recognize such considerations do not lend themselves well to diagnosis specific RCT recruitment these are important clinical considerations. The predominant assumptions of natural science model with the emphasis on quantitative evaluation with predictability may fail to appreciate the role of art therapy in personal well-being.

We must understand that art therapist emphasizes creativity and subjective ways of knowing or reflection. The process has the affinity with the qualitative, descriptive, phenomenological, metaphorical and interpretive methods of inquiry. Accordingly, we need to refine and develop more suitable research methodology and where one can capture these.[29]

PARADIGM SHIFT: TOWARDS A HOLISTIC AND AN INTEGRATIVE APPROACH

There is an emerging trend to combine different classical methods of treatment with the more unconventional or lesser established alternatives to provide a more integrated approach. The focus is on providing a holistic and more person-specific care. Verbal psychological therapies have evolved from classical Freudian analytical approach to Kleinian perspective focusing on human dynamics of relationships. Subsequently with the rise of cognitive and cognitive behavior therapy (CBT), there was an increased emphasis of more structured and manualized approach involving a patient-driven (therapy) self-exploration with measurement of change. While recognizing the advantages of the latter, it is also increasingly appreciated that CBT is not the panacea for all mental illness. Some problems are too deep seated or painful or unique to respond to or even explore in such a standardized approach. Acknowledging the patient's own subjective worldview, beliefs, values, and narratives (which may not always be verbal) are key to providing a more holistic and patient-centered therapeutic-approach. New treatments or variation of old therapies sometimes represent a revolutionary departure from what was done before.[30,31] This paradigm shift lies in the emphasis on "thriving" and "well-being", rather than focusing on symptom relief or a search for a "cure" for illnesses. The focus is shifting from illness to health.[32,33]

Art therapy can be used for enhancement of mental well-being and not limited to treatment of specific diseases. Art therapy therefore works under wide variety of settings including both physical ailments and mental illnesses alike. Art therapy has been tried to help people suffering from specific physical or mental health conditions or groups not defined by diagnostic framework of illness or conditions e.g. victims of torture or refugees fleeing conflicts. It has been used to support people living with human immunodeficiency virus (HIV) or other chronic physical health conditions such as cancer or asthma or mental health conditions such as PTSD, anxiety or mood disorders or in people struggling with addiction and substance misuse. Art therapy is not restricted by age and has also been tried in all age groups ranging from children including young people with learning difficulties to cerebral palsy to autism to adults and older adults with dementia.

SCOPE OF ART THERAPY IN INDIA

The study of visual cultures of different countries has given a new insight about the place of visuality and literacy in specific nations.[34]

We believe there are advantages of using nonverbal communication in addition to conventional methods of psychotherapy which are especially important in a multilingual country like India. In India, social workers have been widely and effectively using art-making in their rehabilitation programs for mentally challenged children and in marginalized populations such as destitute, prisoners and other underprivileged groups of the society. At the same time, we have relative rich resources comprising trained artists, psychologists, psychiatrists, psychotherapists, and educationists though often concentrated in urban settings. Unfortunately, in spite of having a sizeable skilled workforce, our mental hospitals, institutes and clinics do not incorporate art therapy in their model of care. There is a need to form partnerships between these organisations and the institutions to create multidisciplinary teams. Teams can take an innovative skill-based approach as opposed to profession-based structure and may consist of partnerships between artists and psychotherapists or social workers. Resource allocation is critical and this would involve physical space and material to create artwork along with employing professionals. There is little in the form of formal art therapy training in India. Therefore, unlike other methods of psychotherapy, art therapy is sometimes conducted jointly by a trained artist and a competent psychologist or psychotherapist to ensure there is the right "skill mix" in the room.[35]

FUTURE DIRECTION

The inherent conflict and incongruities between the assumptions of the natural science world and the art therapist's personalized approach to human experience has not yet been adequately reconciled. We are still waiting to find the right research framework to explore the effectiveness of art therapy.

Hence, compared with global growth of clinical experience in art therapy, the findings of researchers look meager. We hope in the next decade methodological advances in evaluation of art therapy will lead to stronger link between research and practice.

The degree of professional maturity and acceptance of art therapy across the globe is variable. While recent years have seen increased networking of alternative therapies including art therapy in the western world, development of art therapy networks in India are in its infancy. The Indian Psychiatric Society's setting up a *Task Force on Art therapy* in 2018 can be seen as a small but important step in the right direction. Developing a network among current practitioners would provide a platform of learning and future development. It has been found that a sizeable number of social workers have been using art-making in their rehabilitation programs. Professionals across India have been working using art-work in their effort to support a range of difficulties ranging from children with challenging behavior, destitute populations, people with physical disability, people in prison as well as several others underprivileged groups in society. However, these ventures are often not linked up with academics or professional psychologists or psychiatrists though the projects are working on improving mental well-being. One might argue current psychiatric and psychological practices in India do not incorporate art therapy. We hope the task force and networks can help building some links between these worlds. A comprehensive guideline for art therapy adapted to Indian service provisions may promote better involvement of psychiatrists and psychologists in art therapy. For art therapy to be accepted and flourish there needs to be a provision to train art therapists of the future. There needs to be work to develop a curriculum in art therapy adapted for Indian conditions. A national approach can ensure a degree of standardization in the competencies expected of a dedicated art therapist. In fact, it can comment on the minimal mixed skills needed in the room in a multi-professionally delivered art therapy. Cross-disciplinary working would also need awareness of art therapy as a treatment modality among psychiatrists and therefore recognition within the psychiatric curriculum.

REFERENCES

1. Wolf RI. The Interface of Cognitive and Sensuous Ways of Knowing for Art Therapists. New York, College of New Rochelle: Digital Commons; 1988.

2. Westland G. Verbal and Non-verbal Communication in Psychotherapy. New York: WW Norton and Company; 2015.
3. Kreitler H, Kreitler S. Psychology of the Arts. Durham, NC: Duke University Press; 1972.
4. Arnheim R. Art and visual perception: a psychology of the creative eye (New version). California: University of California Press; 1974.
5. Verstegen I. Arnheim, Gestalt and Art: A Psychological Theory. New York: Springer-Verlag Wien; 2005.
6. De Botton A, Armstrong J. Art as Therapy. London and New York: Phaidon Press; 2013.
7. Rubin JA. Art therapy: an introduction. London: Taylor and Francis Group; 1999.
8. Malchiodi CA. The Art Therapy Sourcebook. New York: McGraw-Hill; 1998.
9. Atlas JD. Logic, Meaning and Conversation: Semantic Indeterminacy, Implication and their Interface. Oxford: Oxford University Press; 2005.
10. Kaplan FF. Art, Science and Art Therapy: Repainting the Picture. London: Jessica Kingsley; 2000.
11. 30,000 Years of Art: The Story of Human Creativity Across Time and Space. London, New York: Phaidon Press; 2007.
12. Berger J. Ways of Seeing. London; British Broadcasting Corporation and Penguin Group; 1972.
13. Naumburg M. Dynamically Oriented Art Therapy. New York: Grune and Stratton; 1987.
14. Wallace E. Creativity and Jungian thought. Art Psychother. 1975;2:181-7.
15. Perls F. Gestalt Therapy Verbatim. Lafayette, CA: Real People Press; 1969.
16. Garai J. New vistas in the exploration of inner and outer space through art therapy. Art Psychother. 1976;3:157-67.
17. McLuhan M. Understanding Media: The Extensions of Man. Cambridge: MIT Press; 1994.
18. Elkisch P. The scribbling game, a projective method. The Nervous Child. 1948;7(3):247-56.
19. Silton NR. Exploring the Benefits of Creativity in Educations, Media, and the Arts. Hershey, United States: Information Science Reference (an imprint of IGI Global); 2016.
20. Groys B. Comrades of time. E-flux J. What is Contemporary Art? Sternberg Press; 2010. pp. 22-38.
21. Uttley L, Scope A, Stevenson M, Rawdin A, Taylor Buck E, Sutton A, et al. Systematic review and economic modelling of the clinical effectiveness and cost-effectiveness of art therapy among people with non-psychotic mental health disorders. Health Technol Assess. 2015;19(18):1-120, v-vi.
22. NICE (2014). Psychosis and schizophrenia in adults: the NICE guideline on treatment and management. NICE Clinical Guideline 178. [online] Available from: https://www.nice.org.uk/guidance/cg178/evidence/full-guideline-490503565 [Last accessed July, 2021].
23. Attard A, Larkin M. Art therapy for people with psychosis: a narrative review of the literature. Lancet Psychiatry. 2016;3(11):1067-78.
24. Crawford MJ, Killaspy H, Barnes TR, Barrett B, Byford S, Clayton K, et al. Group art therapy as an adjunctive treatment for people with schizophrenia: multicentre pragmatic randomized trial. BMJ. 2012;344:e846.
25. Galletly C, Castle D, Dark F, Humberstone V, Jablensky A, Killackey E, et al. Royal Australian and New Zealand College of Psychiatrists clinical practice guidelines for the management of schizophrenia and related disorders. Aust N Z J Psychiatry. 2016;50:410-72.
26. Deshmukh SR, Holmes J, Cardno A. Art therapy for people with dementia. Cochrane Database Syst Rev. 2018;9:CD011073.
27. Bruscia K. Standards for clinical assessment in the art therapies. The Art in Psychotherapy. 1988;15:5-10.
28. Malchiodi CA, Medical Art Therapy with Adults. London: Jessica Kingsley; 1999.
29. Wood M, Molassiotis A, Payne S. What research evidence is there for the use of art therapy in the management of symptoms in adults with cancer? A systematic review. Psycho-Oncology. 2011;20(2):135-45.
30. Christopher L. Out at the edge: Notes on a paradigm shift. Journal of Counseling and Development. 1985;64(3):165-72.
31. Ickovics JR, Park CL. Paradigm shift: why a focus on health is important. J Soc Issues. 1998;54(2):237-44.
32. Junge MB, Linesch D. Our own voices: new paradigm for art therapy research. Art Psychother. 1993;20:61-7.
33. Burt H. Art Therapy and Postmodernism: Creative Healing Through a Prism. London: Jessica Kingsley; 2012.
34. Elkins J. Visual Cultures. United Kingdom: Intellect Ltd.; 2010.
35. Bhattacharya D, Mallick A, Basu H, Banerjee Pal S, Ghosh S. Art therapy as an adjunctive treatment for adult psychiatry patients. Benefits in a multi-lingual and multi-cultural context. Presented at World Psychiatric Society Regional Conference, Kochi in September 2015.

CHAPTER 19

Interface with Law

Vinay B, Shashidhara HN, Suresh Bada Math

INTRODUCTION

Law is not only important for an orderly social life but also for the very existence of mankind by regulating the human behavior. In simple terms, law can be assumed as a system of coded rules and regulations, which a society recognizes it and empowers the authorities to enforce, and violation of which attracts pecuniary action. Law is a binding custom or practice of a community, a rule of conduct or action prescribed or formally recognized as binding or enforced by a controlling authority.[1] Legal system consists of a set of rules and norms to protect and promote a secure living for its citizens in a cultured society. The legal system ensures individual and collective rights, prescribes duties for everyone, and also provides for the ways and means of enforcing them. This law also provides protection to the person with mental illness and disability. Psychiatry is the medical specialty which involves the diagnosis, treatment, and prevention of mental, emotional, and behavioral disorders.[2]

Arboleda-Flórez defined "Forensic Psychiatry" as a branch of psychiatry that deals with the interface between psychiatry and the law. It not only deals with issues at the interface of criminal law but also with the matters arising out of civil law cases.[3] Further, the legal interface also plays a crucial role during the provision of services to person with mental illness, which may be related to professional negligence, deprivation of liberty during the height of mental illness, and safeguards enabled to protect and promote the rights of persons with mental illness during the provision of mental health services.

From the perspective of the persons with mental illness are particularly vulnerable to violation of their fundamental rights. Persons with mental illness are often deprived of their liberty, secluded, stigmatized, discriminated, and marginalized. They often end up wandering homeless mentally ill in the community or in the mental hospitals with increased likelihood of rights violation. If a protective mechanism such as mental health legislation is not in place, they can be susceptible to abuse by anyone in the society.

When a physician agrees to attend to a patient, there is an unwritten contract between the two. Contract can be defined as an agreement between two or more persons which creates an obligation to do or not to do a particular thing.[4] This contract may be expressed or implied in the form of consent. The patient entrusts himself/herself to the physician and the physician agrees to do his/her best. The doctor–patient contract is almost always an implied contract, unless intervention with significant risk is required, during which written informed consent is obtained. In the context of the doctor–patient relationship, the contract obligates the doctor to provide reasonable degree of care and skill, while maintaining the professional secrets and without undertaking any procedure beyond his skill.

Legislation forms an integral component in the implementation of mental health care; forming a dynamic mechanism between the mental illness, treatment of the mentally ill, and the law. The legislation is needed to protect against discrimination of persons with mental illness. As we look back into earlier days, mental health legislation aimed to safeguard members of the public from the perceived danger from the person with mental illness, which led to isolating them from the rest of the society, especially due to inadequate treatment facilities. However, over many decades, the field of psychiatry has seen much advancement with regard to understanding mental illness, assessment, treatment, psychosocial management along with revolution of the human rights movements which has led to significant change in the mental health legislation scenario **(Flowchart 1)**.

The Mental Health Care Act 2017 focuses more from the rights perspective and less from the treatment perspective. It also brings in a paradigm shift from collective rights to individual rights-based Act. The chapter presents a bird eye view of the interface of law and psychiatry with specific focus on the civil and criminal responsibilities along with clinical-related issues.

INTERFACE BETWEEN MENTAL ILLNESS AND THE LAW

Mental illness is defined as collectively all diagnosable mental disorders that are characterized by alterations in thinking, mood, or behavior (or some combination thereof) associated with distress and impaired biological-social-occupational functioning. There lies interface between these two entities (psychiatry and law), which are enormous fields, and these interact in numerous ways. The interface can be categorized into three domains, namely: (1) Law regulating psychiatry profession (mental healthcare services-related interface), (2) psychiatry profession assisting judiciary system in civil law-related interface, and (3) assisting judiciary system in criminal law-related interface **(Fig. 1)**.

Flowchart 1: The paradigm shift noted in the mental health legislations of India.

Indian Lunacy Act, 1912	
Prime concern: Protection of society from person with mental illness	*Limitation:* Custodial care of persons with mental illness

↓

Mental Health Act, 1987	
Prime concern: Treatment to persons with mental illness	*Limitation:* Proxy consent is valid under the Act

↓

Mental Healthcare Act, 2017	
Prime concern: Protecting the individual rights of the patient followed by treatment	*Limitation:* Undermines collective rights

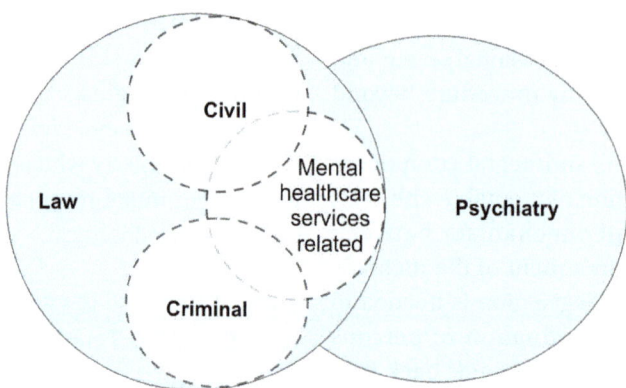

Fig. 1: Psychiatry and law interface.

Law Regulating Psychiatry Profession (Mental Healthcare Services/Clinical-related Interface)

The law governs mental health professionals in their clinical care delivery to safeguard the rights of the person with mental illness. Issues surrounding persons with mental illness in relation to law and mental healthcare services/clinical care are in the specific context of admission, consent, treatment, discharge, disability, rehabilitation, and community treatment. For instance, involuntary admission and treatment infringes on a person's fundamental rights—"Right to Life and Liberty" (Article 21 of the Constitution of India—no person shall be deprived of his life or personal liberty except according to procedure established by law). Courts have held that mental health legislation must impose only reasonable restriction in a least restrictive environment and the procedural law must be just and fair to the purpose of restricting the liberty of person with mental illness. Issues related to curtailing of liberty during admission and treatments are regulated by mental health legislation such as Mental Health Care Act 2017.[5]

Approaches to Mental Health Legislation

The approaches to the mental health legislations can be understood in different perspectives. Depending on the nature of coverage of the legislation, which are usually categorized into the following:[6]

- Consolidated single mental health legislation approach for dealing with persons with mental illness.
- Dispersed mental health rules and regulations approach. In this approach, there is no single legislation. Provisions related to mental health are implanted into various other relevant legislations.
- Combination of above approach.

The mental health legislation approaches in India are a combination approach, which appears to be better than either comprehensive or scattered approach. This mixed approach is facilitated by enacting mental health legislation, which deals effectively in admission, treatment, discharge, research, and protection of rights in a comprehensive legislation. Other relevant legal issues are related to criminal and civil issues in various other legislations. Law pertaining to health can also be understood by the concept and terminology of hard law and soft law. The soft law are referred as quasi-legal instruments (policy) that have no legal force, such as nonbinding resolutions, declarations, and guidelines created by governments and private organizations.[7] Hard law refers generally to legal obligations that are binding on the parties involved and which can be legally enforced before a court. With this regard, mental health legislation in India can be enlisted as follows:

- Hard laws pertaining to mental health legislation are Mental Health Care Act 2017; Rights of Persons with Disabilities Act 2016; The Juvenile Justice (Care and Protection of Children) Act 2015; Protection of Women from Domestic Violence Act 2005; National Trust for Welfare of Persons with Autism, Cerebral Palsy, Mental Retardation and Multiple Disabilities Act 1999; Narcotic Drugs and Psychotropic Substances Act 1985.
- Soft law pertaining to mental health legislation are mental health policy and mental health programs such as National Mental Health Policy 2014 and the National Mental Health Programme (with its operational arm, the District Mental Health Programme); National Programme on Non-communicable Diseases. Depending on the implication on person with mental illness, there are three varieties of legal interface such as:
  - *Legislations having direct implication*: Mental Health Care Act 2017;[5] Rights of Persons with Disabilities Act 2016;[8] National Trust for Welfare of Persons with Autism, Cerebral Palsy, Mental Retardation and Multiple Disabilities Act, 1999.[9]
  - *Legislations having indirect implication*: Narcotic Drugs and Psychotropic Substances Act 1985[10]; Protection of Women from Domestic Violence Act 2005[11]; The Juvenile Justice (Care and Protection of Children) Act 2015.[12]
  - *Legislations having general implication*: The Constitution of India,[13] The Protection of Human Rights Act 1993;[14] National Human Rights Commission, Criminal and Civil Code Procedures (Contract Law, Tort Law), Indian Penal Code (IPC), and case laws.

Mental Health Legislations in Mental Healthcare Services or Clinical Scenario

- Admission, treatment, and discharge are regulated in Section 86–90 chapter XII of the Mental Healthcare Act (MHCA) 2017. The admission is categorized into the following:
  - Admission of person with mental illness as independent patient (Section 85, 86, and 87)
  - Admission of person with mental illness as with high support needs (Section 89-Supported admission up to 30 days)
  - Admission of person with mental illness as with high support needs (Section 90-Supported admission beyond 30 days).
- *Emergency treatment*: In Section 94 of the chapter XII in MHCA 2017, it states that any medical treatment including treatment for mental illness provided by any registered medical practitioner to prevent death or irreversible harm to health of the person or in care of serious harm to self or others. The period of treatment in case of emergencies should be limited to 72 hours or till the person with mental illness has been assessed at a mental health establishment.
- The MHCA 2017 prohibits certain treatment or procedures on person with mental illness (Section 95, chapter XII) which are:
  - Electroconvulsive therapy without the use of muscle relaxants and anesthesia
  - Electroconvulsive therapy for minors
  - Sterilization of person with mental illness if it is intended as a treatment for mental illness
  - Chained in any manner.

- The MHCA 2017 in Section 96 restricts performance of psychosurgery for person with mental illness without informed consent and approval from the concerned board.
- The procedures such as seclusion or solitary confinement should not done, wherever such measures are required, only physical restraint can be used:
  - To prevent imminent and immediate harm to self or others
  - Should be authorized by psychiatrist in charge.
- The MHCA 2017 in case of attempt to commit suicide states in Section 115 that, unless proved otherwise it shall be presumed that the person having severe stress and shall not be tried and punished under IPC 309 but provide care, treatment, and rehabilitation to such person.

The Narcotic Drugs and Psychotropic Substances Act 1985 (NDPS Act 1985): The Narcotic Drugs and Psychotropic Substances Act 1985 is a law relating to narcotic drugs, to make stringent provisions for the control and regulation of manufacturing, transportation, selling, and using of narcotic drugs and psychotropic substances. The amended NDPS rules of 2015,[15] brought in paradigm shifts in the perspective of the legislation. Rule 52N of the amended rules gives all government hospitals shall be deemed to be a recognized medical institution. These recognized institutions need to have at least one registered medical practitioner possessing a minimum qualification of a degree in medicine or dentistry and who has undergone training in pain relief and palliative care for prescription of essential narcotic drugs for pain relief and palliative care or training in opioid substitution therapy.

The Indian Medical Council Act 1956 (102 of 1956): The Medical Council of India, with the previous approval of the Central Government, has notified regulations relating to Professional Conduct, Etiquette and Ethics for registered medical practitioners 2002 (Amended in 2016).[16] According to the Medical Council of India (MCI) Regulations 2002 guidelines:[16] Inpatient records should be maintained in a standard proforma for 3 years from commencement of treatment. If any request is made for medical records either by the patients/authorized attendant or legal authorities involved, the same may be duly acknowledged and documents shall be issued within the period of 72 hours. Also, to maintain a register of certificates with the full details of medical certificates issued with at least one identification mark of the patient and his signature. Further, the MHCA 2017 under Section 25 discusses about the "Right to basic medical records" for person with mental illness. Hence, mandates all mental health professionals to maintain basic medical records both for inpatient and outpatient.

Law in organ transplantation and role of psychiatrist: The Transplantation of Human Organs and Tissues Rules, 2014[17] mandates for every proposed live voluntary donor to undergo psychiatric evaluation by a psychiatrist to certify the applicant's mental condition, awareness, absence of any overt or latent psychiatric disease, and ability to give free consent.

Psychiatrist Assisting Judiciary System

Before we move on to the second aspect of interface, brief overview of civil and criminal law is put forward for better understanding. Civil law and criminal law serve different purposes in the legal system. The primary purpose of civil law is to resolve disputes and provide compensation for someone injured by someone else's acts or behavior. The primary purpose of criminal law is to prevent undesirable behavior and punish those who commit an act deemed to undesirable by the society.

In civil law, it is the injured person who brings the lawsuit. However, in criminal law, the government files charges. The injured person may file a complaint, but it is the government that decides whether criminal charges should be filed or not. A violation of criminal law is considered a crime against the state and is a violation of public law rather than private law. In some instances, a person may be entitled to file a complaint, trusting the legal system to punish the wrongdoer with prosecution, while bringing a civil lawsuit to receive compensation for the damages done by the wrongdoer.

Another key difference between civil and criminal law is the standards of proof required to reach a verdict. A plaintiff need only prove his civil law case by a "preponderance of evidence." This standard requires that the plaintiff convince the court that, based on the evidence presented at trial, it is "more likely than not" that the plaintiff's allegation is true.

In contrast, the standard of proof is higher in criminal law proceedings. The state must prove their case "beyond a reasonable doubt." The reason for this higher standard is because a person's freedom is at stake, and the fundamental belief that convicting an innocent person is worse than allowing a guilty person to go free. The psychiatry professional with relation to law interface (civil and criminal) requires specific skills, knowledge, and the ability to assist legal bodies in determining the significance of psychiatric issues.

Civil Law-related Interface

Civil law is defined as a body of rules that protects the private rights of citizens, offers legal remedies that may be sought in a dispute, and covers areas of law such as contracts, torts, property, and family law. In civil law, it revolves around the factors, which determine the capacity to perform particular function by the person with mental illness. Capacity refers to an assessment of the individual's psychological abilities to form rational decisions, specifically the individual's ability to understand, appreciate, and manipulate information and form rational decisions while competency is a legal term that refers to the mental ability and cognitive capabilities required to execute a legally recognized act rationally and it is a judicial decision.[18]

The interface of the professionals with the law will be with regard to assessing the individual's capacity to make decisions aiding the judicial system to decide on the competence of the individual in various civil cases such as:

- *Testamentary capacity*: The test for determining whether a person possesses testamentary capacity is well established and was set out by Cockburn CJ in Banks v Goodfellow.[19] In determining whether a testator has the capacity to make a will, the court laid out four broad criteria[20]: It is essential to the exercise of such a power that a testator shall:
  - Understand the nature of the act and its effects
  - Understand the extent of the property of which he is disposing
  - Be able to comprehend and appreciate the claims to which he ought to give effect
  - That no disorder of the mind shall poison his affections, pervert his sense of right, or prevent the exercise of his natural faculties—that no insane delusion shall influence his will in disposing of his property.[18,19]

Further, two more criteria were included for testamentary capacity as follows— intact cognitive function and the will to be executed in the absences of any coercion. Often, psychiatrist or a medical officer is called to assess the testamentary capacity of the person executing the will.

- *Marriage and divorce:* Family law is the branch of civil law that deals with marriage, divorce, annulment, child custody, maintenance, adoption, child support, and any other issues affecting families. Depending on religion of practice, various acts govern the marriage and divorce in India. Understanding the law governing marriage and divorce is crucial as it varies across the existing family laws. There are two questions with reference to the marriage. Is the marriage a valid one? Is it possible for the relationship to continue?

According to Hindu Marriage Act and Special Marriage Act, consent and understanding are essential legal requirements whether marriage is considered a contract or a sacrament. Marriage between two Hindus is not solemnized only if at the time of the marriage,[21,22] if neither party is incapable of giving a valid consent to it in consequence of mental illness. Although capable of giving consent but been suffering from mental illness of such a kind or extent by which individual unfit for fulfilling obligation of the marriage for 2 or more years. Further, other factors which need to be considered are: Attempts to treat the person with mental illness and the individual's response to treatment, both of which play a crucial role in determining the divorce or ability to fulfill the obligations of the marriage.

Under Muslim law, persons of unsound mind and minors can be validly contracted into marriage by their legal guardian. While in Parsi Law, mental illness is not a ground for nullity of the marriage but for divorce, it is similar to the Hindu Marriage Act.

Tort law: It is a branch of civil law that is concerned with personal injury and civil wrongdoing. Tort law deals with the remedies for civil wrongs, and frequently involves monetary compensation to the injured party. There are two categories of torts: Unintentional tort (negligence) and intentional tort.

Intentional tort: The classic intentional tort in medical practice is forcing unwanted medical care on a patient. Other intentional torts are assault, battery, fraud, invasion of privacy, and intentional infliction of emotional distress.

Unintentional tort: "Medical negligence" means breach of contract with regard to professional health services rendered. The standard of skill and care required of every healthcare provider in rendering professional services or health care to a patient shall be that degree of skill and care ordinarily employed in the same or similar field of medicine as defendant, and the use of reasonable care and diligence.[23] Cause of action for negligence arises only when damage occurs; for, damage is a necessary ingredient of this tort. Thus, the essential components of negligence are three: "duty," "breach," and "resulting damage." To succeed in proving liability, you need to prove that the doctor or nurse was negligent and acted in a manner that no other medical provider would have done. In the UK, there are two tests of liability: The Bolam test and the Bolitho test. The Bolam test was developed by the Bolam v Friern Hospital Management Committee,[24] an English tort law case that develops rules for assessing standards of reasonable care in negligence involving professionals. The test states that if doctors failed to reach the standard of a responsible body of medical opinion, they are negligent. In the Bolitho test, on the other hand, the court should not accept a defense argument as being "reasonable", "respectable", or "responsible" without first assessing whether such opinion is susceptible to logical analysis. In simple words, if a judge is not satisfied that the body of expert opinion cannot be logically supported at all. Aftermath of "Bolitho test", clinical negligence claims have become more difficult to defend because this test gives greater effects to judicial discretion when determining liability in medical negligence.

Criminal Law-related Interface

Criminal law is the body of law that relates to crime. *"Actus Non Facit Reum Nisi Mens Sit Rea"* is a Latin maxim which means that for an act to be illegal, the person should do it with a guilty mind.[25] In law, crime consists of two elements: Actus Reus (actual conduct) and Mens Rea (mental element of the act). Conviction of a crime requires proof of a criminal act and intent. With regards to person with mental illness implicated in criminal law, the role of the psychiatrist will be in assessing the case for the fitness to stand trial and in case of insanity plea, psychiatrists are often called for conducting mental health evaluations and providing treatment.

Insanity plea: Insanity plea is a defense by excuse in a criminal case, arguing that the defendant is not responsible for his or her actions due to an episodic or persistent psychiatric disease at the time of the criminal act. In India under Section 84 of the IPC (IPC ACT 45 of 1860) states that *"nothing is an offence, which is done by a person, who at the time of doing it, by reason of unsoundness of mind, is incapable of knowing the nature of the act or that he is doing what is either wrong or contrary to law."*[26]

The court of law is concerned with the legal insanity not in the medical insanity. Any person, who is suffering from any kind of mental illness, is called "medical insanity," however "legal insanity" means person suffering from mental illness should also have a loss of reasoning power.[27]

As noted in case of Bapu @ Gajraj Singh vs. State of Rajasthan in Supreme Court, mere abnormality of mind or partial delusion, irresistible impulse or compulsive behavior of a psychopath affords no protection under Section 84 IPC.[28] To establish insanity plea under Section 84, the burden of proof lies with the person with mental illness and requires establishing that:

- The person was suffering from mental illness during the commission of crime
- The person was not aware of the nature of the act
- The person was not aware of the consequence of the act
- The person was not aware that act was wrong or contrary to the law.[28]

Psychiatrists may be asked to assist the court in determining whether accused was suffering from mental illness, and that mental disorders affected a person's capacity or he/she had the clear intent and making him/her legally culpable.

Fitness to stand trial: Person with mental illness may incapacitate their cognitive, emotional, and behavioral faculties. A person with mental illness may not be in a position to defend his case. If a person is suffering mental illness and not in a position to defend his case, the court will postpone the proceedings of the case and they will be referred to treatment.

Person with mental illness is said to fit for trial if:

- Has the ability to understand and to respond rationally
- Is aware of the charge and the consequences of the charges if proven guilty
- Has the ability to assist the lawyer to defend the case
- Has understanding in the procedure of the court

- Demonstrates expected behavior in the court.

The standard for determining whether a person is fit to stand trial is in fact a very low one when compared to previous one where the standard for proving that a person was insane when an offense was committed is usually a high one.

Subpoenas and Expert Witness

Subpoenas: A subpoena or witness summons is a legal document, usually issued by the clerk of a court, which requests that a party (e.g., a psychiatrist) does one of the two things: Provide documents or appear and give testimony. Subpoenas are usually issued by the clerk of the court in the name of the judge presiding over the case.

On receiving the subpoena, one should[29] not ignore it. A subpoena is part of a court's legal process. The nature of subpoena determines whether it requires production of records, the appearance of the therapist in court, or both. Subpoenas are formal legal documents that should be taken seriously. A person who receives a request for the production of documents or a request to appear in court should take the necessary steps to comply with the demand sought. Failure to comply with a subpoena order may result in contempt of court charges.

Expert witness: An expert witness is a person whose opinion by virtue of education, training, certification, skills, or experience is accepted by the judge as an expert. The Indian Evidence Act under Section 45[30] enumerates the law relating to opinion of experts or commonly known as expert opinion/expert evidence. The definition of an expert may be referred from the provision of Section 45 of Indian Evidence Act that an "expert" means a person who has special knowledge, skill, or experience in any of the following: Foreign law, science, art, handwriting or finger impression, and such knowledge has been gathered by him by practice, observation, or proper studies. Duty of the expert would not be as a witness of fact but to depose his evidence as an advisory character with necessary scientific criteria for testing the accuracy of the conclusion so as to enable the judge to form his independent judgment by application of the criteria to the facts proved by the evidence.

The court may summon a psychiatrist to testify as either a "fact witness," or an "expert witness."[31] An expert witness as per definition who has special knowledge that the average person may not possess may testify in the form of an opinion about facts directly related to the profession of psychiatry whereas a fact witness testify about direct observations such as treating psychiatrist testifying about his or her patients illness and treatment.

ROLE OF JUDICIARY IN PROTECTING RIGHTS OF THE PERSON WITH MENTAL ILLNESS

A person with mental illness is entitled to treatment with the same dignity and decency as any other human being. A mentally ill person does not become a nonperson merely on account of certain disabilities. Persons with mental health illness are exposed to a range of human rights violations[32] which can occur inside institutions, through inadequate and harmful care and treatment, but also outside, with people experiencing stigma, discrimination, and limitation to the exercise of civil liberties and rights. The Apex and High Courts are thus inevitably called upon to consider cases of violation of fundamental rights of persons with mental illness. The judiciary roles pertaining to protection of rights of the person with mental illness are noted in the following cases:

- *Sheela Barse (II) and Others vs. Union of India and others,*[33] *filed under:* Articles 21 and 32 of the Constitution of India.
- *Sheela Barse vs. Union of India,*[34] *filed under:* Article 21 and 32 of the Constitution of India; Mental Health Act, 1987; Mental Health Authority Rules, 1990; Section 13 of the Lunacy Act 1912.
- *RD Upadhyay vs. State of AP and others,*[35] *filed under:* Articles 21 and 32, Constitution of India.
- Rakesh Chandra Narayan v. State of Bihar 1989 AIR 348,[36] 1988 SCR Supl. (3) 306, "In a welfare State—and we take it that the State of Bihar considers itself to be one such—it is the obligation of the State to provide medical attention to every citizen. Running of the mental hospital, therefore, is in the discharge of the State's obligation to the citizens..."

CONCLUSION

Psychiatric and legal approaches toward the persons with mental illness have changed over time and will undoubtedly be changed in future. This interface between law and psychiatry is a specialized branch of psychiatry which deals with the assessment and treatment of persons with mental illness. From the perspective of the persons with mental illness are particularly vulnerable to abuse and violation of their fundamental rights. If a protective mechanism is not in place, they can be susceptible to abuse by anyone in the society. Legislation is an important mechanism to ensure appropriate, adequate, timely and humane healthcare services. Further, it also plays crucial role in upholding the rights of the persons with mental illness.

REFERENCES

1. Merriam-Webster. Definition of Law. [online] Available from: https://www.merriam-webster.com/dictionary/law. [Last accessed April 2022].
2. American Psychiatric Association. What is psychiatry? [online] Available from: https://www.psychiatry.org/patients-families/what-is-psychiatry. [Last accessed April 2022].
3. Arboleda-Flórez J. Forensic psychiatry: contemporary scope, challenges and controversies. World Psychiatry. 2006;5(2):87-91.
4. Contract LII/Legal Information Institute. (2007). Staff LII. [online] Available from: https://www.law.cornell.edu/wex/contract. [Last accessed April 2022].
5. Mental Healthcare Act, 2017. [online] Available from: http://www.prsindia.org/uploads/media/Mental%20Health/Mental%20Healthcare%20Act,%202017.pdf. [Last accessed April 2022].
6. World Health Organization. (2003). Mental health legislation and human rights. (Mental Health Policy and Service Guidance Package). [online] Available from: http://www.who.int/mental_health/policy/services/7_legislation%20HR_WEB_07.pdf. [Last accessed April 2022].
7. Druzin BH. Why does soft law have any power anyway? Asian J Int Law. 2017;7(02):361-78.
8. Rights of Persons with Disabilities Act, 2016. [online] Available from: http://www.disabilityaffairs.gov.in/upload/uploadfiles/files/RPWD%20ACT%202016.pdf. [Last accessed April 2022].
9. National Trust for the Welfare of Persons with Autism, Cerebral Palsy, Mental Retardation and Multiple Disabilities Act, 1999. [online] Available from: http://thenationaltrust.gov.in/upload/uploadfiles/files/act-englsih.pdf. [Last accessed April 2022].
10. Narcotic Drugs and Psychotropic Substances Act, 1985. [online] Available from: https://indiacode.nic.in/bitstream/123456789/1791/1/198561.pdf. [Last accessed April 2022].
11. Protection of Women from Domestic Violence Act, 2005. [online] Available from: http:// ncw.nic.in/acts/TheProtectionofWomen from DomesticViolenceAct2005.pdf. [Last accessed April 2022].
12. Juvenile Justice (Care and Protection of Children) Act, 2015. [online] Available from: http://wcd.nic.in/sites/default/files/JJ%20Act%2C%202015%20_0.pdf. [Last accessed April 2022].
13. The Constitution of India. [online] Available from: http://www.legislative.gov.in/sites/default/files/COI-updated-as-31072018.pdf. [Last accessed April 2022].
14. The Protection of Human Rights Act, 1993 [online] Available from: http://nhrc.nic.in/sites/default/files/PHRA_Bilingual_2018.pdf. [Last accessed April 2022].

15. Narcotic Drugs and Psychotropic Substances (Third Amendment) Rules, 2015. [online] Available from: https://pharmexcil.com/uploadfile/ufiles/NarNot05_0515sl06.pdf. [Last accessed April 2022].
16. The Indian Medical Council (Professional conduct, Etiquette and Ethics) Regulations, 2002. [online] Available from: https://www.mciindia.org/documents/rulesAndRegulations/Ethics%20Regulations-2002.pdf. [Last accessed April 2022].
17. The Transplantation of Human Organs and Tissues Rules, 2014. [online] Available from: https://mohfw.gov.in/sites/default/files/THOA-Rules-2014%20%281%29.pdf. [Last accessed April 2022].
18. Leo RJ. Competency and the capacity to make treatment decisions: a primer for primary care physicians. Prim Care Companion J Clin Psychiatry. 1999;1(5):131-41.
19. Banks v Goodfellow [1870] 5 LR QB 549. [online] Available from: https://www.lexiswebinars.co.uk/legal/hot-topics/vulnerable-clients/supporting-materials/Banks-v-Goodfellow.PDF. [Last accessed April 2022].
20. Shulman KI, Himel SG, Hull IM, Amodeo S, Barnes C. BANKS V GOODFELLOW (1870): TIME TO UPDATE THE TEST FOR TESTAMENTARY CAPACITY. 1870;95:17.
21. The Hindu Marriage Act, 1955. [online] Available from: https://highcourtchd.gov.in/hclscc/subpages/pdf_files/4.pdf. [Last accessed April 2022].
22. The Special Marriage Act, 1954. [online] Available from: http://keralaregistration.gov.in/pearlpublic/downloads/The%20Special%20Marriage%20Act.pdf?tok=49sddh3ss34ff4. [Last accessed April 2022].
23. The Delaware Code. Title 18. Insurance Code, Chapter 68. Health-care Medical Negligence-insurance and Litigation. available online at https://delcode.delaware.gov/title18/c068/sc01/index.html[Last accessed on 03 May 2022].
24. Bolam v Friern Hospital Management Committee [1957] 1 W.L.R. 582. [online] Available from: https://www.lawteacher.net/cases/bolam-v-friern-hospital-management.php. [Last accessed April 2022].
25. Actus Reus Non Facit Reum Nisi Mens Sit Rea Definition [online] Available from: http://www.duhaime.org/LegalDictionary/A/ActusReusNonFacitReumNisiMensSitRea.aspx
26. The Indian Penal Code, 1860. [online] Available from: http://ncw.nic.in/acts/theindianpenalcode1860.pdf. [Last accessed April 2022].
27. Math SB, Kumar CN, Moirangthem S. Insanity defense: past, present, and future. Indian J Psychol Med. 2015;37(4):381-7.
28. Bapu @ Gajraj Singh vs State Of Rajasthan on 4 June, 2007. [online] Available from: https://indiankanoon.org/doc/673880/. [Last accessed April 2022].
29. Mossman D. 'You've been served': What to do if you receive a subpoena. [online] Available from: https://www.mdedge.com/psychiatry/article/104566/practice-management/youve-been-served-what-do-if-you-receive-subpoena. [Last accessed April 2022].
30. The Indian Evidence Act, 1872. [online] Available from: http://ncw.nic.in/acts/THEINDIANEVIDENCEACT1872.pdf. [Last accessed April 2022].
31. Being an Effective Psychiatric Expert Witness | Psychiatric Times [online] Available from: http://www.psychiatrictimes.com/risk-assessment/being-effective-psychiatric-expert-witness. [Last accessed April 2022].
32. Agarwal SP, Goel DS, (Eds). Mental health: An Indian perspective, 1946-2003. New Delhi: Published for Directorate General of Health Services, Ministry of Health & Family Welfare. Gurugram: Elsevier; 2004. p. 532.
33. Sheela Barse vs. Union of India, (1993) 4 Supreme Court Cases 24. [online] Available from: https://indiankanoon.org/doc/451948/. [Last accessed April 2022].
34. Sheela Barse (II) and Others vs. Union of India and others, (1986) 3 Supreme Court Cases 632. [online] Available from: https://indiankanoon.org/doc/525548/. [Last accessed April 2022].
35. R.D. Upadhyay vs. State of A.P. and others, (2001) 1 Supreme Court Cases 437. [online] Available from: https://indiankanoon.org/doc/1258611/. [Last accessed April 2022].
36. Rakesh Chandra Narayan v. State of Bihar 1989 AIR 348. [online] Available from: https://indiankanoon.org/doc/1505647/. [Last accessed April 2022].

CHAPTER 20

Interface with Parapsychology

PK Singh

INTRODUCTION

The interface of psychiatry with parapsychology must be examined objectively and rationally because they both deal with experiences which are out of the ordinary and are therefore, either deviant or different. They are of great theoretical as well as practical value because it is incumbent upon the therapist to decide as to when, how and how much to intervene to bring relief to the suffering individual in great mental distress and consequential dysfunction and danger. Psychiatry has so far associated itself only with the disciplines of psychology, neurophysiology, sociology, and a few others. Parapsychology has so far remained completely marginalized, even though it deals quite intimately with the phenomena that psychiatry deals with. Parapsychology does not find a place even in the standard textbooks of Psychiatry. A major basic difference between the two should be understood. Parapsychology deals with paranormal experiences, whereas psychiatry deals with abnormal experiences. Paranormal refers to experience of real events and entities through unknown channels whereas abnormal refers to experience of nonexistent events and entities through seemingly known channels. This provides the rationale for examining the interface between psychiatry and parapsychology. The first step would be not to dismiss it straightway or to consider it psychopathic by default.

DEFINITIONS

Psychiatry is a medical discipline which deals with the study of causes and treatment of mental disorders. Psychology is the scientific study of behavior and experience. Parapsychology refers to supposedly scientific study of behavior and experience which manifest independent of or without subservience to the known laws of space, time, and causality. Paranormal phenomena are also referred to as Psi phenomena. From a purist perspective, parapsychology should also be considered an integral part of psychology itself because paranormal experiences also find their expression through the medium of mind only, which is in the domain of psychology.

Parapsychology is divided into two main branches: (1) extrasensory perception (ESP) which is the study of communications ostensibly without participation of the known sensory organs and (2) psychokinesis or the study of physical events that apparently occur without involvement of any recognized motor organs.[1] Parapsychology has gained wider recognition primarily because of JB Rhine's pioneering work in experimental parapsychology at the laboratory of Duke University where researchers successfully used statistical tools to demonstrate that psychic phenomena are dormant in ordinary people, and not necessarily confined to people who overtly demonstrate such gifts.[2] It was only after his contributions that this word has gained access in common parlance.

DIFFERENCES

Most of the things in this universe are more similar than different, which obviously will depend on the perspective from which we are examining the said entities. The same applies more appropriately to psychiatry and parapsychology also. As has been mentioned earlier, there may be phenomenological similarities between parapsychological experiences and psychiatric conditions. However, with adequate knowledge and training a detailed evaluation would show that the two conditions are entirely different and require different approaches to deal with. A psychiatrist who is not open-minded about the possibility of paranormal experiences will almost certainly be unable to distinguish psychopathological from paranormal and equally unable to assist the occasional person who is perplexed about unusual paranormal experiences, that he would like to report and discuss with someone outside his family.[1] Unless and until more and more professional attention by larger and larger number of mental health workers is given to the possibility of encountering the generally fleeting parapsychological events in their day to day clinical and paraclinical works, the expansion of this interface and emergence of newer relevant insights would not occur. Parapsychological entities have not found any formal place in any of the nosological systems of psychiatry.

Certain points which can help in differentiating between paranormal experiences and psychopathological states of mind have been mentioned in the literature, which can help in differential diagnosis of various psychiatric conditions. Points of differentiation[1] are as follows:

- The difference lies in the correspondence between the content of the claimed experience and independently verifiable occurrence of that event at a distant place. The details of parapsychological experiences correspond with an actual event whereas hallucinations or delusions of psychotic patients do not.
- Paranormal experiences usually last for a few minutes and rarely recur or do so only infrequently whereas psychopathological events occur on a sustained basis and recur quite frequently.
- Paranormal exper iences are more commonly visual than auditory, psychopathological hallucinations on the other hand are more auditory than visual.
- Patients experiencing psychopathological hallucinations are usually strongly convinced of their reality and have no interest in having them verified while this is not so with people having paranormal experiences.
- Similarly, psychopathological delusions have no relation with reality but are expressed and experienced with inflexible conviction associated at times with inappropriate emotions.

Paranormal experiences do not always have a pathological significance. It has been part of anecdotal personal experience of many.

INTERFACE

The famous psychiatrist and philosopher Karl Jaspers, in his book General Psychopathology (Jaspers, 1913/1997), stated that all claimed paranormal phenomena could really only be manifestations of psychiatric symptoms. However, later advances of Psi research based on scientific protocols and the resultant changes in epistemology of parapsychology that occurred in the 19th and 20th century, modified to some marginal extent at least, psychiatrists' opinions about Psi phenomena.[3]

It has been opined that "parapsychology helps us to develop a deeper understanding of mind, affording us fresh insights into psychopathology. A notable example is that it enables analysis of near-death experiences (NDEs), assisting in the study of the process of dying and it also illuminates the inner psychological life of the individual. Survival research has notable usefulness on account of its applicability in counseling grieving families and helping suicidal patients. Furthermore, it is relevant in a number of issues that are currently matters of debate, such as euthanasia. Parapsychology can also function as an effective mediator between religion and psychiatry. It is conceivable that it may assist in the testing out of some of the contentious aspects of religious belief."[2]

VARIETY

A variety of different types of paranormal phenomena have been described in different types of literature from time immemorial and surprisingly in almost all cultures and countries of the world. Some of the major types are given here.

Telepathy

Telepathy refers to mind-to-mind communication through means other than the normal senses. The apparent communication between two minds without the use of known sensory channels was initially called "thought transference" and later came to be known as telepathy. Telepathic communications usually occur between persons who share a bond of affection or love. Such experiences most commonly have been reported among members of the same family and close friends; marital partners experience telepathic communications as frequently as do members of the same biological families. In other words, the bond between the persons concerned is emotional rather than physical or genetic one. Sometimes even physical symptoms have been reported to be precipitated by telepathic communications. Apart from family members and close friends, a few psychiatrists have reported telepathic links with their patients. Jung has reported to having unexpectedly experienced severe headache when his patient shot himself in the head.[1]

Precognition

Precognition refers to knowledge of an event that has not yet occurred, or information that appears to have been transferred from the future into the present. In this form of ESP, an individual experiences awareness of future events in the absence of the possibility of having access to any kind of source of rational inference. It may occur while awake or in dream and vary in the quantum of precise details perceived about the future event. Precognitive experiences are usually unpleasant when they occur and are generally concerned with accidents, deaths, or other disastrous events. This may lead to severe distress, depression, and sometimes to marked guilt feelings due to irrational self-blame. This has both diagnostic and therapeutic implications. Precognition per se may not be pathogenic. On the contrary, there are a number of instances recorded in the literature which show that because of these experiences some persons were forewarned of the impending dangers and could be saved from them and hence may be regarded to serve an adaptive function.[1]

Retrocognition is a related phenomenon wherein individual displays the knowledge of a past event that could not have been learnt or inferred by normal means.

Clairvoyance

Clairvoyance or Remote viewing refers to knowledge of objects, people, or events that are hidden via space or time. For example, an object hidden in a box in a different room, a photograph sealed in an envelope, an event that is occurring to a loved one who is thousands of miles away, or the characteristics of a room that only existed in the past.

Psychokinesis

Psychokinesis or telekinesis is an alleged psychic ability allowing a person to influence a physical system without physical interaction. It is like mind interacting with matter at a distance without an intervening physical link. The word "psychokinesis" was coined in 1914 by an American author Henry Holt in his book "On the Cosmic Relations".[4] On closer scrutiny, it appears that some phenomena very similar to psychokinesis is constantly in operation within the mind-brain system of every individual. The nonphysical component of the mind influences the brain through "internal psychokinesis" to allow the execution of voluntary motor actions and various executive mental functions. Every time we decide to carry out a task or speak out a thought, this phenomenon of mind acting upon the matter, takes place. Even though qualitatively and contextually different, it is also a kind of psychokinesis. Paranormal healing or faith healing is also sometimes included in this category.

Reincarnation

Reincarnation is one example of the survival of consciousness in a disembodied or discarnate form. Other examples of paranormal survival of consciousness even after death of physical form are apparitions, NDEs, out-of-body experiences (OBEs), ghost activities including poltergeist phenomena and mediumship phenomena.

Spontaneous cases of reincarnation, mostly seen in children, have been repeatedly observed and reported from almost all cultures and countries of the world. Nearly 2,600 reported cases of the reincarnation type have been scientifically investigated in several cultures over the past about five decades. In 64–80% cases, a deceased person matching the statements of child was identified. Cross-cultural comparisons have shown that certain features recur across cultures, which are: age of speaking about a previous life (between 2 and 4 years), age of discontinuation of talk about previous life (usually between 5 and 8 years), high incidence of violent death (63%) of the previous personality, far beyond the rate of violent death in the general populations of the respective countries, and high frequency of mention, by the subjects, of mode of death (78%) in the previous life, other features such as sex change and intermission between two lives vary between cultures.[1]

However, no case should be taken as a case of reincarnation type without carefully excluding normal and paranormal explanations. The phobias and philias of infancy, unusual play in early childhood, a child's idea of having parents other than its own or nonacceptance of parents, differences in temperament manifested soon after birth, unusual birthmarks and their correspondence with wounds on a deceased person, unusual birth defects, cognitive, physical and behavioral differences between monozygotic twins reared together, gender identity disorder, and similar disorders or abnormalities reported in psychology, child psychiatry or medicine that cannot be explained in terms of known influences of genetics or environment, either alone or in combination might find an explanation in the hypothesis of reincarnation.[1]

Apparitions

"A visual appearance, usually manifesting only once or rarely, which suggests the presence of a deceased person or animal or of a living person or animal not within the sensory range of the percipient. Such communications are perceived in visual and auditory modalities and occur usually in a state of altered consciousness. A considerable number of authentic cases have been documented wherein images (apparitions) of persons in crisis have been perceived by their close relatives or friends."[1]

Near-death Experiences

Many people when they are close to death, report later on, that they had undergone profound, transcendent experience of having moved out of their body and the ordinary constraints of time and space.

"Although NDEs occur to psychologically healthy individuals, they have been mistaken for psychopathological conditions." NDEs have been compared with depersonalization, autoscopy, psychoactive substance-induced hallucinations, post-traumatic stress disorder, and brief psychotic disorder. Regardless of their cause, the after effects of NDEs have been, by and large, beneficial to the experiencers in personal growth in the form of increased spirituality, generosity and concern for others, decrease in fear of death and forgiveness.[1]

Out-of-body Experiences (OBEs)

An OBE is an experience that typically involves a feeling of floating outside one's body and, in some cases, the feeling of perceiving one's physical body as if from a place outside one's body (autoscopy). OBEs can be induced by brain traumas, sensory deprivation, NDEs, dissociative and psychedelic drugs, dehydration, sleep, and electrical stimulation of the brain, among others. It can also be deliberately induced by some. One in ten people have an OBE once, or more commonly, several times in their life.

Neuroscientists and psychologists regard OBEs as dissociative experiences arising from different psychological and neurological factors.

Poltergeists

This German word literally means a "noisy ghost". It refers to a type of ghost or other supernatural entity which is responsible for physical disturbances, such as loud noises and objects being moved or destroyed.[4] "Such occurrences have been reported even in ancient literature. However, in the past century, a number of authentic cases have been recorded by the investigators of such phenomena that they were able to witness themselves, at first hand."[1]

VALIDITY

Future of parapsychology will depend on whether or not the issue of validity for paranormal phenomena gets unquestionably established in a manner that is comparable to the definitiveness of scientific methods. A considerable number of cases of paranormal experiences have been carefully investigated, found authentic by independent investigators, and published in the scientific books and journals of high standards. Suffice it to say that enough evidence is available on the authenticity of the phenomena to understand its relevance to psychiatry. Independent surveys of general populations have shown that between 10 and 15% of persons reported having had communications from persons not in contact with them; perception of such communications generally occurs in visual or auditory modalities. Such visions usually occur during an altered state of consciousness (dozing or daydreaming) and the person perceived is usually a close relative or a friend in a crisis or stressful situation, often in a life-threatening situation. Some of the persons having such experiences may be confused or perplexed.[1]

The issue of validity applies also to psychiatric categories. The validity of nearly all nosological psychiatric categories remain to be established. However, there has been good progress as far reliability in identifying these categories is concerned. Parapsychological entities have difficulty with both validity and reliability in terms of replicability. However, both psychiatry and parapsychology deal with entities which are not amenable to direct observation in the same way that other worldly and natural phenomena are available to sensory cognition.

The argument of theoretical implausibility of paranormal phenomena gets contradicted by the observations of the modern physics subsumed under the rubric "Paraphysics". "The view held by classical physicists that two objects cannot occupy the same space at the same time has given way to the observations made by Klauber that two subatomic particles can exist together just as two waves rolling over the ocean heading in opposite directions and passing through each other unhindered, occupy the same area of water surface for a time."[2] This generates the stage for possible theoretical acceptance of coexistence of material brain and subtle mind within the same space. The discovery of physical properties of Neutrino and similar other subatomic particle has raised the hope that the Physics of subatomic particle might provide answers to at least some of the mysteries of mind and may be of other occult phenomena. To understand this, one has to go back to the era of discovery of X-rays for which Roentgen was awarded Nobel Prize in 1901. For the first time in history of mankind, people came to know that there are rays which can cross through human flesh and cast shadow of his bones on a photographic plate. This was miraculous at that point of time but it was very much within the laws of nature. The relevance and utility of X-rays continues to be maintained even after more than a century. It is possible therefore that there may be subtler rays and particles with other more differentiated functions. "Trillions of neutrinos are passing through one's body every second and yet no one is able to detect them. They pass through matter virtually without our being aware of their presence. One can only imagine the existence of similar unknown particles not coupling with physical fields, constituting other worlds coexisting with ours. The right-handed electrons and quarks have been proven to exist. Thus, there may be a variety of neutrino-like particles, in the sense that they are tenuous and imperceptible and it may be conjectured that the extracerebral component of the 'mind stuff' may be partly or fully composed of such diverse particles. Our bodies are made up of leptons and quarks, unobservable with the present-day instrumentation. Subtle realms may be made of such 'particle families', coexisting with our physical world without our being aware of their existence. Thus, extra dimensions have been postulated based on elementary-particle physics evidence and the possibility of our consciousness drifting over to other dimensions has been speculated."[2]

Inspired by the shadow matter theory of astrophysics, Wassermann proposed a shadow matter theory for living beings as having a twin body made of heavier "Matter Proper" along with lighter "Shadow Matter". Given that the density of Shadow Matter universe is much less than the ordinary matter, the shadow matter body is immensely lighter than ordinary matter body. According to this theory, every quark in the nucleus of an atom can bind a corresponding shadow matter quark. So, also every electron can bind a shadow matter electron. From this hypothesis, it follows that every atom made up of quarks and electron can bind a shadow matter atom. Our ordinary matter brain will have a corresponding shadow matter brain bonded with the ordinary brain. The binding force of shadow matter body and physical body is supposed to be the gravitational force.[2] The subtler shadow matter brain may be the bearer of mental functions. The "new" physics may bring in more answers for the psychiatric patient in future than their modern doctors of science have today. Therefore, all the possibilities that the validity of paranormal experiences may get established as a natural or supernatural phenomena have not exhausted as yet.

Carl Jung, who was deeply interested in parapsychological events, has described the collective unconscious, which serves as man's repository for all history's archetypes. He comments in "Psychology and the Occult" (1977) that "anyone who has the least knowledge of the parapsychological material which already exists and has been thoroughly verified will know that so-called telepathic phenomena are undeniable facts". He describes how synchronicity occurred in his own life and served to guide him to his discoveries, very much like those Nobel Prize winning physicists noted in Koestler's book "The Roots of Coincidence", who believed they had been guided to answer scientific problems via synchronistic events, even while attempting to discern the phenomena "scientifically".[5] Jung coined the word "synchronicity" to describe "temporally coincident occurrences of acausal events". The theory of synchronicity is culmination of Jung's lifelong engagement with paranormal phenomena.[4]

CRITICISM

Just as there are strong and committed believers in the reality of paranormal phenomenon, there are equally strong critics and opponents of this concept, who consider this whole area as full of fraud and deception. Many doyens and stalwarts of parapsychology were found to be resorting to deception as reported by a few other authors. However, there are also many die-hard and honest believers who are committed on the basis of personal experience and anecdotal evidences.

All such criticisms of parapsychology must be understood against the backdrop that one of the basic flaws of science of parapsychology and also psychology is that it applies the methods of scientific investigation to a field where it is not strictly applicable. Scientific methods are applicable to observable phenomenon. Neither Mind nor Psi are phenomena which are observable in the traditional sense by the perceptual apparatus.

The philosopher Raimo Tuomela has summarized as to why much of parapsychology is considered a pseudoscience in his essay "Science, Protoscience, and Pseudoscience":[6]

- Parapsychology relies on an ill-defined ontology and typically shuns exact thinking.
- The hypotheses and theories of parapsychology have not been proven and are in bad shape.
- Extremely little progress has taken place in parapsychology on the whole and parapsychology conflicts with established science.
- Parapsychology has poor research problems, being concerned with establishing the existence of its subject matter and having practically no theories to create proper research problems.
- While in parts of parapsychology there are attempts to use the methods of science there are also unscientific areas; and in any case parapsychological research can at best qualify as prescientific because of its poor theoretical foundations.
- Parapsychology is a largely isolated research area.

One very important criticism of this field is the lack of predictability and replicability of paranormal phenomena. However, lack of predictability should not be taken as foolproof evidence for lack of validity. It simply indicates that the phenomenon cannot be brought under predictable voluntary control. There are many other normally available human abilities which are not under strict voluntary control, such as creativity and innovativeness. They are different from the "standard" psychological phenomena or processes such as attention, perception, or memory. Creativity cannot be commanded at will. It is a transcendental expression based on inspiration. It is possible therefore that glimpses of paranormal experiences that many reasonable people authentically report, may actually be true and valid. The subtle phenomenon of Psi cannot be brought down to the level of crude matter. Across the whole of science, rates of successful replications are relatively low. According to one 1994 survey, the success rate for replication across all social and physical sciences was only 41%. In other words, it appears that the replication criteria applied to ESP experiments are unduly harsh.[7]

The mental and the material are qualitatively different and therefore cannot be measured by the same yardstick. They are likely to exhibit different properties and characteristics. Taken together also, they cannot be conceptualized to represent the whole truth. It would be irrational therefore to assume that human beings have an objective and complete awareness of total reality, and that there are no natural laws or phenomena or forces beyond those we can presently detect or conceive of.[7]

IMPLICATIONS

Scientists and philosophers have both ventured to conjecture on the nature of mind from time immemorial but have not made any progress of such nature that can be understood by people of all pursuits of knowledge. The moment we accept that parapsychic phenomena are valid and real, we lay the foundation of its relevance to psychiatry.[8-10] Acknowledgment of the validity of paranormal phenomenon will very fundamentally change the mindset and explanatory models of psychiatrists as they will not jump to inference of psychopathology at every mention of paranormal experience. Their schemas of conclusion will allow them to accept that so-called paranormal experiences might at times be experiences of normal people with normal mental processes. Examination of the interface with parapsychology is likely to be the most fertile interface to explore from the point of innovations and breakthrough to understand the mysteries of mind.

"It is important to emphasize that when an individual with Psi abilities lives in a culture that may not believe in or recognize his claimed paranormal or otherwise exceptional experiences, this rejection may cause him to react in several ways. The experiment may deny his own experiences and consciously or unconsciously suppress them; this may lead to a variety of compensatory behaviors. The subject may become distressed due to social rejection. This, again, may interfere with his functioning and manifest itself with anxiety or other neurotic features and, at the same time, he may find his subjective experience quite difficult to handle. Therefore, he may become uncertain as to whether his experiences are indeed real or just a figment of his imagination. This may disturb his reality testing, since he does not have anything that he might compare personal experiences with. Consequently, Psi experiences could potentially precipitate into psychiatric diseases, into psychosis in particular. In some ways, a personal Psi experience can variously produce fear of insanity due to the misunderstanding of one's subjective experiences that leads to a morbid preoccupation with psychic experiences, feelings of isolation, psychosomatic symptoms, anxiety, and affective disorders."[3]

FUTURE

Future is full of immense potentials emanating out of this interface between psychiatry and parapsychology.[9,10] Only a few centuries ago, psychiatry was not a known branch of science even though psychiatric phenomena were described millennia ago. Parapsychology too is poised for a leap. In the 1970s, this field of research was known as Metapsychiatry. With increasing validation of parapsychology as an acknowledged and established branch of knowledge, the doors would be flung wide open for completely new, integrated and comprehensive nosology for psychiatric conditions, for clinical parapsychology, for parapsychopharmacology, for parapsychological counseling and psychotherapy, for interfacing with spiritual therapy, prayer healing, faith healing and many more which hitherto fall in the despicable basket of occult and magic. One of course must be honest, selective, and objective.

CONCLUSION

However, it should be kept in mind that although it is important to be alert to the possibility of paranormal experiences being presented independently or as an integral or coexistent part of other psychopathologies, the psychiatrists should be extremely careful in evaluation of such experiences. Because there may be boasters, braggers, and imposters presenting or claiming credit for pseudoparanormal experiences. Satwant Pasricha summarizes that parapsychology is relevant to psychiatry in the following spheres: First, its knowledge would assist mental health professionals in differentiating paranormal experiences from psychopathological phenomena leading to adequate treatment strategies. Second, it would enhance understanding of certain medical, psychological, and psychiatric disorders that cannot be explained in terms of currently available theories of the genetic or environmental influences. Third, it would facilitate advancement of knowledge in brain/mind relationship.[1] Furthermore, this is the best way to emphasize the wholeness of mental health and the deep value of considering the patient as a full human being even if he or she has a paranormal experience. This is a very important starting point for the emerging development of a person-centered psychiatry.[3]

Parapsychology lies in the borderland between science and spirituality. Any major breakthrough in this area might prove to be the much sought-after providential bridge between the two.

REFERENCES

1. Pasricha SK. Relevance of para-psychology in psychiatric practice. Indian J Psychiatry. 2011;53(1):4-8.
2. Pandarakalam J. Aspects of parapsychology relevant to spirituality and psychiatry. [online] Available from https://www.researchgate.net/publication/255613667 [Last accessed July, 2021].
3. Iannuzzo G. (2012). Clinical parapsychology and parapsychological counseling in psychiatric practice. [online] Available from https://www.anomalistik.de/images/pdf/sdm/sdm-2012-01-iannuzzo.pdf [Last accessed July, 2021].
4. Wikipedia. [online] Available from https://en.wikipedia.org [Last accessed July, 2021].
5. Mark B. Telepathy, parapsychology and psychiatry. [online] Available from www.rcpsych.ac.uk/pdf/markbeddow1.11.04.pdf [Last accessed July, 2021].
6. Tuomela R. Science, protoscience, and pseudoscience. In: Joseph C Pitt, Marcello Pera (Eds). Rational Changes in Science: Essays on Scientific Reasoning. Springer, Netherlands, 1987. pp. 83-102.
7. Taylor S. From psychology to parapsychology: are psychologists right to be skeptical about

ESP? Out of the darkness. [online] Available from https://www.psychologytoday.com/us/blog/out-the-darkness/201405/psychology-parapsychology [Last accessed July, 2021].
8. Taylor S. Do psychic phenomena exist? Why my mind is open to telepathy and precognition. [online] Available from https://www.psychologytoday.com/us/blog/out-the-darkness/201404/do-psychic-phenomena-exist-0 [Last accessed July, 2021].
9. Alvarado CS. His torical writings on parapsychology and its contributions to psychology. [online] Available from www.pflyceum.org/85.html [Last accessed July, 2021].
10. Ullman M. Psychiatry and parapsychology: the consummation of an uncertain romance. In: Schmeidler GR (Ed). Parapsychology: Its Relation to Physics, Biology, Psychology, and Psychiatry. Metuchen, NJ: Scarecrow Press, Inc.; 1976.

CHAPTER 21

Interface with Technology and Mental Health

Koushik Sinha Deb, Preethy K

INTRODUCTION

The Encyclopædia Britannica describes technology as the practical application of scientific knowledge for the change and manipulation of human environment.[1] The term technology has been used in many different senses over time, indicating manufacturing, fabrication, and industry to symbolizing knowledge, technique, or procedure.[2]

Technology, however understood, is omnipresent in today's world and is intimately entwined in our everyday life. Human life, therefore, is inescapably influenced by the technology we generate and consume. Social, occupational, physical, or psychological interfaces with technology, all influence the mental health of an individual. Conversely, the mental health of an individual can influence the way a person uses and interfaces with technology (e.g., use of mobile phones to call suicide helpline or use of phones to search for ways to commit suicide). Technology is therefore a culture tool,[3] to be wielded for benefit or harm. Therein lies the importance of understanding the role of technology in mental and holistic health in today's world.

Of particular interest is the sub-branch of "information technology (IT)" which deals with the collection, transport, storage, processing or transformation, retrieval, and presentation of data or information, in all its forms".[4] IT has the potential to promote positive mental health and improve resilience at a large scale previously not possible. Dissemination of universal preventive information, identification of individuals at risk, and delivery of low intensity interventions have opened avenues of mental health service delivery at scale through the use of IT. Newer areas of research in mHealth,[5] eHealth,[6-8] Ecological Momentary Assessment (EMA),[9,10] and digital phenotyping[11,12] have gained intense traction in the last decade and are showing some early promising results.

TECHNOLOGY AND ITS EFFECT ON A CHILD AND AN ADOLESCENT

The brain and the mind of children and adolescents are at a stage ongoing rapid development. The environmental experiences which a person goes through during childhood and adolescence can have a profound impact over learning and behavior, as it is the period of high neuroplasticity. Children can start imitating actions that they see on screen after around 6 months of age. By 2 years of age, they are able to understand the content shown on screen.[13] Studies suggest that by viewing age-appropriate content under supervision, toddlers can improve speech and language function.[14] Watching television can increase knowledge, racial attitudes, and imagination in preschoolers.[15] Use of interactive applications such as "learn-to-read" can improve language and mathematical skills as it helps in practicing phonics, word recognition, letters, and numbers.[16,17] Exposure to socially contingent media with appropriate content, timing, and intensity have been found to be effective in improving language among adolescents.[18,19] Video games have been found to enhance the aspects of attention, working memory, and visuospatial skills, which are related to performance in science, technology, engineering, and mathematics.[20] Specific digital learning tools can be effective in improving the recognition of facial expression and emotions among children[21,22] and specially in those with autism.[23]

Conversely, the use of screen for long duration or without appropriate supervision can lead to detrimental effects. Introduction to screen viewing at an early age has been associated with poor language development,[24] aggression, increased externalization behavior, and poor social interaction.[25] Mobile use by parents during their interaction with the child causes decreased parental responsiveness, which in turn can lead to poor bonding and poor self-regulation by the child.[26-29] Use of mobile devices as a "shut-up" toy for children[30] has been implicated with conduct[31] and attention deficit disorders.[32,33]

In adolescents emerging to adulthood, the important developmental tasks of identity formation, relationship building, trust, and intimacy are influenced by their interaction with the digital virtual world. Adolescents experiment with different identities and roles in the virtual world, through online forums, posts, social media profiles, by creating "Avatars". While the virtual world provides a safe space to explore sensitive topics such as sexuality, negative experiences such as cyberbullying, exposure to emotionally charged or inappropriate content can induce significant stress and psychiatric morbidity.[34,35] Students who use the Internet predominantly for studies have been found to have a higher academic performance compared to those who use Internet predominantly for socialization.[36]

TECHNOLOGY AND MENTAL HEALTH

Our online identity differs significantly from our offline self; and is an ever ongoing experiment with values, morals, gender and identity, culture, and ethos.[37] This has sometimes resulted in technology anxiety and compulsive behavior.[38] Inability to continuously keep updated with social networking pages[39] has been labeled as FOMO (fear of missing out) or the "Zeigarnik" effect,[40] which describes the individual's desire for closure, explaining why the unfinished conversations over the Internet draw our attention more. "Phantom vibration syndrome" refers to the constant checking of one's smartphone because of the feeling that it has vibrated.[41]

With time and increased Internet bandwidth, social media have become more intimate, often blurring the lines between private and public. Instagram, snapchat, and dating applications such as Tinder have resulted in new social behaviors of sexting, online dating, and zoom bombing. Social media have also been highly criticized for artificially swaying public opinion by spreading falsehood and furthering conspiracy theories. Incorrect advice, or too much contradictory information, can deter people from taking right health decisions often with devastating results.[42] The interface of technology with daily life has moved beyond the realm of scientific speculation into reality, with vaccine hesitancy for COVID-19 in developed countries being the most eye-opening example.[43,44]

INTERFACE OF TECHNOLOGY IN PATIENT CARE IN PSYCHIATRY

Technology has the potential to bring about tremendous changes in the field of psychiatry with respect to patient care. Technology can help in diagnosis, assessment, prevention, early intervention as well as treatment of mental illness. Mental illness is a complex disorder that not only has a multifactorial etiology, but also the symptoms of the certain illnesses such as depression and anxiety disorders can vary at different times of the day and in different situations. Assessment in such cases should preferably be done at that moment, when the patient is experiencing symptoms to understand the patient better. "Digital phenotyping" offers an advantage in such scenario by capturing the information from the patient at that moment.[12,45] It can capture the behavior and physiological response of an individual a (e.g., avoidance of crowded places in agoraphobia or approaching a place such as alcohol shop), using global positioning system (GPS) or biosensors and can help in objectively assessing the extent of problem behavior. Apart from this, call and text logs, proximity of a person to another person (analyzed using Bluetooth), and extent of use of social media applications can also inform the clinician about the extent of social interaction of the person.[46] Digital phenotyping has also been useful in predicting symptoms of depression and anxiety and in predicting relapse in psychosis.[47]

Apart from this, use of screening and diagnostic instruments that have been adapted for use through electronic devices has helped in faster and easy capture of data and for faster analysis. Usefulness of such technology-enabled decision making was realized long back and the CATEGO program, a computer based system for diagnosis of symptoms of schizophrenia, was developed as part of International Pilot Study for Schizophrenia.[48] Assessment of brain structure and function using neuroimaging modalities such as magnetic resonance imaging (MRI), functional magnetic resonance imaging (fMRI), and diffusion tensor imaging (DTI) and electrophysiological studies such as electroencephalogram (EEG) has also led to significant advancements in the understanding of the neurobiological basis of the mental illness. Technology has made it easier to assess the role of genetics in the development of mental illness. The genome-wide association studies can analyze a large amount of genetic data from a large population to find the association of common genetic variants with mental illness. The response of an individual to treatment to a particular drug—whether he is at a higher risk of side effects or at a higher probability of response—can be predicted with the help of pharmacogenomics.[49,50] Individualized medicine is now possible for mental disorders, due to the technological advancements of the last decade.

Technology not only helps in assessment or diagnosis, but also can help in early intervention as well as in treatment. For example, In India, Alcohol Web India—an online screening website provided free of cost brief intervention following an online screening about alcohol use disorder and its management. The availability of helpline numbers, e.g., "Suicide Prevention Helpline Number" helps an individual with suicidal ideas to contact the helpline with just a phone call to discuss their problems and reduces the risk of completed suicide. Text-based automated reminders for appointments have been found to be effective in reduction of missed appointments. Applications can now provide medication reminders, find peer support, and provide cognitive remediation in people with severe mental illness.[51] Computer-based and Internet-based psychotherapy modules developed for mental illness such as depression and anxiety,[52] post-traumatic stress disorder (PTSD),[53] social phobia,[54,55] and obsessive-compulsive disorder (OCD) have been found to be effective and cost-effective.[56] Avatar therapy, in which computer-generated images of faces are created to interact with patients, has been used to reduce persistent auditory hallucinations.[57] Application-guided therapy has been found efficacious for stimulation in patients with dementia, as a relaxation tool for patients with anxiety disorder, for exposure and response prevention in PTSD and phobia and as a tool to reduce craving in substance use disorders.[58] reSET (Pear Pharmaceuticals) is a Food and Drug Administration (FDA)-approved mobile application for substance use disorder that has been found to be effective as an adjunct to conventional in-person treatment.[59]

Applications based on artificial intelligence such as "chat bots" are recently being tried in the field of mental health and initial results have been promising. Some chat bots such as Woebot (Stanford University) deliver self-guided cognitive behavioral therapy (CBT) principles in a conversational format.[60] The Indian start-up, Wysa (Touchkin), has shown remarkable growth during the pandemic. In Wysa, artificial intelligence (AI)-based emotionally intelligent bots can provide CBT and dialectical behavior therapy to improve mental resilience. "Ginger", another Indian mental health start-up that originally began at the MIT Media Lab, provides application-based psychiatrists and health coaches for subjects.

However, a limitation of these applications is that it requires a person to have a device which can download this software and the person should be capable of reading, or typing, or at least speaking in the language the application has been designed. India, being a large country, with different languages and with different dialects, the use of these applications remains restricted. Also, due to the wide variation in the socioeconomic status across the country, having a smartphone or advanced electronic device to download such applications becomes a challenge. While on one hand, such applications can help in providing quality services round the clock, on demand by the patient, which a human therapist or psychiatrist may not be able to, the actual utility in the Indian context may get restricted to few people because of the challenges mentioned.[61]

Telemedicine, which has come to the forefront during the lockdown associated with COVID-19 pandemic provides a useful synergy of technology and professional involvement. Telemedicine has lot of advantages in a resource-poor country such as India, where it can help to provide services to people suffering from mental illness at a far-off location. Service delivery through tele-psychiatry has been reported to be highly efficacious in treating all age-groups, from children and adolescents, up to the geriatric population.[62,63] The benefits of telepsychiatry have culminated in initiation of the National Tele Mental Health Program by the Government of India in 2022.[64]

INTERFACE OF TECHNOLOGY IN DIGITALIZATION OF HOSPITAL DATA

Hospital IT can help in managing the flow of patients in the hospital. It can help in monitoring the treatment retention of patients, as well as longitudinal course and outcome of illnesses. Electronic health records (EHRs), patient/personal health records (PHRs), and electronic medical records (EMRs) are all various paradigms for using technology to manage medical data. EHR and EMR are systems of hospital managed data, with hospital ownership and are intended for managing cost and for improving storage and retrieval of records. In contrast, PHR is a system where health data is managed by the patient and is owned by the person, and access is provided to physician or hospital as required. PHR offers advantage over the older EHR from a patient rights perspective and additionally has the benefit of intersystem operability, in that the information is not limited to one hospital or clinician.

Most western hospitals and national health systems currently employ some form of health data, which has opened newer ways of analysis using machine learning and artificial intelligence. Such "Big Data" analysis has gained traction in the field of mental health and illnesses, very recently due to the difficulties in coding and objectifying mental health data. Furthermore, the rapid and continuously generated data quickly becomes difficult to analyze by using traditional statistical approaches. Therefore, several techniques, including natural language processing (NLP), vision computing, and various neural network topology (convolutional neural network, recurrent neural network) have been used to find patterns from such data and have shown encouraging early results.[65,66]

Increase data portability patient health record comes associated with the problems of data authority, data security, and data ownership.[67] To prevent misuse of such personal data, governments of various countries have come up with data privacy rules and laws. Most notable of these are the Health Insurance Portability and Accountability Act (HIPAA) rules of the United States and the General Data Protection Regulation (GDPR) rules of the European Union (EU).[68] HIPAA, the acronym for the Health Insurance Portability and Accountability Act of 1996, is a series of rules that apply to all healthcare providers using digital patient data. "Individually identifiable health information", including demographic data (name, address, birth date, mobile, etc.), that relates to the individual's past, present, or future physical or mental health, or its payment cannot be shared between any entity without expressed consent of the patient. De-Identified Health Information, where such personal data have been removed, can be shared or disclosed for clinical, legal, or public health needs. The GDPR is a similar regulation of the EU that safeguards the privacy and human rights of citizens. The GDPR additionally provides guidelines for international transmission of such data outside the EU.

In 2017, the Supreme Court of India declared the right to privacy as a fundamental right under the constitution of India. The proposed data protection framework suggested by the government is known as the Personal Data Protection Bill-2019 (PDPB), which is the first step toward India's data privacy journey. The PDPB, similar to the GDPR, defines private data and sets up guidelines on their storage, retrieval, and use by all concerned parties.[69] Mentally ill patients need data privacy protection, possibly even more than others, due to their unique cognitive vulnerabilities affecting their capacity to consent. However, in absence of governmental framework and support, implementing such systems for patient data collection and protection will remain an uphill task for resource constrained counties.[68,70]

WHERE ARE WE HEADING WITH TECHNOLOGY?

Technology can be used as a force for democratization, spreading mental health services to the people. Technology can also be elitist and divide the country into the technologically suave and the technology have-nots. The recent COVID-19 epidemic has shown that telepsychiatry services are mostly used by people who are educated and city dwellers, compared to those who are from rural India or are uneducated. Online appointment booking systems are often out of reach for many patients who do not have access to computers. Smartphone-based and application-based resources are available to only to those who can purchase a smartphone, as well as having an understanding of English. Patient health data, which started as an individual rights approach, require familiarity with computer systems, which rules out a huge proportion of the country's population.

Technological solutions should not come at the cost of elimination of traditional human resource-based services. The middle path of triage needs to be developed where technology-enabled services are provided to those who can receive it, while maintaining conventional services for all. Technological solutions need to be matched with the use-capacity of not only patients, but also health service providers, from psychiatrists to community care workers. India needs to develop its indigenous digital infrastructure, from data storage servers to applications that are useful to patients, clinicians, and researchers. India as a country, patients' rights groups, and academic societies need to collaborate to devise guidelines for mental health application development. Finally, the rapid progress of technology requires clinicians to stay agile and remain abreast of the recent developments. Continuing Medical Education (CME) and workshops on such technology interfaces of psychiatry are the need of the day to bring all stakeholders on to the same platform.

REFERENCES

1. Encyclopaedia Britanni. Technology | Definition, Examples, Types, and Facts | Britannica. [online] Available from: https://www.britannica.com/technology/technology. [Last accessed June 2022].
2. Kline SJ. What is technology? Bull Sci Technol Soc. 1985;5(3):215-8.
3. Bijker WE. How is technology made? That is the question! Camb J Econ. 2010;34(1):63-76.
4. Onn CW, Sorooshian S. Mini Literature Analysis on Information Technology Definition. [online] Available from: https://core.ac.uk/download/pdf/234671309.pdf. [Last accessed June 2022].
5. WHO Global Observatory for eHealth. MHealth: new horizons for health through mobile technologies. Geneva: World Health Organization; 2011.
6. Ben-Zeev D. Technology in mental health: creating new knowledge and inventing the future of services. Psychiatr Serv Wash DC. 2017;68(2):107-8.
7. Deady M, Choi I, Calvo RA, Glozier N, Christensen H, Harvey SB. eHealth interventions for the prevention of depression and anxiety in the general population: a systematic review and meta-analysis. BMC Psychiatry. 2017;17(1):310.
8. Naslund JA, Marsch LA, McHugo GJ, Bartels SJ. Emerging mHealth and eHealth interventions for serious mental illness: a review of the literature. J Ment Health Abingdon Engl. 2015;24(5):321-32.
9. Smith KE, Juarascio A. From Ecological Momentary Assessment (EMA) to Ecological Momentary Intervention (EMI): Past and Future Directions for Ambulatory Assessment and Interventions in Eating Disorders. Curr Psychiatry Rep. 2019;21(7):53.
10. de Vries LP, Baselmans BML, Bartels M. Smartphone-based ecological momentary assessment of well-being: a systematic review and recommendations for future studies. J Happiness Stud. 2021;22(5):2361-408.
11. Washington P, Park N, Srivastava P, Voss C, Kline A, Varma M, et al. Data-driven diagnostics and the potential of mobile artificial intelligence for digital therapeutic phenotyping in computational psychiatry. Biol Psychiatry Cogn Neurosci Neuroimaging. 2020;5(8):759-69.
12. Chia AZR, Zhang MWB. Digital phenotyping in psychiatry: a scoping review. Technol Health Care Off J Eur Soc Eng Med. 2022.
13. Canadian Paediatric Society DHTF Ottawa, Ontario. Screen time and young children: promoting health and development in a digital world. Paediatr Child Health. 2017;22(8):461-8.
14. Olson KB, Wilkinson CL, Wilkinson MJ, Harris J, Whittle A. Texts for talking: Evaluation of a mobile health program addressing speech and language delay. Clin Pediatr (Phila). 2016;55(11):1044-9.
15. Thakkar RR, Garrison MM, Christakis DA. A systematic review for the effects of television viewing by infants and preschoolers. Pediatrics. 2006;118(5):2025-31.

16. Pitchford N. Development of early mathematical skills with a tablet intervention: a randomized control trial in Malawi. Front Psychol. 2015;6:485.
17. Kucirkova N. iPads in early education: separating assumptions and evidence. Front Psychol. 2014;5:715.
18. Kirkorian HL, Choi K, Pempek TA. Toddlers' word learning from contingent and noncontingent video on touch screens. Child Dev. 2016;87(2):405-13.
19. Roseberry S, Hirsh-Pasek K, Golinkoff RM. Skype me! Socially contingent interactions help toddlers learn language. Child Dev. 2014;85(3):956-70.
20. Uttal DH, Meadow NG, Tipton E, Hand LL, Alden AR, Warren C, Newcombe NS. (2013). The malleability of spatial skills: a meta-analysis of training studies – PsycNET. APA PsycNET. [online] Available from: https://doi.apa.org/record/2012-14754-001?doi=1. [Last accessed June 2022].
21. Uhls YT, Broome J, Levi S, Szczepanski-Beavers J, Greenfield P. Mobile technologies and their relationship to children's ability to read nonverbal emotional cues: a cross-temporal comparison. Cyberpsychology Behav Soc Netw. 2020;23(7):465-70.
22. Uhls YT, Michikyan M, Morris J, Garcia D, Small GW, Zgourou E, et al. Five days at outdoor education camp without screens improves preteen skills with nonverbal emotion cues. Comput Hum Behav. 2014;39:387-92.
23. Zhang S, Xia X, Li S, Shen L, Liu J, Zhao L, et al. Using technology-based learning tool to train facial expression recognition and emotion understanding skills of Chinese pre-schoolers with autism spectrum disorder. Int J Dev Disabil. 2019;65(5):378-86.
24. Karani NF, Sher J, Mophosho M. The influence of screen time on children's language development: a scoping review. S Afr J Commun Disord. 2022;69(1):825.
25. Karki U, Sravanti L. Excess screen time-impact on childhood development and management: a review. Med Phoenix. 2021;6(1):40-5.
26. Radesky J, Miller AL, Rosenblum KL, Appugliese D, Kaciroti N, Lumeng JC. Maternal mobile device use during a structured parent-child interaction task. Acad Pediatr. 2015;15(2):238-44.
27. Radesky JS, Kistin CJ, Zuckerman B, Nitzberg K, Gross J, Kaplan-Sanoff M, et al. Patterns of mobile device use by caregivers and children during meals in fast food restaurants. Pediatrics. 2014;133(4):e843-9.
28. Braune-Krickau K, Schneebeli L, Pehlke-Milde J, Gemperle M, Koch R, von Wyl A. Smartphones in the nursery: Parental smartphone use and parental sensitivity and responsiveness within parent-child interaction in early childhood (0-5 years): A scoping review. Infant Ment Health J. 2021;42(2):161-75.
29. Radesky JS, Silverstein M, Zuckerman B, Christakis DA. Infant self-regulation and early childhood media exposure. Pediatrics. 2014;133(5):e1172-8.
30. Radesky JS, Peacock-Chambers E, Zuckerman B, Silverstein M. Use of mobile technology to calm upset children: associations with social-emotional development. JAMA Pediatr. 2016;170(4):397-9.
31. Radesky JS, Schumacher J, Zuckerman B. Mobile and interactive media use by young children: the good, the bad, and the unknown. Pediatrics. 2015;135(1):1-3.
32. Hosokawa R, Katsura T. Association between mobile technology use and child adjustment in early elementary school age. PLOS ONE. 2018;13(7):e0199959.
33. Tamana SK, Ezeugwu V, Chikuma J, Lefebvre DL, Azad MB, Moraes TJ, et al. Screen-time is associated with inattention problems in preschoolers: results from the CHILD birth cohort study. PLOS ONE. 2019;14(4):e0213995.
34. George MJ, Odgers CL. Seven fears and the science of how mobile technologies may be influencing adolescents in the digital age. Perspect Psychol Sci J Assoc Psychol Sci. 2015;10(6):832-51.
35. Gray SL. How technology interacts with emerging adulthood psychosocial developmental tasks: an examination of online self-presentation and cell phone usage. 2014. [online] Available from: https://trace.tennessee.edu/cgi/viewcontent.cgi?article=3193&context=utk_graddiss. [Last accessed June 2022].
36. Kim SY, Kim MS, Park B, Kim JH, Choi HG. The associations between Internet use time and school performance among Korean adolescents differ according to the purpose of Internet use. PLoS One. 2017;12(4):e0174878.
37. Lemma A. An order of pure decision: growing up in a virtual world and the adolescent's experience of being-in-a-body. J Am Psychoanal Assoc. 2010;58(4):691-714.
38. McCord B, Rodebaugh TL, Levinson CA. Facebook: Social uses and anxiety. Comput Hum Behav. 2014;34:23-7.

39. Rosen LD, Whaling K, Rab S, Carrier LM, Cheever NA. Is Facebook creating "iDisorders"? The link between clinical symptoms of psychiatric disorders and technology use, attitudes and anxiety. Comput Hum Behav. 2013;29(3):1243-54.
40. Perry B, Singh S. A virtual reality: technology's impact on youth mental health. Indian J Soc Psychiatry. 2016;32(3):222-6.
41. Rosenberger R. An experiential account of phantom vibration syndrome. Comput Hum Behav. 2015;52:124-31.
42. Kuss DJ, Griffiths MD. Social networking sites and addiction: ten lessons learned. Int J Environ Res Public Health. 2017;14(3):311.
43. Garett R, Young SD. Online misinformation and vaccine hesitancy. Transl Behav Med. 2021;11(12):2194-9.
44. Naeem SB, Bhatti R, Khan A. An exploration of how fake news is taking over social media and putting public health at risk. Health Inf Libr J. 2021;38(2):143-9.
45. Huckvale K, Venkatesh S, Christensen H. Toward clinical digital phenotyping: a timely opportunity to consider purpose, quality, and safety. NPJ Digit Med. 2019;2:88.
46. Torous J, Onnela JP, Keshavan M. New dimensions and new tools to realize the potential of RDoC: digital phenotyping via smartphones and connected devices. Transl Psychiatry. 2017;7(3):e1053.
47. Moshe I, Terhorst Y, Opoku Asare K, Sander LB, Ferreira D, Baumeister H, et al. Predicting symptoms of depression and anxiety using smartphone and wearable data. Front Psychiatry. 2021;12:625247.
48. Helzer JE, Brockington IF, Kendell RE. Predictive validity of DSM-III and Feighner definitions of schizophrenia: a comparison with research disgnostic criteria and CATEGO. Arch Gen Psychiatry. 1981;38(7):791-7.
49. Yassin W, Nakatani H, Zhu Y, Kojima M, Owada K, Kuwabara H, et al. Machine-learning classification using neuroimaging data in schizophrenia, autism, ultra-high risk and first-episode psychosis. Transl Psychiatry. 2020;10(1):1-11.
50. Ross CA, Margolis RL. Research Domain Criteria: strengths, weaknesses, and potential alternatives for future psychiatric research. Complex Psychiatry. 2019;5(4):218-36.
51. Firth J, Torous J. Smartphone apps for schizophrenia: a systematic review. JMIR MHealth UHealth. 2015;3(4):e102.
52. Spek V, Cuijpers P, Nyklícek I, Riper H, Keyzer J, Pop V. Internet-based cognitive behaviour therapy for symptoms of depression and anxiety: a meta-analysis. Psychol Med. 2007;37(3):319-28.
53. Spence J, Titov N, Dear BF, Johnston L, Solley K, Lorian C, et al. Randomized controlled trial of Internet-delivered cognitive behavioral therapy for posttraumatic stress disorder. Depress Anxiety. 2011;28(7):541-50.
54. Carlbring P, Nordgren LB, Furmark T, Andersson G. Long-term outcome of Internet-delivered cognitive-behavioural therapy for social phobia: a 30-month follow-up. Behav Res Ther. 2009;47(10):848-50.
55. Andersson G, Carlbring P, Furmark T. Internet-delivered treatments for social anxiety disorder. In: The Wiley Blackwell Handbook of Social Anxiety Disorder. Hoboken: Wiley Blackwell; 2014. pp. 569-87.
56. Ebert DD, Zarski AC, Christensen H, Stikkelbroek Y, Cuijpers P, Berking M, et al. Internet and computer-based cognitive behavioral therapy for anxiety and depression in youth: a meta-analysis of randomized controlled outcome trials. PloS One. 2015;10(3):e0119895.
57. Craig TK, Rus-Calafell M, Ward T, Leff JP, Huckvale M, Howarth E, et al. AVATAR therapy for auditory verbal hallucinations in people with psychosis: a single-blind, randomised controlled trial. Lancet Psychiatry. 2018;5(1):31-40.
58. Park MJ, Kim DJ, Lee U, Na EJ, Jeon HJ. A literature overview of virtual reality (VR) in treatment of psychiatric disorders: recent advances and limitations. Front Psychiatry. 2019;10:505.
59. Campbell ANC, Nunes EV, Matthews AG, Stitzer M, Miele GM, Polsky D, et al. Internet-delivered treatment for substance abuse: a multi-site randomized controlled clinical trial. Am J Psychiatry. 2014;171(6):683-90.
60. Fitzpatrick KK, Darcy A, Vierhile M. Delivering cognitive behavior therapy to young adults with symptoms of depression and anxiety using a fully automated conversational agent (Woebot): a randomized controlled trial. JMIR Ment Health. 2017;4(2):e19.
61. Deb KS, Tuli A, Sood M, Chadda R, Verma R, Kumar S, et al. Is India ready for mental health apps (MHApps)? A quantitative-qualitative exploration of caregivers' perspective on smartphone-based solutions for managing severe mental illnesses in low resource settings. PLOS ONE. 2018;13(9):e0203353.

62. Myers K, Valentine J, Morganthaler R, Melzer S. Telepsychiatry with incarcerated youth. J Adolesc Health Off Publ Soc Adolesc Med. 2006;38(6):643-8.
63. Norman S. The use of telemedicine in psychiatry. J Psychiatr Ment Health Nurs. 2006;13(6):771-7.
64. Sagar R, Singh S. National Tele-Mental Health Program in India: a step towards mental health care for all? Indian J Psychiatry. 2022;64(2):117-9.
65. Figueroa CA, Aguilera A. The Need for a Mental Health Technology Revolution in the COVID-19 Pandemic. Front Psychiatry. 2020;11:523.
66. Aguilera A. Digital technology and mental health interventions: opportunities and challenges. Arbor. 2015;191(771):a210.
67. Ness RB, Joint Policy Committee S of E for the. Influence of the HIPAA Privacy Rule on Health Research. JAMA. 2007;298(18):2164-70.
68. Staunton C, Slokenberga S, Mascalzoni D. The GDPR and the research exemption: considerations on the necessary safeguards for research biobanks. Eur J Hum Genet. 2019;27(8):1159-67.
69. Singh RG, Ruj S. A Technical look at the Indian personal data protection bill. arXiv; 2020. [online] Available from: http://arxiv.org/abs/2005.13812. [Last accessed June 2022].
70. Clarke N, Vale G, Reeves EP, Kirwan M, Smith D, Farrell M, et al. GDPR: an impediment to research? Ir J Med Sci 1971. 2019;188(4):1129-35.

CHAPTER 22

Interface with Education

Alka Subramanyam

SCOPE OF MENTAL HEALTH

Mental well-being is an integral part of this WHO definition of health. Further, mental health can be described as: *"a state of well-being in which the individual realizes his or her own abilities, can cope with the normal stresses of life, can work productively and fruitfully, and is able to make a contribution to his or her community"*. Therefore, it is needless to say that mental health is much more beyond absence of mental illness.

A person's childhood and adolescence are the foundation years of future well-being. A child receiving social-emotional and mental health support achieves better academically and is better equipped in dealing with glitches of life. There is a growing and unmet need for mental health services for children and youth worldwide and more so in less developed countries. It has long been acknowledged that a variety of psychosocial and health problems affect learning and performance in profound ways. Developmental conditions such as autism and learning disorders have better outcomes when identified and intervened in early years. Identifying different stressors, inculcating healthy coping skills, dealing with difficult behavior and emotional issues are of concern during years of schooling. As countries are moving toward the commitment of universal education, educational institutions seem to have an unprecedented opportunity to bring changes. They even have significant influence on families and community; and in collaboration with them and the mental health services can thus be an important source of intervention. They can play a pivotal role in dealing mental health issues in terms of identification, prevention, intervention, positive development, and regular communication between school and families. Mental health issues and corresponding interventions are dealt with in subsequent sections.

INDIAN EDUCATION SYSTEM

Indian education system (representative image) has been shown in **Figure 1**.

Preschool

This includes kids from around 3–6 years of age wherein the child receives informal or kindergarten education. Different mental health aspects in this stage are as follows, which it is important to sensitize the teachers to:

Neurodevelopmental Disorders

These are group of disorders associated with improper functioning of brain and neurological system, manifesting in early in development. It is characterized by deficits in the normal development and thereby causing impairment

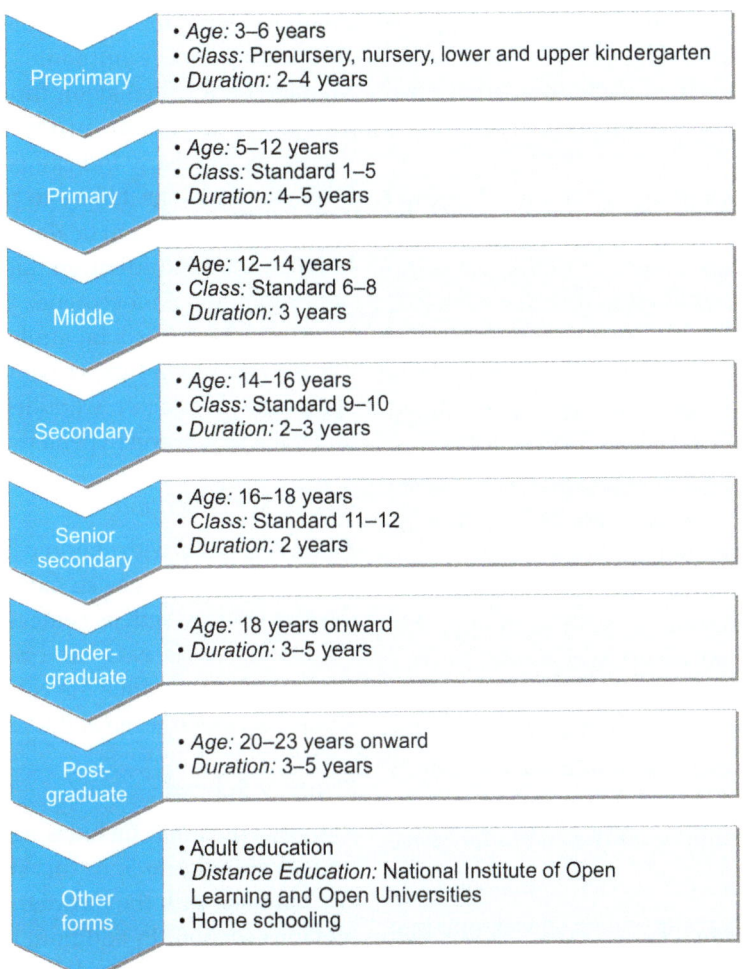

Fig. 1: Indian education system.

in one or the other domain including personal, social, academic or later on occupational. Children with neurodevelopmental disorders can have specific limitations of language and speech, motor skills, behavior, memory, learning or global impairments in social skills or intelligence. The Diagnostic and Statistical Manual of Mental Disorders, 5th Edition (DSM-5) includes intellectual disability, language and speech disorder, autism spectrum disorder, attention deficit hyperactivity disorder (ADHD), and specific learning disorder (SLD).

Intellectual disability: It is defined as a disability with significant limitations in both intellectual functioning (reasoning, learning, and problem solving) and adaptive behavior (conceptual, social, and practical skills) that commences before the age of 18 years. The majority of population-based prevalence estimates for intellectual disability (previously termed as mental retardation) in developing countries range from 10/1,000 to 15/1,000 children. The prevalence of intellectual disability at any one time is estimated to range from 1 to 3% of the population in Western societies.

The intellectually disabled child often has associated behavioral problems. The child is a problem to the school, as she/he cannot grasp as readily as normal children do. Around 40.7% of intellectually disabled children between 4 and 18 years of age have an additional psychiatric disorder. Academic performance is an important source of identification of such children. If it appears to teachers that the child is delayed impairment by 2 or more years below his grade placement and age placement, one may consider the likelihood of intellectual impairment. In addition, physical factors such as growth delay may act as an aid in recognizing the child with a lag in mental development. Some children with syndromal diagnosis and are found to have physical abnormalities, such as dysmorphic facies, abnormal stature and physiques, etc., and can be screened easily. The early stages of growth and development of the child are also important clues. For example, the teachers in schools can easily notice issues with speech elaboration, dentition, and socialization skills.

Autism spectrum disorder: It is a phenotypically heterogeneous group of neurodevelopmental syndromes, with polygenic heritability, characterized by a wide range of impairments in social communication and restricted and repetitive behaviors. Increasingly diagnosed over the last two decades, with the current prevalence estimated at approximately 1% in the United States. Autistic disorder, based on DSM-IV-TR criteria, is believed to occur at a rate of about 8 cases per 10,000 children (0.08%). Screening autism early in life is important in many ways. Autism spectrum disorder has a significant heritable contribution; the risk of a second child having autism when the first has the diagnosis is 5% (100 times the reported prevalence). There is also the possibility that early diagnosis followed by appropriately targeted intervention may improve outcome, especially in management of behavior, functional skills, and communication problems. Some of the noticeable early indicators are isolation from surroundings, failure to play like other children, and apparent deafness, empty gaze, failure to attract attention, lack of smiling, poor imitation of movements, poor response to others, lack of social smile, and lack of appropriate facial expression. Two other symptoms of concern were delayed speech, and restlessness and hyperactivity.

Role of Sex Education

In today's world, with children being exposed to schools and places so early one such as daycare centers, activity centers, and cocurricular classes as early as preschool, it is important to introduce the concept of "good touch-bad touch" even at this stage.

Primary School

Primary education includes ages 5–12 years from standard 1 to 5. At this stage, children can manifest with the disorders discussed in previous section. In addition, they can have symptoms of ADHD and learning difficulties. In this section, impact of social media and role of social media is also discussed.

Attention Deficit Hyperactivity Disorder

It is characterized by a pattern of diminished sustained attention, and increased impulsivity or hyperactivity. Symptoms start coming into notice by early childhood years. Rates of ADHD have been reported to be 7–8% in prepubertal elementary school children. These children are easily distracted, jump up in class, shout out into the classroom, are unable to focus their attention, miss important information in class, disrupt their fellow students, drop class materials, or topple over with their chairs.

The school report or the teacher's diagnostic assessment has a special role in evaluation of ADHD. In view of the high rate of school dropouts (10–12%) and the increased risk of such youngsters for further mental health problems—e.g., conduct disorders in combination with delinquent behaviors, and subsequently substance abuse, it is necessary that ADHD should be identified early and managed.

Specific Learning Disorder

It is produced by interactions of heritable and environmental factors, and characterized by persistent difficulty learning academic skills in reading, written expression, or mathematics, beginning in early childhood, that is inconsistent with the overall intellectual ability of a child. It affects approximately 10% of youth. Repeated failures lead to very poor self-esteem, low motivation, further failure and rejection. Early intervention presupposes early identification. The checklist for SLD in the Sarva Shiksha Abhiyan Manual (SSA, 2003) for initial screening by teachers and NIMHANS battery for assessment by psychologists are helpful tools. DALI or Dyslexia Assessment for Languages of India is a recently developed package that contains screening tools for school teachers and assessment tools for psychologists in Indian Languages to identify dyslexia. All of these can easily be adapted by the school, and trained teachers can screen the same.

The academic problems in children are often misidentified as child's careless behavior or unwillingness to study. Mostly these children are referred for assessment by the school/teacher for reasons of failure, underachievement or behavioral problems. However, there is a long referral gap. Teachers need to be aware of such issues and teacher's training program should include screening of such disorders in the class.

Possible preventive measures in school: As a preschool intervention, focus should be on language development, development of fine motor and visual motor skills and synthetic and analytic phonics. At primary school level, efforts should be made to develop and strengthen language and basic skills of reading, writing, and arithmetic. A reading strategy developed by Das based on the PASS (Planning-Attention-Simultaneous-Successive) theory of cognitive development (Das JP, 1998) may be used. This program is being used at the Maharashtra Dyslexia Association in conjunction with other remedial measures.

Training of teachers: Teachers are generally trained in "teaching methodology"; mostly teaching the verbatim from the textbook rather than identifying the concept to be taught. While teaching language, stress is on grammar, rather than communication. In India due to overcrowded classes and the stress on examination-oriented learning and large curriculum, multisensory teaching, experiential learning and encouragement of thinking has not found a place on a regular basis. NIOS (National Institute of Open Schooling) has benefited many children with SLD, but in addition, children should be exposed to various prevocational skills early in school and then be allowed to choose other subjects from lower standards itself. Adequate number of psychologists, special and regular school teachers need to be trained in understanding SLD. Awareness about SLD can be provided in the Bachelor of Education (BEd) curriculum and short-term "add-on" courses for psychologists can fill the need and availability gap. In addition, policy makers, parents, and community bodies should be sensitized about the issue.

Role of Life Skills

Life skills taught in schools are required by a child to develop his or her own coping resources and thus competence in the face of a challenge, which would otherwise lead to negative consequences. A core set of life skills that have cut across multiple programs are:
- Decision making and problem solving
- Critical and creative thinking
- Communication and interpersonal relationship skills
- Self-awareness and empathy
- Skills for coping with emotions and stressors

Children are made to actively participate in the learning process, based on problem-solving and decision-making skills (e.g., finding an alternative solution to the given problem, weighing the advantages and disadvantages). These programs can impact at various levels: Promoting positive health behavior of child (prevention from addictions and risky sexual behavior); improving teacher and student relationship, thus having fewer problem behaviors in class; and improving the overall academic performance, reducing risk of future mental health issues and behavioral disturbances.

Introduction of life skill teaching in teaching curriculum and manuals in BEd or small courses would significantly affect a huge population of students.

Impact of Social Media

Social media, a powerful educational tool, has various positive influences such as increasing social connections, sharing one's creativity and providing support in times of distress. However, there is a growing concern about its usage especially in adolescents. As per the data, 45% of teens use internet "almost constantly", a figure that has nearly doubled since 2014–15 survey. Another 44% go online several times a day, implying that around 99% teens go online at least multiple times per day. This kind of usage is associated with various risks. A student spending excessive time online starts neglecting the studies; there is sometimes too much of sharing of personal information which can be detrimental; with the advent of smartphone cameras, and the development of online filters and image-manipulation techniques, there has been a rise in the popularity of "selfies" and disturbance in body image; a number of inappropriate and occasionally harmful content and advice is freely available; and there have been recently an increase in incidences of cybercrimes. Parents have adopted different approaches to manage children's internet use. Teachers may also take initiatives to educate about beneficial and safe use of digital media, help build children resilience to cope with upsetting online experiences and on occasions strict measures to tackle cyberbullying and related issues. In Mumbai, a group called "Responsible Netism" is liaising actively with schools to create awareness and promote safe use of social media among school-going children.

Role of Play

According to Piaget, play has an important role in development of child's cognitive development. Evidence suggests that play helps in formation of secure emotional attachments, regulation of emotions, ability to show empathy and form emotional relationship (including friendship) and emotional resilience. Secure emotional attachments, in turn, have been shown to be vital in supporting children's ability to cope with stress and anxiety. In last few decades, there has been huge reduction in the area where children could roam unsupervised around their homes has shrunk. Simultaneously, the change in education policy has substantially restricted the play activity in view of excessive pressure on academics and the amount of learning done through it.

A study in an Indian orphanage of the introduction of a structured play regimen mentioned improved motor, cognitive, and social functioning measures, as compared to children not included in the study. In another review (2017) use of play therapy in children with autism showed improvement in building friendships, social interactions and social competence, family relationships, coping, and reductions in the time spent playing alone. Schools in Finland, which have an average academic time of 4 hours per day, the rest being dedicated to play and free time, have some of the best academic results worldwide, and least dropouts, substance users, and criminal records. Thus, it seems essential to incorporate adequate time and appropriate type of play in the school curriculum and should be given importance similar to academics.

Role of Sex Education

Once again, sex education can continue in primary school too, with a little elaboration about body parts and reinforcing good touch-bad touch with a few age-appropriate examples of each. It is imperative for primary schoolers to understand that even members of the family, close family friends, etc., who indulge in bad touch, must be reported. The fact that there may be use of bribes such as sweets, mobiles, or threats etc. should be ideally demonstrated through audiovisual (AV) shows or pictorial representation.

Middle School

Middle school in India commences at the age 11–14 or standard 5–8. Children in middle school are faced with unique changes; they are looking for a place to belong, and often take paths that negatively affect academic outcomes and their overall health. Apart from common mental disorders which will be discussed further, in high schools, other critical issues faced by them are curricular stress and manifestation of underlying learning problems.

Academic or Curricular Stress

It is defined as distress regarding upcoming academic activities and/or failure or even possibility of failure. School-related situations such as tests, grades, studying, pressure to succeed are the main sources. It may manifest in several domains of child's life such as home, school, peer or neighborhood and affects physical health, nutrition, substance taking behavior, and self-care. Furthermore, curricular stress is a risk factor for mental health issues, e.g. middle school girls who had higher levels of academic stress had higher risk of experiencing depression.

In Indian education system, worth of student is mostly evaluated by performance in studies, and not by vocational, sports or other abilities. Social lives of Indian children and parents are sacrificed in the name of homework and studies. Nearly 63.5% of the students complain of significant academic pressure which was uniform across gender, age, class, and other factors; one-third have diagnosable mental health problems and approximately 6 students in India die due to suicide due related to such stress everyday. This questions the efforts of school system toward well-being of children. Moreover, excess parental vigilance and pressure on child's academic performance leads to added stress.

Both parents and teachers should be made aware that each child is different, and academic proficiency may differ from child to child. Government authorities and school

Specific Learning Disorder

As already mentioned, SLD can be diagnosed even later at middle school stage. Here, the foundation for Sciences and Social Sciences are laid, which child find difficult to memorize and retrieve. Interventions must focus on teaching of concepts, critical thinking, and problem solving while encouraging creativity and divergent thinking.

Children must be provided with ways and means to complete school successfully so they can grow into confident, motivated individuals with their self-esteem intact. Accommodations (Accommodations provide different ways for children to take information or communicate their knowledge back, e.g., tape recorder or word processor) and modifications (Modifications are changes in the delivery, content, or instructional level of subject matter or tests. They result in changing or lowering expectations and create a different standard for kids with disabilities than for those without disabilities) of curriculum are essential for this.

Role of Sex Education

At this stage, knowledge of the reproductive system, including the sexual drive, hormones, puberty, masturbation, menstruation, and sexual orientation can be imparted. At this stage, it is important to hold small and large group discussions to break inhibitions, facilitate open discussions, and inculcate a healthy attitude toward sexuality, so as to break the myths and taboo and hope to create a sexually healthier society.

High School

Mental Health Issues

This phase involves rapid physical and psychological growth, commencing from puberty to complete growth and development. Children go through a numerous physical, hormonal, psychological, behavioral, and social changes. Due to lack of literacy, awareness and social taboos, health of millions of children in this age group is neglected globally. High-risk sexual behavior is one of the major concerns (4% in female, 15% males). At least 20% of youngsters are likely to experience some form of mental illness, such as depression, mood disturbances, substance abuse, suicidal behaviors, eating disorders, and others. A 6-year follow-up study in Chandigarh showed incidence rate of psychiatric disorder to be 0.18% per year among the 10- to 17-year-old. Prevalence of depression varied from 0.1 to 18.5%, conduct disorders from 0.2 to 9.2%, and anxiety disorders from 0.1 to 24.4% across different studies. Considering the prevalence of mental health-related issues at this age, utmost need of efforts on front of mental health education, awareness, and screening sensitization is evident.

Awareness

Mental health education should be a part of general health education and can also be coupled with life skills lessons, and inclusive of information about mental health and mental illness, psychological and emotional development, stress and its effects, positive coping strategies, common mental health problems at their age, importance of healthy relationships and where and how to seek help in need. Educational activities may include school teachers, psychologists, mental health physicians and social workers, and active participation from students and parents to make it more relevant.

authorities both need to ensure that sufficient time is allowed for activities which develop skills for overall well-being rather than only academic ones.

High-risk Behaviors

Identification of psychosocial problems and high-risk behavior/mental health problems.

Certain high-risk behaviors at this level such as smoking, indulgence in substance use or early involvement in sexual behaviors are indicators of current or impending serious underlying problems. Learning disability and even psychosocial problems can manifest as either change in emotions or behavior and indicators include poor attendance and/or academic performance, poor peer relationship, extreme shyness or aggression, mood swings and denial to attend school.

Teachers require specific training in recognition of these disorders. Depression in this age group may present with atypical symptoms such as irritability, conduct problems, substance use, poor academic performance, eating disorders, etc. Suicidal thoughts and attempts require extra vigilance on part of both parents and teachers. Anxiety in this age may be expressed in the form of reluctance to participate in any school activities, school refusal, extreme shyness, unreasonable anxiety, excess somatic concerns, etc. Psychotic disorders also commonly start during this period and have typical sign and symptoms. Substance use in adolescents occurs due to variety of reasons such as peer pressure, depression or anxiety, conduct disorder, substance use in family, etc. It becomes evident generally through another mental condition, poor attendance, poor school performance or delinquency, etc. Conduct disorder will manifest as repetitive and persistent pattern of destructive or hostile behavior which violates rights of others and deviates from age-appropriate norms.

Liaising with Schools for Screening Mental Health Problems

There are certain screening instruments available either self-administered or teacher or parent rated to screen for common behavioral and mental issues in this age group. The instruments can either look for any disorder in general or can focus on specific disorder or group of disorders. Pediatric Symptom Checklist (PSC-17 and 35) is useful in children to assess general psychosocial functioning and problems of attention and externalizing, and internalizing symptoms. Strengths and Difficulties Questionnaire (SDQ) is a 25-item scale which can be self-reported by children and looks into general psychosocial functions as well as emotional symptoms, conduct problems, hyperactivity/inattention, peer relationship problems, and social behavior. Child Behavior Checklist (CBCL), a 113-item questionnaire looks into emotional and behavioral problems which can be reported by either teacher, parent or adolescent. It assesses domains such as anxiety/depression, somatic complains, social problems, thought problems, attention problems, rule-breaking behavior, aggressive behavior, etc. Apart from this, there are specific scales like for anxiety disorders: Revised Children's Anxiety and Depression Scale Youth and Parent Versions (RCADS 2000); Screen for Child Anxiety Related Emotional Disorders (SCARED 1997), etc. For depression, CES-D (Center for Epidemiological Studies-Depression scale) modified version for children and adolescents, Childhood Depression Inventory (CDI), Short Mood and Feeling Questionnaire (SMF-Q), and Patient Health Questionnaire (PHQ)-9 and 2 can be used. In addition to depressive symptoms, suicide-specific questions can also be used to assess presence of suicidal ideation in adolescents. CRAFFT (Care, Relax, Alone, Freely Forget, Friends, Trouble) is another freely available self-administered screening instrument for substance abuse having high sensitivity.

Apart from this Child and Adolescent Disruptive Behavior Inventory-Parent and

Teacher Version (CADBI) for disruptive behavior Eating Disorder Screening questionnaire for eating disorders, Post-traumatic Stress Diagnosis Scale (PDS) for impact of stressful event.

Related Laws and Mental Health

Awareness about laws relating to adolescents can also be imparted, as high-risk behaviors such as sexual behavior, indulgence in drug-related activities, involvement in criminal activities or as victims or perpetrator in childhood sexual abuse activities may land them in legal scuffle. Cigarette and Other Tobacco Products Act (COTPA, 2003) deals with public consumption of nicotine products, Excise Acts with alcohol use, and Narcotic Drugs and Psychotropic Substances Act (NDPS Act, 1985) with consumption and dealings of substance of abuse.

The Protection of Children from Sexual Offenses (POCSO, 2012) Act is concerned with various types of sexual offenses, sexual harassment and pornography against minors and their punishments. The Juvenile Justice Act (care and protection of children), 2015 makes an effort to consolidate the law in relation to children in conflict with the law or in need of care and protection by addressing their basic needs and aiming at their protection, development, treatment, and social integration. Children with substance use problems and conduct disorder may find themselves in conflict with this law at times.

Role of Sex Education

High school is where hormonal changes are at the peak, and the turbulence and impulsivity of adolescence often leads to risky sexual behavior. At this stage, youth must be introduced to healthy and dysfunctional relationships including partner abuse, sexual abuse, coercive sex or sex under the influence of substances; emotional blackmailing, sexually transmitted diseases (STDs), pregnancy, same sex orientation; and options to approach respective authorities in case needed for any of the above stated.

Professional College

Mental Health Issues

Professional college can be a demanding place for many students. Many students may have to first time deal with task of separation from their family. In addition to academic stress, students may have to take up more adult-like responsibilities without having yet learned the skills and maturity of adulthood, such as working, being in relationship, or having friends from different cultures and belief systems.

Around 20% of young adults experience some form of mental health problems such as depression, anxiety, other mood disturbances, substance abuse, suicidal behaviors, eating disorders, and others. A meta-analysis of major epidemiological studies in India reported an estimated prevalence of such morbidity of 22.2/1,000 population in age group of 15-24 years.

A longitudinal study showed the incidence rate of psychiatric disorder to be 0.18% per year among old adolescents. Considering specific mental disorders, prevalence of depression is reported to be 0.1-18.5%, conduct disorders 0.2-9.2%, and anxiety 0.1-24.4% across different studies. Suicide is the third leading cause of death among young adults, and a study reported suicidal ideation in 6.7%, 1.6% reported having a suicide plan, and 0.5%—a suicide attempt in the previous year. Suicidal ideas and attempts were also found to be high in Indian studies two in which 6% youth of 11-17 years and 15.8% adolescents aged 14-19 years reported suicidal ideas, while 0.4% aged 11-17 years and 5.1% aged 14-19 years reported suicidal attempts.

Eating disorders often have their onset during adolescence and are seen in greater proportion of females than males (13.5 vs. 3.6%, respectively). ADHD may persist into adulthood, is seen in 2-8% of college students and is associated with poor academic performance, social difficulties, and an increased risk for alcohol and drug use. There is a paucity of literature regarding prevalence of schizophrenia among college students; however, prodromal or early symptoms of psychotic disorder are commonly experienced in youth.

The alcohol and illicit drugs use have their peaks during young adulthood and hence one of the most prevalent problem among college students. Data from 24 States of India revealed a prevalence of 21.4% of alcohol use among men aged 12-18 years. Further the National Family Health Survey (NFHS-3) showed that 1% women and 11% men aged 15-19 years and 1.4% women and 28.8% men aged 20-24 years consumed alcohol. Alcohol consumption is associated with motor vehicle accidents, accidental injuries, high-risk sexual behavior, sexual assaults, and poor academic performance. Apart from alcohol, other common substances in this age group are nicotine (median prevalence of tobacco use 18.2%; 14% males and 6.3% females), cannabis (3%), and opiates (0.1%) misuse of prescription medication (opioids sedative/hypnotics, and stimulants 16.2%).

Possible Steps for Prevention and Early Identification

Steps to increase awareness, changing attitude toward mental illness and destigmatization through inclusion of mental health issues in curriculum and conducting various workshops about high-risk behaviors, substance use, emotional and behavioral issues, with involvement of students, parents and those students who have faced these issues and open discussions should be undertaken to identify the at-risk and help the teenagers. WHO's Mental Health Gap Action Programme (mhGAP) provides guidelines for nonspecialists to enable them identify priority mental health conditions.

Counseling

Counselors in colleges provide individual and group counseling to students in areas such as attitudes and behavior, relationships with peer, family transitions, test-taking and study skills, career and educational planning, decision making, and promoting more healthy coping skills and also recognize and respond to the need for mental health and behavioral prevention, early intervention and crisis services when required. Counseling may also include providing students with individual planning on academic, career and social or emotional fronts. Most boards of education have stated that it is mandatory to have at least one counselor in every school; however, lack of resources (both personnel and financial) has not seen this being implemented yet in ground reality.

Mentoring

It is a one-to-one professional relationship in which an experienced person (mentor) assists another (mentee) in developing specific skills and knowledge that enhances the mentee's professional and personal growth. Mentoring is one of many approaches that may improve the well-being of youth. Mentors can be formal and natural ones. The formal ones include school teachers, counselors, psychologists, social workers, senior students, faculty, while natural ones are nonparent adults, and natural supports like friends or relatives. It works through socioemotional or attachment theory, learning theory, and role modeling.

Mentoring often leads to positive overall development, increased motivation for various activities, improved functioning, decreased symptoms, better acceptance of psychological issues, and compliance to treatment regimens. Recent researches suggest that mentoring programs have positive effects on all categories of outcomes, i.e., internalizing/externalizing symptoms, school/academic, and interpersonal.

Teen Communities

These are groups of teenagers who are similar to each other in terms of age, gender, ethnicity, and social background, as well as in the types of interests and activities in which they engage. Teen communities are important for identity development, feelings of belonging, and social support, regardless of whether or not they are mediated. In situation of rejection, which is quite common in this age group, they get support from members, reducing their sense of isolation.

Screening for Sexually Transmitted Diseases and Substance Use

High-risk sexual practices and substance use are overtly common among youth as seen across various studies. As per the NFHS-3, 4% of young females and 15% men had experienced premarital sex and only 14.1% females used a contraceptive. It is a known risk factor for getting human immunodeficiency virus/acquired immunodeficiency syndrome (HIV/AIDS) and various other sexually transmitted infections such as gonorrhea, herpes, genital warts, chlamydia, syphilis, trichomoniasis, etc. The higher prevalence is due to various barriers in receiving STD-related information and services for STD screening and treatment. A better understanding of effective strategies to promote STD screening and motivations for STD testing could reduce the delay in getting treatment. Similarly, provisions of routine substance screening can also be introduced in colleges.

PROCESS OF INTERVENTION

The process of identification and intervention has been shown in **Figure 2**.

MODEL OF INTERVENTION

Though intervention at each level may be directed toward different problems and also the specific type of intervention may vary from student to student and has been dealt with appropriately, what follows is a general model of intervention which may be pursued in school-based mental health programs (**Figs. 3 to 5**).

Comprehensive school-based intervention   For whom

INDIAN PERSPECTIVE

The World Health Organization has advocated school mental health (SMH) to be an integral

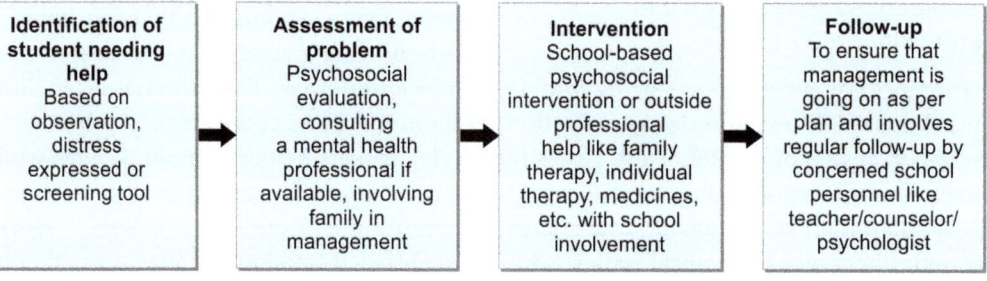

Fig. 2: Process of identification and intervention.

Interface with Education

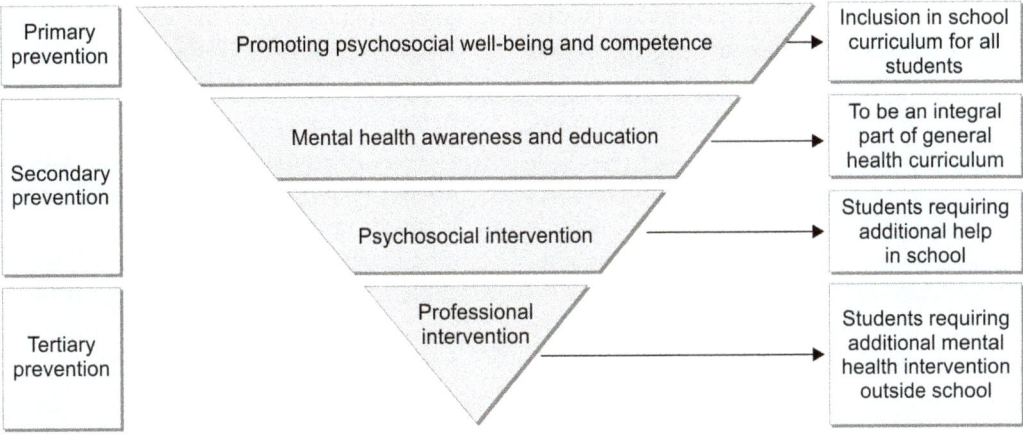

Fig. 3: Comprehensive model of intervention.

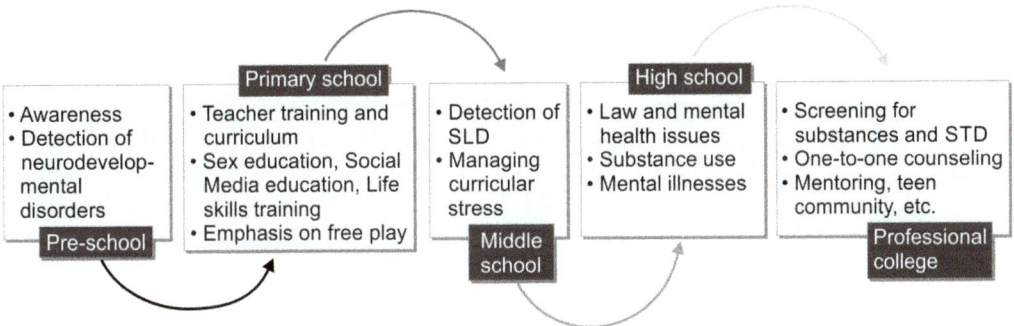

Fig. 4: Specific focus of intervention in various stages of school. (SLD: specific learning disorder)

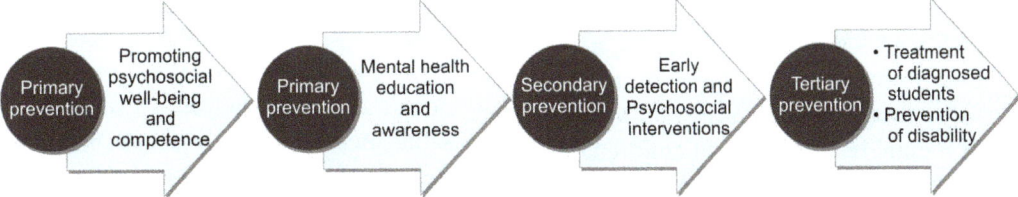

Fig. 5: The preventive model for promotion of school mental health.

part of school health systems. There is growing recognition about need such programs in India as well.

- Central Board of Secondary Education (CBSE) recommends that all secondary and senior secondary schools to employ a counselor. Further, CBSE has also started inclusion of life skills training in curriculum.
- In 2008, a few components of SMH were incorporated in the National Mental Health Programme (NMHP).
- Integrated Child Development Services (ICDS, 1975) was launched with plan of laying basis for proper physical and psychosocial development of the children (Ministry of Women and Child Development, Government of India, 1975).

- Recently, Ministry of Health and Family Welfare has started a program titled "*Rashtriya Bal Swasthya Karyakram*" under the National Rural Health Program. The program aims to screen children with developmental delays, including disabilities and there is provision for a psychologist at the district level for helping such children.

Despite these policies, outcome is not very promising due to inadequate implementation of the same.

SCHOOL MENTAL HEALTH IN INDIA: CURRENT STATUS

- There have been a few efforts toward long-term SMH services where institutions working in school mental health, send multi-disciplinary teams of experts to schools on a periodic basis to conduct awareness programs for teachers and students, as well as helping children with minor or major psychological problems. Though these approaches are noticeable, lack of broader national coverage and reluctance of schools has limited their overall impact.
- *NIMHANS Bengaluru:* In 1970, a two-phase program started to train teachers regarding detection and management of mental health issues in children. First phase—teacher orientation and training in management of child mental health issues thus preventing unnecessary outside referrals. Further, started SMH program for overall psychosocial development of children with the help of various stimulation programs. Simultaneously, in Mumbai, around the same time, SMH clinic was the first truly community-based service started by the Department of Psychiatry at TNMC and BYL Nair Charitable Hospital, where a team consisting of a psychiatrist, psychologist, and social worker actually visited schools to screen children and create awareness of mental health issues in teachers and parents.
- *Health promotion using life skills in adolescent program:* Started at NIMHANS, focused on psychosocial competence by enabling behavioral, emotional, and social skills in adolescents. The teachers were also trained to enable them to integrate this program in school services and the results showed a positive impact.
- *Promotion of wellness for preschoolers:* A structured program involving preschoolers and their mothers to improve mother-child interaction and to enhance prosocial behavior and cognitive skills.
- *Zippy's Friends Program:* Focus on promotion of mental health and mental well-being of children, is currently running in various countries, including India where it was launched with support from an NGO Sangath; however, in India its spread was limited to a single state and needs expansion.

Factors preventing effective collaboration in the growing education-mental health interface in India:
- Lack of a trained mental health professionals and lack of funding.
- Reluctance and apathy of schools including lack of resources and additional responsibility on teachers.
- Parents opposition due to fear of child being labeled by mental health professionals.
- Limited sensitization on promotive mental health.

CONCLUSION AND FUTURE DIRECTIONS

Mental health services if integrated within educational systems create a continuum of comprehensive care that can promote health, mental health, and academic achievement. Strategies to incorporate the different levels of interventions within a school, and use of resources from within the school, are probably the most sustainable. Involvement of all stakeholders will ensure that young people can access preventive and treatment services whenever they are needed. Application of the evidence from global programs and use of technology can ensure quality and accessibility, but public and political partnership will be needed to ensure successful implementation. Focus should be on capacity building, setting of outcome assessments for such programs to measure effectiveness, liaison and interactions on international level for expert help and if required, use of technology for increasing reach of such programs where not feasible otherwise, etc. Proposed model should have both universal and targeted approach to mental health problems in children and adolescents.

SUGGESTED READING

1. Achenbach TM, Edelbrock C. Manual for the Child Behavior Checklist/4-18 and 1991 Profile. Burlington, VT: University of Vermont, Department of psychiatry; 1991.
2. Adam M. Learning disabilities. [online] Available from https://www.scribd.com/document/272044348/ld [Last accessed June, 2021].
3. Agarwal S, Kumar N. Juvenile Justice (Care and Protection of Children) Act 2015: a review. Space Cult India. 2016;3:5-9.
4. Agarwal SP. Child and adolescent mental health: a pragmatic perspective. In: Agarwal SP, Goel DS, Ichhpujani RL, Salhan RN, Shrivastava S (Eds). Mental Health: An Indian Perspective (1946–2003), 1st edition. New Delhi: Directorate General of Health Services, Ministry of Health and Family Welfare (India); pp. 290-2.
5. Ahmad A, Khalique N, Khan Z, Amir A. Prevalence of psychosocial problems among school going male adolescents. Indian J Community Med. 2007;32:219-21.
6. American Psychiatric Association. Diagnostic and Statistical Manual of Mental Disorders (DSM-5). Washington DC: American Psychiatric Publishing; 2013.
7. Anderson GE, Jimerson SR, Whipple AD. Student ratings of stressful experiences at home and school: loss of a parent and grade retention as superlative stressors. J Appl School Psychol. 2005;21:1-20.
8. Anderson M, Jiang J. (2018). Teens, social media and technology. [online] Available from http://www.pewinternet.org/2018/05/31/teens-social-media-technology-2018 [Last accessed June, 2021].
9. Angold A, Costello EJ, Messer SC, Pickles A. Development of a short questionnaire for use in epidemiological studies of depression in children and adolescents. Int J Method Psychiatr Res. 1995;5:237-49.
10. Arnett JJ. Emerging adulthood. A theory of development from the late teens through the twenties. Am Psychol. 2000;55:469-80.
11. Arun P, Chavan BS. Stress and suicidal ideas in adolescent students in Chandigarh. Indian J Med Sci. 2009;63:281-7.
12. Baird G, Charman T, Cox A, Baron-Cohen S, Swettenham J, Wheelwright S, et al. Screening and surveillance for autism and pervasive developmental disorders. Arch Dis Child. 2001;84:468-75.
13. Bansal V, Goyal S, Srivastava K. Study of prevalence of depression in adolescent students of a public school. Ind Psychiatry J. 2009;18:43-6.
14. Beidas RS, Stewart RE, Walsh L, Lucas S, Downey MM, Jackson K, et al. Free, brief, and validated: standardized instruments for low-resource mental health settings. Cogn Behav Pract. 2015;22:5-19.
15. Bej P. Adolescent health problems in India: a review from 2001 to 2015. Indian J Community Health. 2015;27:418-28.
16. Botvin GJ, Baker E, Filazzola AD, Botvin EM. A cognitive-behavioral approach to substance abuse prevention: one-year follow-up. Addict Behav. 1990;15:47-63.
17. Central Board of Secondary Education (CBSE). Counselling in schools. Circular no. 08 of 2008. [online] Available from www.cbse.nic.in/welcome/htm [Last accessed June, 2021].
18. Central Board of Secondary Education (CBSE). Life skills education in class VII. Circular no. 11/04 of 2004. [online] Available from http://cbse.gov.in/circulars/2004/Circulars_11.htm [Last accessed June, 2021].
19. Cheney GR, Ruzzi BB, Muralidharan K. A profile of the Indian education system. Prepared for the

New Commission on the Skills of the American Workforce. 2005.
20. Dalton A. Factors affecting the health of middle school students. (2000, Doctoral dissertation). [online] Available from https://www.google.amanda dalton [Last accessed June, 2021].
21. Deb S, Chatterjee P, Walsh KM. Anxiety among high school students in India: comparisons across gender, school type, social strata, and perceptions of quality time with parents. Australian J Edu Dev Psychol. 2010;10:18-31.
22. Deb S, Strodl E, Sun J. Academic stress, parental pressure, anxiety and mental health among Indian high school students. Int J Psychol Behav Sci. 2015;5:26-34.
23. DuBois DL, Holloway BE, Valentine JC, Cooper H. Effectiveness of mentoring programs for youth: a meta-analytic review. Am J Community Psychol. 2002;30:157-97.
24. Faulstich ME, Carey MP, Ruggiero L, Enyart P, Gresham F. Assessment of depression in childhood and adolescence: an evaluation of the Centre for Epidemiological Studies Depression Scale for Children (CES-DC). Am J Psychiatry. 1986;143:1024-27.
25. First indigenous dyslexia assessment tool launched. [online] Available from http://www.dbtindia.nic.in/first-indigenous dyslexia-assessment-tool-launched/ [Last accessed June, 2021].
26. Flaherty LT, Garrison EG, Waxman R, Uris PF, Keys SG, Siegel MG, et al. Optimizing the roles of school mental health professionals. J Sch Health. 1998;68:420-4.
27. Frith E. (2017). Social media and children's mental health: a review of the evidence. [online] Available from https://dera.ioe.ac.uk/29528/1/Social-Media_Mental-Health_EPI-Report.pdf [Last accessed June, 2021].
28. Froeschle J, Moyer M. Just cut it out: legal and ethical challenges in counselling students who self-mutilate. Prof Sch Couns. 2004;7:231-5.
29. Gaur DR, Vohra AK, Subash S, Hitesh K. Prevalence of psychiatric morbidity among 6 to 14 years old children. Indian J Community Med. 2003;28:133-7.
30. Goodman R, Ford T, Simmons H, Gatward R, Meltzer H. Using the Strengths and Difficulties Questionnaire (SDQ) to screen for child psychiatric disorders in a community sample. Br J Psychiatry. 2000;177:534-9.
31. Gupta K, Arnold F, Lhungdim H. Health and living conditions in eight Indian cities. National Family Health Survey (NFHS-3) India 2005-06. [online] Available from https://dhsprogram.com/pubs/pdf/od58/od58.pdf [Last accessed June, 2021].
32. Gupta N, Aggarwal NK, Bhatia MS. The protection of children from sexual offences (POCSO). Delhi Psychiatr J. 2013;16:429-31.
33. Haase AQ, Boyd D. Teen communities. (2011). [online] Available from https://www.danah.org/papers/2011/TeenCommunitiesDRAFT.pdf [Last accessed June, 2021].
34. Hendren R, Birrell WR, Orley JH. (1994). Mental health programmes in schools. Geneva: World Health Organization. [online] Available from http://apps.who.int/iris/bitstream/handle/10665/62308/WHO_MNH_PSF_93.3_Rev.1.pdf;jsessionid=AA3589B286ADBDBF06AD49B726757214?sequence=1 [Last accessed June, 2021].
35. Hess RS, Copeland EP. Stress. In: Bear GG, Minke KM (Eds). Children's Needs III: Development, Prevention and Intervention, 1st edition. Washington, DC: National Association of School Psychologists; 2006. pp. 255-65.
36. House of Commons Health and Education Committee. Children and young people's mental health—the role of education. First joint report of the Education and Health Committees of Session 2016–2017. [online] Available from https://publications.parliament.uk/pa/cm201617/cmselect/cmhealth/849/849.pdf [Last accessed June, 2021].
37. Jellinek MS, Murphy JM, Little M, Pagano ME, Comer DM, Kelleher KJ. Use of the Pediatric Symptom Checklist to screen for psychosocial problems in pediatric primary care: a national feasibility study. Arch Pediatr Adolesc Med. 1999;153:254-60.
38. Kaffenberger C, Seligman L. Helping students with mental and emotional disorders. In: Erford BT (Ed). Transforming the School Counselling Profession, 2nd edition. Upper Saddle River, NJ: Pearson Merrill/Prentice Hall; 2007. pp. 351-83.
39. Kouzma NM, Kennedy GA. Self-reported sources of stress in senior high school students. Psychol Rep. 2004;94:314-6.
40. Kroenke K, Spitzer RL. The PHQ-9: a new depression diagnostic and severity measure. Psychiatr Ann. 2002;32:509-15.
41. Kumar D, Bharath S, Hirisave U, Agarwal S, Shah H. School mental health programs in India: current status and future directions. In: Kutcher S, Wei Y, Weist MD (Eds). School Mental Health: Global Challenge and Opportunities, 1st edition.

Cambridge: Cambridge University Press; 2015. pp. 95-104.
42. Leekam S, Libby S, Wing L, Gould J, Gillberg C. Comparison of ICD-10 and Gillberg's criteria for Asperger syndrome. Autism. 2000;4:11-28.
43. Lindsay S, Hounsell KG, Cassiani C. A scoping review of the role of LEGO® therapy for improving inclusion and social skills among children and youth with autism. Disabil Health J. 2017;10:173-82.
44. Los Angeles County Department of Mental Health. (2011). RCADS quick guide—child. [online] Available from http://lausdsmh.net/wp-content/uploads/2012/03/RCADS-Child-Quick-Guide1.pdf [Last accessed June, 2021].
45. Malhotra S, Kohli A, Kapoor M, Pradhan B. Incidence of childhood psychiatric disorders in India. Indian J Psychiatry. 2009;51:101.
46. Mental health screening and assessment tools for primary care. [online] Available from https://www.aap.org/en-us/advocacy-and-policy/aap-health-initiatives/Mental-Health/Documents/MH_ScreeningChart.pdf [Last accessed June, 2021].
47. Ministry of Health and Family Welfare, Government of India. (1982). National Mental Health Programme. [online] Available from https://mohfw.gov.in/sites/default/files/9903463892NMHP%20detail_0.pdf [Last accessed June, 2021].
48. Ministry of Health and Family Welfare, Government of India. (2014). Rashtriya Bal Swasthya Karyakram. [online] Available from http://nhm.gov.in/rashtriya-kishor-swasthya-karyakram.html [Last accessed June, 2021].
49. Ministry of Women and Child Development, Government of India. (1975). Integrated Child Development Services Scheme. [online] Available from https://icds-wcd.nic.in/icds.aspx [Last accessed June, 2021].
50. Nair MK, Paul MK, John R. Prevalence of depression among adolescents. Indian J Pediatr. 2004;71:523-4.
51. Narcotic Drugs and Psychotropic Substances Act. Government of India. (1985). [online] Available from http://narcoticsindia.nic.in/upload/download/document_id08b2dbdc9ca941d237893bd425af8bfa.pdf [Last accessed June, 2021].
52. National Family Health Survey (NFHS-3) India 2005-06. [online] Available from https://dhsprogram.com/pubs/pdf/frind3/frind3-vol1andvol2.pdf [Last accessed June, 2021].
53. Ohta M, Nagai Y, Hara H, Sasaki M. Parental perception of behavioral symptoms in Japanese autistic children. J Autism Dev Disord. 1987;17:549-63.
54. Patel V, Flisher AJ, Nikapota A, Malhotra S. Promoting child and adolescent mental health in low and middle income countries. J Child Psychol Psychiatry. 2008;49:313-34.
55. Pedrelli P, Nyer M, Yeung A, Zulauf C, Wilens T. College students: mental health problems and treatment considerations. Acad Psychiatry. 2015;39:503-11.
56. Perlis RH, Smoller JW, Ferreira MA, McQuillin A, Bass N, Lawrence J, et al. A genome wide association study of response to lithium for prevention of recurrence in bipolar disorder. Am J Psychiatry. 2009;166:718-5.
57. Pillai A, Patel V, Cardozo P, Goodman R, Weiss HA, Andrew G. Non-traditional lifestyles and prevalence of mental disorders in adolescents in Goa, India. Br J Psychiatry. 2008;192:45-51.
58. Rai D, Gaete J, Girotra S, Pal HR, Araya R. Substance use among medical students: time to reignite the debate? Natl Med J India. 2008;21:75-8.
59. Raman V, Singhal M. Play therapy with children: its relevance and utility in the Indian context. J Indian Assoc Child Adolesc Ment Health. 2015;11:121-57.
60. Rani PG. Financing primary education and Sarva Shiksha Abhiyan. New Delhi: National Institute of Educational Planning and Administration; 2003.
61. Rao C, Midha R, Midya V, Sumathi TA, Singh N, Oberoi G, et al. (2015). Dyslexia Assessment for Languages of India (DALI). [online] Available from https://www.researchgate.net/publication/323704398_Dyslexia_Assessment_for_Languages_of_India_DALI [Last accessed June, 2021].
62. Rhodes JE, Grossman JB, Resch NL. Agents of change: pathways through which mentoring relationships influence adolescents' academic adjustment. Child Dev. 2000;71:1662-71.
63. Ross JG, Luepker RV, Nelson GD, Saavedra P, Hubbard BM. Teenage health teaching modules: impact of teacher training on implementation and student outcomes. J Sch Health. 1991;61:31-4.
64. Sadock BJ, Sadock VA, Ruiz P, (Eds). Kaplan and Sadock's Comprehensive Textbook of Psychiatry, 10th edition. Philadelphia: Wolters Kluwer; 2017.
65. Sahoo S, Khess CR. Prevalence of depression, anxiety, and stress among young male adults in

India: a dimensional and categorical diagnoses-based study. J Nerv Ment Dis. 2010;198:901-4.
66. Schulte-Körne G. Mental health problems in a school setting in children and adolescents. Dtsch Arztebl Int. 2016;113:183-90.
67. Schwab Learning. (2002). Parent's guide to differences and disabilities in learning. [online] Available from www.schwablearning.org [Last accessed June, 2021].
68. Screen for Child Anxiety Related Emotional Disorders (SCARED) Parent Version. Department of Psychiatry, University of Pittsburgh School of Medicine. [online] Available from http://www.wpic.pitt.edu/research/AssessmentTools/ChildAdolescent/ScaredParent-final [Last accessed June, 2021].
69. Scripture Union. All the right moves: life-skills for an aids-free generation: twelve to fifteen-year programme. Rondebosch, South Africa: Scripture Union; 1994.
70. Sharma R, Grover VL, Chaturvedi S. Suicidal behavior amongst adolescent students in south Delhi. Indian J Psychiatry. 2008;5:30-3.
71. Spence SH. A measure of anxiety symptoms among children. Behav Res Ther. 1998;36:545-66.
72. Srinath S, Girimaji SC, Gururaj G, Seshadri S, Subbakrishna DK, Bhola P, et al. Epidemiological study of child and adolescent psychiatric disorders in urban and rural areas of Bangalore, India. Indian J Med Res. 2005;122:67-79.
73. Stevens GD, Stevens HA. Identifying the mentally retarded child in the rural school. Elem School J. 1947;481:49-54.
74. Sunitha S, Gururaj G. Health behaviours and problems among young people in India: Cause for concern and call for action. Indian J Med Res. 2014;140:185-208.
75. Taneja V, Sriram S, Beri R, Sreenivas V, Aggarwal R, Kaur R. 'Not by bread alone': impact of a structured 90-minute play session on development of children in an orphanage. Child Care Health Dev. 2002;28:95-100.
76. The Cigarettes and Other Tobacco Products (Prohibition of Advertisement and regulation of Trade and Commerce, Production, Supply and Distribution) Act, 2003. An Act enacted by the Parliament of Republic of India by Notification in the Official Gazette. (Act 32 of 2003). [online] Available from http://mohfw.nic.in/index1.php?lang&level=2&sublinkid=671&lid=662 [Last accessed June, 2021].
77. The CRAFFT Screening Tool. Centre for Adolescent Substance Abuse Research. [online] Available from http://www.ceasar-boston.org/CRAFFT/index.php [Last accessed June, 2021].
78. The Delhi Excise Act, 2009. [online] Available from http://delhi.gov.in/wps/wcm/ [Last accessed June, 2021].
79. United Nations Office on Drugs and Crime (UNODC). (2004). National survey on extent, pattern and trends of drug abuse in India. [online] Available from www.unodc.org/india/national_Survey.html [Last accessed June, 2021].
80. Vaidya G, Dhavale HS. Child psychiatry in Bombay: the school mental health clinic. Hosp Med. 2000;61:400-1.
81. Verma S, Gupta J. Some aspects of high academic stress and symptoms. J Pers Clin Stud. 1990;6:7-12.
82. Waxman RP, Weist MD, Benson DM. Toward collaboration in the growing education-mental health interface. Clin Psychol Rev. 1999;19:239-53.
83. Weidner G, Kohlmann CW, Dotzauer E, Burns LR. The effects of academic stress on health behaviors in young adults. Anxiety Stress Coping. 1996;9:123-33.
84. Wenz-Gross M, Siperstein GN. Importance of social support in the adjustment of children with learning problems. Except Child. 1997;63:183-93.
85. Whitebread D. Free play and children's mental health. Lancet Child Adolesc Health. 2017;1:167-9.
86. Williams JR, Zenilman J, Nanda JP, Mark H. Recruitment strategies and motivations for sexually transmitted disease testing among college students. J Am Coll Health. 2008;57:357-60.
87. World Health Organization. (2004). Promoting mental health: concepts, emerging evidence, practice: summary report. [online] Available from https://www.who.int/mental_health/evidence/en/promoting_mhh.pdf [Last accessed June, 2021].
88. World Health Organization. Mental Health Gap Action Programme (mhGAP). [online] Available from https://www.who.int/mental_health/mhgap/en/ [Last accessed June, 2021].
89. World Health Organization. Young people: health risks and solutions. Fact sheet no. 345.2011. [online] Available from http://www.who.int/mediacentre/factsheets/fs345/en/index.html [Last accessed June, 2021].

CHAPTER 23

Interface with Cinema

Sachin Nagendrappa, Shubrata Kalmane

CINEMA AND PSYCHIATRY

Cinema is an important form of art that is a powerful medium of the portrayal of society and culture across the world. Over a century, cinema has grown to a greater extent. Especially over the last few decades, cinema has evolved to an immense extent with improved and advanced audiovisual techniques, which captures attention, evokes emotional response and feelings of people who are watching it, and creates a dream-like experience, and thus making cinema a very influential mode of mass communication.[1] Films with mental health themes (like A Beautiful Mind, Black Swan, Taare Zameen Par, etc.) have grown popular, even though the concepts of mental illness they reflect are frequently either sentimentalized or grossly exaggerated.[2]

Psychiatry and cinema incidentally share some commonalities; both are concerned with human behaviors and motivations. The heart of cinema is the portrayal of characters and stories, whereas mental health professionals share similar interests in human characters and behaviors and both rely on emotions as a core.[3]

While sharing his views, Dr Green considers plenty of reasons to show the importance of the interface between psychiatry and art, and art includes cinemas also. First of all, he considers that mental health research has an immense impact on understanding the cultural aspects of mind and human behavior. It helps in understanding the mind, relationships, and psychological development.[2] Cinema is also considered as an important tool for social change, strengthening human emotions, and as a tool for positive change in the belief system of the community. In the current world, we see mental health issues are on the rise. Hence, it is extremely important to portray mental illness in a way that is accurate and not stigmatizing.

Pathak et al.[4] describe major processes which are involved in the creation of a cinema that brings the concept into a reality and thus helps in disseminating knowledge, making changes in attitudes and beliefs. The three major processes include production, representation, and reception. Production involves creation and execution through audio and video. Representation helps in understanding and analyzing various information portrayed in different media.[5] Reception is the final process where the audience is involved and it deals with how they respond and receive the cinema. The three processes are important interfaces with psychiatry. In this chapter, we will try to understand the interfaces of cinema with psychiatry, the depiction of mental illnesses in cinemas, cinemas as a tool for education about mental health, and changing the perception of public in eradicating the stigma toward mentally ill people and finally about the future directions.

DEPICTION OF MENTAL ILLNESSES AND PORTRAYAL OF MENTAL HEALTH PROFESSIONALS IN CINEMAS

Cinemas about mental health conditions can be a double-edged sword. On one side, it may help in creating awareness about mental health conditions, good portrayal of a psychiatrist, psychologists, and other allied mental health professionals, and creating knowledge about certain mental illnesses, thus helping in increased treatment-seeking behavior. Whereas on the contrary, it may create more stigma, by depicting psychiatric patients as violent, portraying mental health professionals as weird persons, and life-saving treatment such as electroconvulsive therapy (ECT) as inhuman treatment. These may do more harm and create a negative impression toward mental health and mental health professionals. Though it may be argued that it is the viewer's discretion to take the message given by the cinema, but at the same time, the film crew must be aware of the sensitivity and gravity of the mental health condition and not sensationalize violence and substance use.

Mental health professionals are portrayed as lead roles or as supporting characters over a century. However, across cultures, the depiction of mental health professionals is somewhat similar to the unbalanced portrayal of stereotypes. Professionals who are involved in mental health care are subjected to ridicule, criticism, and inaccurate judgment.[6]

The portrayal of mental health professionals notes it to be wrong most of the time. This may be due to a lack of experience and lack of knowledge during various phases of making a cinema. Most often the word "psychologist" is generically used to denote various mental health professionals including psychiatrists, psychiatric nurses, counselors, and psychiatric social workers. These kinds of wrong portrayals may directly or indirectly influence public perceptions on treatment and also mental health professionals. That may result in false expectations, lack of treatment-seeking, or reduce motivation. This also influences people who are willing to enter the profession of mental health negatively. Most movies across the world show mental professionals as people who cross boundaries are manipulative, or with someone who has an internal motive and is corrupted. This is a lack of experience in the field of psychiatry in the filmmakers. Some of the films depict psychoanalysis as the only treatment or the most practiced form in managing psychiatric illness. The majority of the role of the movie included only males as therapists. This trend is changing recently as females are also considered for the role of therapists. In earlier Hollywood movies, there was a racial disparity as only white men were considered for the role of therapists. Movies never discuss the research, which is ongoing in the field of mental health. But recently, movies are increasing in number over the last decade where they portray mental health professionals as balanced people who are motivating, empathic, compassionate, and well-intentioned.[6]

A study was done in India about the portrayal of psychiatrists in Hindi cinemas commonly known as Bollywood. The study found that in movies, 42.4% of psychiatrists were portrayed as clinically incompetent, 30.3% were shown not arriving at a diagnosis, 39.4% of psychiatrists were shown as breaching their professional ethics, 24.2% transgressed nonsexual boundaries, and 15.2% of psychiatrists' word depicted as violating sexual and nonsexual boundaries. This shows the gravity of the negative depiction of the psychiatrists, this which may convey a wrong message to the audience and aversion toward treatment seeking. In the same study, only 23.1% of the movies showed a positive side that is a good treatment outcome.[7] Few movies need special mention. Sumitra Bhave–Sunil Sukthankar duo has produced three movies in Marathi, namely, Devrai, Astu, and Kaasav, having themes of schizophrenia, Alzheimer disease, and depression, respectively. Devrai depicts a story of a man who suffers from schizophrenia and is struggling to come to terms with his illness and the frustration of his helpless sister. Devrai was produced in association with Schizophrenia Awareness Association and KS Wani Memorial Trust. Renowned psychiatrist, Mohan Agashe, has been proactive in making of all these movies from contributing for the story line, getting the right facts, playing a major role in the movie to helping monetarily.[8]

SUBSTANCE USE IN CINEMAS

Substance use disorders are major health concerns of any country in the world. Alcohol, smoking nicotine, and many other substances such as cannabis, cocaine, and many other illicit substances have been portrayed in cinemas across the world. The role of cinema is well-known in influencing the choices of individuals to use substances, especially the young adolescents who tend to use psychoactive substances likely influenced by the favorite characters using a particular substance which can be explained through observational learning theory. One study from India had shown that 90% of the Bollywood movies had one or more depictions of alcohol use.[9] Similarly, another study investigated the drug use representations in scenes from Academy Award (Oscar)-nominated movies from 2008 to 2011. Results were surprising that all the Oscar-nominated movies had at least one scene in the movie where drug use was shown.[10] This is a matter of serious concern. Oscar-nominated movies have a wide range of audiences across the world. It is highly likely to influence society's behavior and acceptance toward substance use. It is a matter of immediate concern that regulatory authorities should cautiously regulate the portrayal of substance use. On the other hand, there are some movies with good themes highlighting the gravity of substance use disorders. These movies also highlight the negative consequences of substance use and also motivate to keep people away from using drugs.[11]

ELECTROCONVULSIVE THERAPY IN CINEMA

Andrade et al. in 2011[12] reviewed 13 Hindi movies which contained referrals or depictions of ECT between 1967 and 2008. ECT was used to punish, obliterate identity, cause insanity, and for a variety of other clinically invalid reasons. ECT was almost often forced upon patients. Premedication was a rare occurrence. Genuine ECT devices were used infrequently. Stimulation with electroconvulsive treatment almost always appeared to induce pain.

In several cases, multiple shocks were delivered in the same session. Usually, the convulsions were strange. Though there was no mortality, the treatment induced mental disturbances, amnesia, weakness, and sometimes a zombie-like state; clinical improvement was rare. Unfortunately, even the newer releases did not show any improvement in the accuracy of the depiction of ECTs.

The Scenario is not so Bleak!

Though we see the stigmatized portrayal of mental health issues in the majority of the movies, there are few ones, which portray the same sensitively and truthfully. National Alliance on Mental Illness list contains movies such as "A Beautiful Mind" (on Schizophrenia), "Matchstick Men" (on the obsessive-compulsive disorder), "It's Kind of a Funny Story" (on depression and suicidal ideation), and many more.[13]

Even in India, we have very good examples of cinemas with sensitive and realistic portrayals of mental health themes. "Taare Zameen Par" is one such cinema that describes the difficulties of a child with dyslexia very well. It can be used to educate parents of children with dyslexia. Likewise, cinemas such as "My Name is Khan" and "The Spirit" have made a positive impact.

In India, we have our psychiatrists as producers of movies with mental health themes. Late Dr Ashok Pai is one such psychiatrist, who produced movies such as "Kaadina Benki" and "Prathama Ushakirana" in the local language, Kannada, which went to win National and State awards.[14] There are producers and scriptwriters who take the help of mental health professionals while planning for a cinema.

CINEMA AS A TOOL FOR EDUCATION AND CHANGING PUBLIC PERCEPTION

Cinemas can be used as a tool for education and changing public perceptions. Several studies analyzed cinemas as a tool for learning and concluded that cinemas enhance reasoning, critical thinking, retention, understanding, abstract thinking, and self-regulation. It also opens and promotes social thinking and awareness of social perspectives. It has also shown an impact on decision-making capacities. Practical implementation of cinema in the learning curriculum is known to be effective as it generates creativity and involvement.[15,16] Cinema can be called a universal language, there may be 100 different languages, it is often noted that the scenes can invoke emotions, and the person watching the movie can relate to themselves. Cinema can be a strong tool when used wisely. Parents should teach their younger ones to critically evaluate and take positive points, and teach how to evaluate critically with the utmost sensitivity, respect, and validate others' emotions.

In his book, Mad Tales from Bollywood,[17] Dr Bhugra looks at the interface of psychiatry and popular Bollywood cinema culture. Dr Bhugra says "Cinema not only reflects the society it is set in but also acts as a reflector to the society." He believes cinema leaves an impression on society, and society reacts to it in different ways. The consistency of portrayal may bring changes in society's perceptions over a while according to him. Thus, we believe it holds good not only in Indian cinema but also in cinemas across the borders in any language. The audience expects entertainment; there needs to be a social message and better depiction of humanity, justice, and nonviolence. Movies play a major role in reducing harms related to substance use, reducing in crime rate when values and ethics are portrayed well. This also motivates in improving the quality of life, decision-making, and in turn formation of a better society to live in.

NOVEL APPROACHES IN TEACHING PSYCHIATRY THROUGH MOVIES

Cinemas can be used as a tool to teach mental health professionals, especially the residents in psychiatry. A team can select a movie and it can be shown in presence of psychiatry residents and faculty. It is practiced in some colleges in India. After a short introduction, the positive and negative aspects of the movie are discussed, this will enhance the critical examination skills of the trainees and give a window for novel perspective to mental illness in public perspective, this innovative idea is called as cine clubs and Dr Gurvinder has described in his article about the novel way to teach the psychiatry trainees.[18] Movie clubs also help in understanding the stigma surrounding mental illness in public perspective how the mental health professionals themselves are facing the stigma and approach to destigmatize and ways to approach can be effectively delivered through cine clubs.[19] Apart from the social perspective, we can use cinema to identify the signs and symptoms of illness, how to approach a patient in correct fashion, how cinema has portrayed, is there a wrong depiction movie can also be discussed, thus trainee can learn arriving at diagnosis overcoming the diagnostic dilemma effectively.[20] It can also be used effectively in creating interest in ungraduated students.[21] Thus, it can be effectively used and the success of such clubs can be successfully replicated in other institutes.

Media Guidelines for Cinema: Need of the Hour!

World Health Organization published media guidelines for reporting suicides in 2008. Since then, several other organizations including the Indian Psychiatric Society have further modified those guidelines and come up with a clear set of criteria for reporting suicides. Though implementation of this has not been complete, we see that there has been a positive change after this. With cinema being a very powerful media influencing people's mindset and with frequent mental health aspects being seen in almost one in every three movies, it is high time we have a clear guideline, dos, and don'ts about the portrayal of mental health issues in cinema. It is vital that we need to be sensitive to the local culture and geographic location while chalking out these guidelines.

ADVOCACY

As mental health professionals, we need to be proactive in recognizing the negative portrayals in cinemas and strongly advocating for change. In 2019, the promo of a movie was released with the title "Mental Hein Kya?." The Indian Psychiatry Society took it seriously, objected to the title and wrote in public domain (Social Media) which went Viral. They asserted that the film's title is discriminative, stigmatizing, degrading, inhumane in projecting mental disorders and people who suffer from mental disorders. Then print and visual media started taking interest and many newspapers published statements of film maker and IPS officials. IPS wrote to film maker but there was no response. IPS did a massive press conference with Indian Medical Association at IMA HQs, which got wide coverage. IPS wrote to PM, IB Minister, Health Minister and NHRC but there was no progress. IPS filed a PIL in Ahmadabad high court. Honorable High Court directed CBFC to call IPS leaders and listen them. President and Hony General Secretary explained the reasons and suggested the CBFC. They were requested not to issue a certificate without giving proper thought to it and also suggested to invite two mental health professionals including a psychiatrist. Film was reviewed by CBFC with a psychiatrist and a psychologist on Board. Film makers informed honorable High Court regarding change of title from "Mental Hai Kya" to "Judgemental Hai Kya".[22]

FUTURE DIRECTIONS

Psychiatry and cinema will continue to evolve and share common aspects of understanding individual characters and stories. Cinemas can be used as an effective tool to bring changes in public perception about mental illness and to educate about misconceptions related to mental illness. It is a positive trend; there is increased positive portrayal about mental health conditions and roll off mental health professionals in managing the psychiatric illness. The representation of mental illness in cinema should contain the right information, which represents mental health professionals with sensitivity and empathy. Before making a movie on mental illness and mental health aspects, the team involved in scriptwriting and direction should acquire knowledge by discussing with the mental health professional and caregivers of the person suffering from the condition. Cinemas should discourage stigmatizing and stereotyping particular conditions instead they should educate about early intervention and management. There should be research on the impact of cinemas on the attitude toward mental health and mental health professionals across the world. There need to be policies by the government, which involve mental health professional to regulate the wrong depiction of mental illness and management aspects. It is equally important for the audience to critically think before changing their attitude or behavior based on the portrayal in cinemas.

REFERENCES

1. Damjanović A, Vuković O, Jovanović AA, Jašović-Gašić M. Psychiatry and movies. Psychiatr Danub. 2009;21(2):230-5.
2. Green J. Psychiatry and the arts: new interfaces? Adv Psychiatr Treat. 2008;14(3):163-6.
3. Beachum L. (2010). The psychopathology of cinema: how mental illness and psychotherapy are portrayed in film. Honor Proj. [online] Available from: http://scholarworks.gvsu.edu/honorsprojects/56. [Last accessed April 2022].
4. Pathak A, Biswal R. Mental illness in Indian Hindi cinema: production, representation, and reception before and after media convergence. Indian J Psychol Med. 2013;43(1):74-80.
5. Seale C. Health and media: an overview. Sociol Heal Illn. 2003;25(6):513-31.
6. Niemiec RM, Louis S, Louis S. The portrayal of psychologists. 2006.
7. Banwari GH. Portrayal of psychiatrists in Hindi movies released in the first decade of the 21st century. Asian J Psychiatr. 2011;4(3):210-3.
8. Gosh T. Why Marathi short film Still Alive, screened at 51st IFFI, is a timely take on mental health. [online] Available from: https://indianexpress.com/article/lifestyle/art-and-culture/marathi-short-film-still-alive-51st-iffi-mental-health-suicide-prevention-7156186/. [Last accessed April 2022].
9. Rao R, Panda U, Gupta S, Ambekar A, Gupta S, Agrawal A. Portrayal of alcohol in Bollywood movies: a mixed methods study. Indian J Psychiatry. 2020;62(2):159-66.
10. Castaldelli-Maia JM, Gil F, Ventriglio A, Torales J, Florio L, Moura HF, et al. Substance use portrayal in Oscar-nominated movies. Curr Drug Res Rev. 2021;13(3):230-5.
11. Das S, Doval N, Mohammed S, Dua N, Chatterjee SS. Psychiatry and cinema: what can we learn from the magical screen? Shanghai Arch Psychiatry. 2017;29(5):310-3.
12. Andrade C, Shah N, Venkatesh BK. The depiction of electroconvulsive therapy in Hindi cinema. J ECT. 2010;26(1):16-22.
13. Greenstein L. (2017). The Best Movies about Mental Health. [online] Available from: https://www.nami.org/Blogs/NAMI-Blog/December-2017/The-Best-Movies-About-Mental-Health. [Last accessed April 2022].
14. Rajadhyaksha A, Willemen P. Encyclopedia of Indian Cinema. London: Routledge; 1999.
15. Moskovich Y, Sharf S. Using films as a tool for active learning in teaching sociology. J Eff Teach. 2012;12(1):53-63.
16. Marcus AS. "It Is as It Was": Feature film in the history classroom. Soc Stud. 2005;96(2):61-7.
17. Bhugra D. Mad Tales from Bollywood: Portrayal of Mental Illness in Conventional Hindi Cinema. East Sussex: Psychology Press; 2006.
18. Kalra G. Psychiatry movie club: a novel way to teach psychiatry. Indian J Psychiatry. 2011;53(3):258-60.
19. Kalra G. Talking about stigma towards mental health professionals with psychiatry trainees: a movie club approach. Asian J Psychiatr. 2012;5(3):266-8.
20. Kalra G. Teaching diagnostic approach to a patient through cinema. Epilepsy Behav. 2011;22(3):571-3.
21. Datta V. Madness and the movies: an undergraduate module for medical students. Int Rev Psychiatry. 2009;21(3):261-6.
22. Kaur G. (2019). 'Mental Hai Kya' Renamed as 'Judgemental Hai Kya'. [online] Available from: https://www.sinceindependence.com/mental-hai-kya-renamed-as-judgemental-hai-kya/. [Last accessed April 2022].

CHAPTER 24

Interface with Dance, Music, and Theater

Pavitra KS

INTRODUCTION

Dance, theater, and music are creative expressions of human beings and remain universal. Yet they can be uniquely individualized. Dance is more than just exploring different ways of moving the body to music; it is a way of moving that uses the body as an instrument. It helps bringing out our inner expression. In other words through the medium of body, one tries to communicate the feelings of mind. We all use gestures, facial expressions, and nonverbal body behaviors while communicating and hence dance lies in each of us. According to Sangita Ratnakara an ancient treatise by Sarangadeva Sangita—music is stated as a composite performance art consisting of *Gita* (melodic forms, song), *Vadya* (instrumental music), and *Nritta* (dance, movement).[1] Music has also been described as the art of sound in time, expressing ideas and emotions in significant forms through the elements of melody, harmony, and color.[2] Though both dance and music can be both seen in the nature in diverse forms, the creativity in dance and music appears unique to human beings. There are numerous forms of music and dance. Be it classical—meaning which has an established system of studying pattern and has sound theoretical construct or one of the several other forms, dance and music are interwoven in human culture worldwide.

The interface of psychiatry with dance and music will be discussed under the following subsections:
- Dance and music and their relationship to mind and brain
- Dance and music as expressive therapies for mental illnesses
- Dance and music therapy for mental health problems in children and adolescents
- Mental health problems in dancers and musicians
- Dance and music in school mental health programs
- Dance and music therapies in India.

A brief discussion on theater and psychiatry also will be done at the end of the chapter.

When we talk about dance and music therapies, the contributor, herself an established professional dancer can remember the workshop which she conducted on dance therapy some time back. The questions and the doubts which most of the clinicians and postgraduates have, can lead to the therapeutic nihilism in using dance or music therapy for mental illnesses. Many agree that it is quite interesting but not practical. Most of them think listening to music or dancing is very beneficial for relaxation but at the same time doubt its efficacy in therapy of mental illnesses. Majority appeared concerned about double-blind randomized controlled trials (RCTs) for music and dance therapy were lacking and how to prescribe them as treatment either as monotherapy or in combination with medications for their patients. They were unsure about who should or can do dance and music therapy, what should be the protocol, patient's and therapist's continued motivation, the duration of therapy. Finally, a minority of them totally rejected these therapies as something which "do not work" and said they would prescribe medications instead which they said were easily supported through the RCTs and hence they felt confident in prescribing them. We also should note here that the difficulties for the doctors in Indian setting are plenty. Any kind of psychotherapeutic intervention is difficult in Indian setting because of the patient overload, patient difficulties with the compliance of the sessions, and psychiatrist's comfort levels with prescribing medications. Hence, the present chapter on the interface of psychiatry and performing arts tries to look at the studies available for using dance and music therapies for mental illnesses as well as their role in the promotion of mental health. The author being a consultant psychiatrist and a dance performer-choreographer herself would also attempt to present her perspective on how Indian dance and music can be used in the field of mental health in the Indian setting.

DANCE, MUSIC AND MIND

Dance is generally believed to be an entertainment. Though most of us agree that entertainment is beneficial for mental health we doubt the therapeutic value of dance. Interestingly each and every dance form of India finds its roots in Bharata's Natyashastra[3] which is dated probably in 2nd century BC. In the first chapter of Bharata's Natyashastra titled "Natyotpatti", Bharata himself narrates how actually dance came into existence. According to this, dance was created by Brahma in order to alleviate stress, negative feelings such as fear, anger, lust, jealousy and to calm the mind. Brahma's this new creation was in response to the plea made by Indra and his associates when the whole universe was full of these negative feelings and the people were suffering.

Whether Brahma really created it or the dance came into practice by a collective effort is a different question. But what is important for this discussion is that the original purpose of dance was not just providing entertainment as it is often thought today. Its main purpose was therapeutic which was to alleviate the suffering of mind, an art form with body as a medium was chosen. Mind-body relationship thus is integral to Indian dance forms. The basic emotions in dance as mentioned in Natyashastra[3] are eight. They are called "Rasas. *Sringara*—love, *veera*—valor, *karuna*—compassion, *adbhuta*—wonder, *hasya*—humor, *bhayanaka*—fear, *bibhatsya*—disgust, and *raudra*—anger are the eight rasas cited in Bharata's Natyashastra".[3]

The benefits of dance physically are quite well known. There have been various studies which have proven the physical benefits of dance—dance increases physical fitness, strengthens cardiovascular health, and flexibility. Researchers have found the increased awareness of our body through dancing.[4] Cognitive skills such as art appreciation, creativeness, imagination, musicality, sense of rhythm, and body control are increased by the medium of dance.[5] It is evident that dance has impact on the mental health aspects of an individual too. According to Alpert, elevated endorphin levels during dancing lead to elevated mood. He observes that emotional awareness is achieved because of the body going to a "self-awareness mode". This helps in stress reduction.[6]

Let us now look at the connection between music and mind. A detailed discussion on history of connection between music and mind can be found in an excellent review—"Psychiatry and music" by Nizamie and Tikka.[7] Only a few important ones will be mentioned here. Ancient Greek philosopher Plato (428-347 BC) considered that different music tunes aroused different emotions.[8] During Vedic times, there are references to seven "swaras"—basic notes being related to eight basic moods—*Ashta rasas*.[3] The musical notes *Madhyama* and *Panchama* are associated with *sringara* (emotion of love) and *hasya* (humor). The notes *Shadja* and *Rishabha* are associated with *raudra* (anger), *adbhuta* (wonder), *veera* (Valor). *Swaras nishada* and *Gandhara* with *karuna* (pathos) and *Dhaivata* with *bhayanaka* (fear) and *bibhatsya* (disgust).

We, through our own experiences, know that in times of stress, soothing music calms our mind. Certain tunes may evoke emotions of sadness and may bring tears. We may feel like dancing with joy to certain tunes. The lullabies put us to sleep. There have been studies which have shown that music benefits for physical health. Music played during surgery has shown to lessen pain and anxiety related to surgery.[9] Music has shown to reduce blood pressure, pulse, heart rate and aid in cardiovascular recovery from stress.[10]

BRAIN AND MUSIC-DANCE

It is now evident that music and dance both have an intrinsic connection with mind and hence with the brain. Human nervous system processes music in different ways. It can include perceptual processing, emotional processing, autonomic processing, cognitive processing and behavioral or motor processing.[11-13]

The link between dance and brain has been looked at two different dimensions in the research—dance observation and active dancing. The very nature of dancing makes it difficult to study the brain through imaging experiments. Dance perception has been studied based on "activity observation network—mirror neuron system" of the human and primate brain. This concept developed around the possibility that this neural system upholds the perception and reproduction of activity performer's actions.[14] This system is thought to include premotor and parietal cortices which might be associated with activity re-enactment in human beings. It also involves the supplementary area, superior temporal sulcus, and primary motor cortex. Neuroimaging in dancers has revealed important and interesting findings. They are: (1) dance performers show active movement observation and simulation neuronal networks—premotor cortex in particular. This may be because of increased motor representation of the observed movement, (2) the difference in action observation system in dancers correlates positively with the level of dance training, (3) dance training even for short duration is correlated with cerebral functional plasticity, and lastly (4) perception of recorded versus live dancing brings about differential cerebral activity.[15]

As observed earlier, there have been difficulties in studying active dancing. Motion artifacts involved during neuroimaging pose a problem. Even then, there have been attempts to overcome this barrier too. Brown et al. attempted studying some aspects of dance performance when artists were dancing. They observed amateur tango dancers performing tango steps (involving only the leg movements) while in a positron emission tomography (PET) scanner.[16] Dance performance was correlated with gray matter thickness in the superior temporal gyrus and white matter diffusivity in the corpus callosum. This indicates the importance of these regions in dance performance. The investigation shed some light on the specificity of dance training on brain structure and function, tested the existence of a sensitive period in the context of dance, and provided neuroimaging support for dance-based interventions.[15]

Thus, research on link between dance and brain and music and brain provides a better understanding regarding the basis of its therapeutic use in psychiatry. This will support the mounting scientific evidence for both dance and music therapies. It will provide new insights into the field of dance and music therapies.

DANCE, MUSIC AS EXPRESSIVE THERAPIES FOR MENTAL ILLNESSES

Dance and music therapies are essentially conceptualized as the branches of psychotherapy for mental illnesses. Even in other psychotherapy sessions, we should remember that the nonverbal behaviors of both the therapist and the client are considered important. We know that the art we realize that the fine arts and craftsmanship activities like drawing, drumming, singing, innovative movements—dance and drama permit the people of all age groups, from different cultural backgrounds, to communicate their musings, sentiments, and feelings in a way different from the typical methods of verbal expressions. Hence, they have unique utility as mental health interventions.

While expressive therapies can be considered a unique domain of psychotherapy and counseling, within this domain exists a set of individual approaches. Hence, music therapy and dance therapy are defined as follows.[17]

Music therapy uses music to effect positive changes in the psychological, physical, cognitive, or social functioning of individuals with health or educational problems.[18] Dance/movement therapy is based on the assumption that body and mind are interrelated and is defined as the psychotherapeutic use of movement as a process that furthers the emotional, cognitive, and physical integration of the individual. Dance/movement therapy effects changes in feelings, cognition, physical functioning, and behavior.[19]

A detailed discussion on expressive therapies can be found in the book on expressive therapies by Cathy A Malchiodi.[17] There are important differences between each expressive therapy. The type of expressive therapy which should be used in a particular patient depends on several factors—therapist's expertise in that particular area, patient's comfort levels, nature of illness, and severity of emotional distress. According to Knill et al.,[20] while the entirety of the expressive treatments includes activity, each has characteristic contrasts. For instance, visual art forms are helpful for more private, segregated work. They may be suited better in the process of individuation; music regularly touches on a feeling as well as promote socialization when individuals team up in group singing, at the same time playing instruments. Dance of movement offers chances to respond and shape connections. Thus, expressive treatments present themselves as a new extension of psychotherapy. They have a few explicit attributes not generally found in stringently verbal treatments like self-articulation, active participation creative mind or imagination and mind-body associations.[17]

Creativity in therapy has the potential to impact clients in memorable ways that traditional interventions do not. When therapists choose to use expressive therapies, they give their clients the opportunity to become active participants in their own treatment and empower them to use imagination in productive and corrective ways. Whether through art, play, music, movement, enactment, or creative writing, expressive therapies stimulate the senses, thereby "sensitizing" individuals to untapped aspects of themselves[21,22] and thus facilitating self-discovery, change, and reparation.

Goodman[2] distinguished three stages that portray the recuperating capacity of music, namely magical, religious, and scientific. In the magical phase, the primitive men believed that the natural sounds in nature acted as the medium of communication between man and the invisible power above him. The second phase of religious healing phase was one where man accepted that music and instruments are endowments from God and he utilized them in ritualistic purification ceremonies. The scientific stage is characterized by logic and reasoning. This stage began with Greek savants like Socrates, Aristotle, and Plato. Despite the fact that Aristotle was quick to perceive the soothing force and the cathartic ability of music, Plato recognized explicit symphonious rhythms and modes for various feelings.

The beginning of current music therapy has its origin in post-the Second Great War period. Then artists visited different hospital settings in United States of America and played music for individuals experiencing post-war physical and emotional injuries.[23] Following this, clinicians began employing artists at their facilities as they noticed huge advantages of music on the well-being of post-war victims.

Dance or movement therapy as a treatment for mental illnesses began as early as 1940, by Marian Chace. She was one of the spearheading figures in the field of dance therapy.[24] She waltzed with people with mental illness in the backyard of a medical clinic and tracked down the restorative impacts that dance had on the patients. It was discovered particularly helpful in patients who cannot utilize words to communicate their sentiments. In dance therapy, methods like reflecting, acknowledging, and intensification are embraced. The space and objects around the clients are given explicit consideration to. Later Marian Chace, Mary Whitehouse, and Trudy Schoop shaped the therapeutic framework for dance therapy through the expansion of perception, understanding, the control and modification of dance components into the training.[24]

Later Marian Chace, Mary Whitehouse, and Trudy Schoop formed the foundation for dance therapy through the addition of observation, interpretation, and the manipulation of dance elements into the practice.[24]

MUSIC THERAPY IN INDIA

Descriptions of music as a treatment—*Raga chikitsa* for both physical and psychological ailments can be found in ancient Indian systems of Ayurveda and Yoga.[25] Expression of devotional feelings in different ways known as "Bhakti" is a fundamental factor for Indian music of most genre, classical in particular unlike the West. "Raga" in Indian music is application of *swara* patterns in a particular manner. This element can evoke different emotions and can be stimulating, anxiolytic and calming. The approach based on these "Ragas" has been used as the fundamental unit of music therapy in Indian settings. This is known to increase attention. The aim is to chart out the musical preference and listening pattern. Though music therapy has a strong theoretical framework, traditional backup, it still remains in an infantile stage. One of the important reasons appears to be lack of scientific evidence.[7]

DANCE THERAPY IN INDIA

Though dance as an art form is quite popular in India and has remained so for centuries, its therapeutic usefulness has been neglected. Today there have been numerous self-proclaimed dance therapists, or dance therapy centers which claim that they can cure any illness through dance therapy. Lack of scientific evidence, lack of knowledge of clinical psychiatry, the psychiatrists not liaising with these therapists for the betterment of patients have earned a bad name for dance as a "fancy-nonworking treatment"! However, there are few centers which have been using dance therapy. Delhi-based dancer Tripura Kashyap who has been in training and research, and has written books on dance therapy.[26] Her latest guidebook being, "Contemporary Dance: Practices, Paradigms and Practitioners".[27] In Delhi, at the Bhoomika Creative Dance Centre, Tripura offers movement training capsules over 6 months—a total of 40 hours training spread out so that special education and regular classroom teachers can try out an activity for body coordination, trust building, etc. during the training period.

Apart from this, there have been several dancers who have been experimenting with different types of mental illness ranging from mentally challenged to dance therapy for marital problems as well. But the psychiatrists need to step into the field and strengthen these experiments with appropriate methodologies so that we have a strong scientific foundation for dance therapy in India.

USE OF DANCE AND MUSIC IN A PSYCHIATRIC SETTING

Nizamie and Tikka suggest numerous applications for music within a psychiatric setting.[7] It can be in the form of background music, group-singing sessions and music to accompany dance apart from music therapy per se. There are numerous benefits of the application of music in a therapeutic environment such as making positive alteration in mood and emotional states, improving concentration and attention span, developing coping and relaxation skills, exploring self-esteem and personal insight, enhancing awareness of the self and the environment and improving social interactions.[28] Central Institute of Psychiatry (CIP), Ranchi, which held weekly dance and music "socials" since its establishment in 1918.[29] Specifically such facility makes the ward environment socially more interactive. It is opined that every psychiatric inpatient facility should have such a commodity.

Similarly, use of dance in psychiatric settings can be done from the paradigm of Marian Chace who danced for the inmates of mental hospital. A regular dance class as an activity needs to be started in each psychiatric ward.

MUSIC AND DANCE AS THERAPIES IN PSYCHIATRY

It is common in psychiatry or any medical illness, the treatment includes both pharmacological and nonpharmacological interventions. For example, in diabetes, along with medications, one advises dietary modification and physical exercise. In psychiatric disorders, psychotherapeutic approaches are part of treatment in every disorder. The principles from psychotherapy are used in establishing a good rapport with the patient which is vital for drug compliance throughout the treatment course. Psychoeducation itself is an important component which is crucial in eliciting the cooperation of patient and family. Hence, search for innovative methods to make the patient better is not anew to psychiatry.

One important hurdle in using dance and music therapy in psychiatry has always been lack of scientific, methodologically strong studies. Though studies on dance therapy have begun as early as 1940, well before chlorpromazine was discovered 1952[30] and the documented evidences for both music and dance therapies are lacking in the scientific world. The formal report on music as a treatment modality was first published in 1964.[31] Until the mid-1990s, larger part of studies were contextual investigations and published largely as case reports. Hence, they lacked sound evidence for implications to treatment settings.[23]

But there has been a renewed interest in the last 20 years and there have been several clinical studies, reviews and meta-analyses although not found in recognized journals of psychiatry, but in the journals related to allied sciences like nursing, psychology, sports medicine.

Evidence in Different Psychiatric Disorders

In a Cochrane review,[32] dance therapy was found to have no evidence for its therapeutic effect on depression.[32] In this review, the databases till 2014 were searched for both published as well as unpublished RCTs on dance-movement therapy for depression in people of all backgrounds. Three investigations with a total of 147 members met the inclusion criteria. This included two studies with both adult males and females and one with adolescent girls. Though there was some evidence that dance therapy was somewhat better efficacious than standard treatment methods in adults, it was not significant. In the study with adolescents, there was no difference. In one more study, the dropout rates from dance therapy were insignificant. The study reported an improved social functions, self-esteem, and quality of life. Another study of low methodological quality reported similar findings. However, it needs to be kept in mind that both of them lacked methodological soundness.

After this Cochrane review, one more study appears worth mentioning. The team led by Pylvänäinen et al.,[33] researched the impacts of dance-movement therapy in a mental health care setup. They studied persons suffering from depression attending the outpatient facility. The researchers hypothesized that dance which incorporates both physical and emotional components should provide relief to psychiatric symptoms. The participants had a diagnosis of moderate-to-severe depression with chronicity or recurrence. They were assessed at 3 months after the therapy. The authors concluded that addition of dance therapy improved the effect of the treatment. Notably this effect was observable irrespective of the antidepressant treatment. Role of dance therapy in schizophrenia has been reviewed in a Cochrane review.[34] This review included a one single blind study with a sample of 45 patients. One group was administered routine treatment alone and the other both routine care and dance therapy. Dropout rate was 40% in both the groups by 4th month. Cochrane audit on dance treatment and schizophrenia[34] included one single visually impaired investigation (absolute n = 45) of sensible quality. It contrasted dance treatment in addition to routine consideration and routine care, the Positive and Negative Syndrome Scale (PANSS) average endpoint scores as well as the positive subscores were found to be similar in both. Toward the end of treatment period, significantly more number of people who received dance therapy along with routine treatment had around 20% decrease in PANSS negative symptom scores. Their average negative endpoint scores were lower too. No difference was found in satisfaction and quality of life scores.

A later study in schizophrenia on dance therapy along with medications,[35] showed significant decrease in state anger and depression compared to the control group (on only medications) after treatment. For psychotic symptoms, the dance/movement therapy group showed a significant decrease of negative psychotic symptoms compared to the control group after treatment.

A systematic review was conducted on the effectiveness of dance therapy on reducing symptoms of mental illnesses recently.[36] All of the twelve studies were aiming to observe the effectiveness of dance-movement therapy on mental illnesses. More than half of the reviewed studies approved the effectiveness of dance/movement therapy on mental illnesses. The studies reported a decrease in test anxiety symptoms, significant decrease of depression symptoms, significant higher vitality, and lower negative symptoms in schizophrenia, better body image in eating disorders and fewer signs of body dissatisfaction, and so on. Overall, dance-movement therapy was an effective treatment technique for mental illnesses.

Interestingly, Leeder et al. studied a group of female victims of domestic violence.[37] Here drama as a mode of therapy was utilized to make them ventilate their feelings. The women were able to look at their futures in a different way. It was important to note that they were being viewed here as not just "victims" but as talented artists who had great potential for the society. Hence, authors felt that drama therapy can change lives from the viewpoint of one's self-esteem, the way one relates to herself to the society and can have benefits for their future mindset is the study quoted a participant "...you get to express it, however, whatever, you want to say. No judging. That's what was really amazing for me, that your drama is your therapy."[37]

Another Cochrane review[38] examined studies on dance therapy for people with dementia. It looked at 102 studies. After studying all the studies, it was opined that good methodological design, bigger sample size and clear intervention details are required to infer whether dance therapy is an effective treatment for dementia. According to the available data, it was concluded that there exists no evidence for or against dance-movement therapy as an effective intervention for dementia.

The research suggestions given by the Karkou et al.[38] are important for anyone who is interested in conducting high-quality research in the field of music and dance therapies. Further studies are required keeping in focus what interventions, comparison factors, and outcome assessments are used. It is advisable that a selection of sample subjects is done meticulously using a standard screening tools. This should be followed by careful randomization. It is important to describe the steps of intervention which needs to be uniformly done with all the participants. It would be beneficial to identify primary outcomes too. This will help us avoid paying attention solely to cognitive skills. As suggested by qualitative findings, dance therapy as a type of psychotherapy, almost certainly, will significantly affect emotional and social components.[38]

Another interesting study is worth mentioning. This study examined the effectiveness of hip-hop dancing on participants' cognitive skills.[39] Some of these abilities like working memory and critical thinking are connected to a better performance in STEM (science, technology, engineering, and mathematics) disciplines. Participants were challenged with asset of digital tasks which assessed key areas like working memory, speed of mental rotation, problem-solving skills, and the process of theory of mind. The authors controlled confounding factors such as demographics and dance-style experience other than hip-hop dancing. The hip-hop dancers had much faster mentally rotating images of hands at greater angle disparities. They also displayed greater accuracy in identifying human facial images with positive emotions.

MUSIC THERAPY FOR MENTAL ILLNESSES

The evidence for music therapy for mental illnesses appears much stronger. Again seeing from Cochrane reviews, findings of the meta-analysis demonstrate that music used as a therapeutic modality has useful effects in individuals with depression albeit for a short period. Music therapy along with the routine treatment appears to give better results as compared to routine treatment alone. Added to this music therapy did not have any adverse events. It also was efficacious in decreasing anxiety levels and improving functioning levels in depression.[40]

Likewise in schizophrenia, the benefits were noticed. However, the conclusions were that moderate- to low-quality evidence suggests that music therapy as an addition to standard care improves the global state, mental state (including negative and general symptoms), social functioning, and quality of life of people with schizophrenia or schizophrenia-like disorders. However, effects were inconsistent across studies and depended on the number of music therapy sessions as well as the quality of the music therapy provided. Further research should especially address the long-term effects of music therapy, dose-response relationships, as well as the relevance of outcome measures in relation to music therapy.[41]

MUSIC AND DANCE THERAPIES IN CHILDHOOD PSYCHIATRIC DISORDERS

There have been several therapists who have been conducting therapy sessions in special schools, nongovernmental organizations. These interventions are usually activity sessions to engage the children with mental health problems—most likely autism spectrum disorders (ASDs), mental retardation, and attention deficit hyperactivity disorders. However, there have been many studies recently looking at the role of dance and music therapy in childhood mental disorders. The Cochrane review findings suggest a fairly large Cochrane review has been conducted on the efficacy of music therapy on ASD.[42] This review included 10 investigations with 165 children. They analyzed both the short- and long-term benefits of music therapy in ASD with sessions ranging widely from 1 week to 7 months. The positive impact was noticed in several areas compared to either routine care or placebo treatment. Improvement in social interaction, nonverbal and verbal communication, social skills and initiation were noticed behaviorally which stood significantly. Compared to both placebo and routine care significant improvement was noticed in the areas of quality of parent-child relationships. There were no side effects in any of the studies.

In attention deficit hyperactivity disorder, the data from studies remains inconclusive.[43]

Surprisingly though many therapists use music and dance therapy in mentally challenged children and adults, studies are not many. Cameron[44] did a review of available studies which revealed some positive findings. Instituting music therapy for long term was found to be efficacious in components of communicating skills, expressing oneself, social skills, and developmental changes.

Another review, which was presented as a conference paper and available online by Paušić et al.,[45] assessed the benefits of dance and movement therapy in child mental health. It is understandable that a performing art form like dance helps active expression of emotions. In addition to this dance as a therapy was found to be useful in improving body image, perception of self and others. Increase in the tolerance toward others and improved ability toward others were the other advantages. It was also seen to be effective in reducing problematic behaviors. Dance led to a better parent-child bonding and made parenting much easier in the case of children with special needs. It helped children in perceiving both their as well as others' competency. As commonly seen by the dance trainers, through dance a gradual welcome transition takes place in body stance, balance, and movement control. This was reported by the authors even in children with disabilities. It acted as a remedy for initiating and maintaining motivation for physical exercise especially in adolescents avoiding physical exercises and having increased weight.

School Mental Health Programs–role of Music, Dance and Theater to Promote Mental Health of Children

Surprisingly despite the evidence available from the studies about the usefulness of music and dance in the cognitive and social development of children, attention has not been paid into inculcating dance and music into the school mental health programs. In India, generally music and dance are parts of cocurricular activities, but seldom they are viewed as important. Rather they are many a time perceived as hurdles to scholastic performance of the children. But the research findings have proven otherwise. Continuous music learning in children is reported to be advantageous in enhancing linguistic and literacy skills. This is demonstrated by several studies correlating these two domains.[46] These studies have also tested whether the training in music correlates directly with the enhancement of literacy skills. Results of these investigations are both mixed. Their interpretation becomes more complicated because of the different literacy-related outcome measures. The review by Gordon et al. has identified a total of 13 studies with a total of 901 children. The factors which played a role in enhancement of literacy skills were duration of training, age of the child and the type of control used while studying the intervention. These studies support the hypothesis that training in music can be beneficial for children in terms of literacy and phonological awareness skills.

Studies indicate that music as a therapy has positive impact on different skills in childhood. They stand as guidelines to further research as to what benefits music can have for scholastic abilities and developmental aspects in children.[47] Dumont et al. reviewed the findings from 46 studies. Important components of development—motor, social, cognitive, language, and academic were analyzed through these studies. Some studies included listening to music, instrumental playing as part of music therapy. Others defined designed music intervention in a precise way. Thus, there was wide difference in the conceptualization as to what is the intervention.

In conclusion, although the underlying mechanisms are not always clear, evidence of reviewed studies seems suggestive of some beneficial effects.

Music and dance are interwoven with the life in most of the cultures of the world. And hence it becomes important to study their importance and their contribution to health first in its natural environment. However, for any modality be it a process or medication to be advocated as a treatment, it needs to be proven through methodologically sound studies. But good qualitative research is required to understand the characteristics of the process. This will help to set hypotheses and test them through quantitative methods. As rightly noted by Dumont et al., a combined approach of qualitative and quantitative research methods can give great and practical insights into dance and music as therapies in mental illnesses as well as mental health promotion.[46] In addition, having a more clear view of the effects and influencing variables, would help in focused research on the influence of music and dance on the child development.

MENTAL HEALTH PROBLEMS IN MUSICIANS AND DANCERS

The interface of psychiatry and music and dance not only involves the use of dance and music for mental health problems, but also concerns with the study of mental health problems in musicians and dancers. Studies have shown higher incidences of substance use and mood disorders in musicians.[48] However, this needs to be examined with caution. Professional dancers and musicians face very different problems because of their need to perform for their livelihood. whereas dancing and music as hobbies might not have these difficulties. Dance classes as a routine make the students practice for perfection and hence the physical discipline also remains the foremost. It is possible that the students, majority of who are in their childhood will be benefited by this and do not perceive this as a burden. But as they progress into adolescence, the body image issues become important. Though dance may offer benefits in physical fitness and correct posturing in adolescence, it may also pressurize the adolescent population on maintaining figure and remaining "thin". There have been few studies which have examined these issues. A positive attitude toward one's own body image may develop by initiation into dance for adolescents in particular. This is probably because of the strong physical component of dance. The person who dances would certainly feel empowered with the development of control over her body. Young people also are exposed to some form of socialization through their dance training from the beginning. This also is thought to improve their self-esteem and lessen their social fears and hesitancy. This appears true even for adolescents attending elementary training in dance with no earlier knowledge of dancing.[49,50]

No studies from India have been reported.

The studies have shown a link between higher substance use and particular choice of music and dance in adolescent population.[51] The research also showed higher preponderance of alcohol and nicotine use among musicians as compared to general population. However, the study of professional musicians found that musicians had a better mental health profile when compared with general population.[48]

MUSIC AND DANCE THERAPY IN INDIAN SETTINGS

There have been projects running in premier institutions like CIP-Ranchi and NIMHANS for dance therapy using Indian dance forms and music therapy using Indian music forms are underway. There have been postgraduate dissertations which have been studying these therapies. We hope that in the near future data will be available for the evidence of dance and music therapy for mental illnesses becomes available.

In the meantime, every clinician should try to use music and dance as complementary therapies in his or her patients. In the Indian setting, unless the mental health professionals step in this area, dance and music therapies will be used in unstandardized ways by untrained, over enthusiastic therapists who may be well trained in music and dance but may not have any knowledge on mental illnesses, which may mislead the patients in overestimating the benefits of therapy and discontinuing medications. This may also lead to discontinuing therapy prematurely. This may result in higher dropout rates from studies too.

There are dancers and musicians with adequate expertise in their field for dance/ music therapy available in most of the cities throughout India. Psychiatrists need to liaise with them. They can refer selected, motivated patients initially under their guidance for weekly sessions at least for 3 months. Any finding either positive or negative should be documented. Wherever possible simple assessments can be carried out. Qualitative data from patients on the quality of life, their own perception of mood, improvement need to be documented.

Dance and music as useful tools in scholastic development as well as for mental health promotion have been proven well through the research as we have seen earlier. In schools, these activities need to be inculcated as part of the curriculum. In schools where these already exist, they need to be strengthened. The parents and teachers need to be made aware of the benefits of these toward child and adolescent mental health.

THEATER AND PSYCHIATRY

A discussion of different dimensions of theater and psychiatry is beyond the scope of this chapter. However, an attempt will be made to describe the connection between theater and psychiatry briefly. The word "Drama" has its origin in the Greek root "dran" meaning "to act". The Indian text on dance actually has an element of pure emotional enactment with supportive body gestures called "Natya" which can be seen as today's drama. Popularly drama uses dialogues, body gestures, costumes suiting the roles and at times stage sets to enact a story. Natyashastra, the Indian text on dramatics by Sage Bharata says that everything in drama is nothing but imitation of life. In daily life too, our feelings are expressed through verbal and nonverbal behaviors. Thus, our lives, emotions, and drama are interwoven!

In psychiatry, drama as a treatment tool was first conceptualized by Jacob Moreno, a psychiatrist himself. He named the technique as "Psychodrama". Contrary to modern psychology focusing on the past, psychodrama concentrated on the present and the future. A detailed discussion on the sessions of psychodrama can be found elsewhere.[52] Briefly, in psychodrama, the session is kept focused primarily on one person, the protagonist. The participants the feelings as a reaction to others behaviors, both verbal and nonverbal. The techniques of mirroring, role reversal are used to make one understand self as well as others. Psychodrama encourages spontaneity and creativity in its participants as important paths to one's own understanding of self and others.

The drama therapy which uses theater appears to its origin in Moreno's Psychodrama. It is natural to notice that the theater facilitates and provides a channel for the ventilation of difficult feelings. This may be true not only for the artists who enact drama, but also the viewers who watch the theater shows. Further, drama which enacts emotions, life events which is common to all human beings, provides a safe method to distance oneself from the difficult, "afraid to face" event and watch it as a third person. This helps working through the emotions. Thus, the advocates of drama therapy seem to have applied these observations from the theater experiences to the realms of therapeutic ways in treating mental illnesses. Unlike psychodrama, the modern-day drama therapy can focus on groups or individuals with similar experiences. This will open up opportunities to express and share their emotions in the session. The field truly started to become an independent therapeutic entity when the American Dance Therapy Association came into existence in 1966 which was soon followed by the American

Art Therapy Association in 1969. Finally, the North American Drama Therapy Association was setup in 1979, giving drama an important status as a therapeutic tool for mental illnesses, which encouraged and created opportunities to gain knowledge, insights, practice, and sharing of data in drama therapy.[53] However, in India though theater has evolved into a strong art form, the practice and research in theater with reference to mental illness are still very less. Having a large artist strength and wide variety of theatrical forms, both artistic community and mental health professional force need to come together for Indian theater to be used as therapy in various ways.

The goals of drama therapy in current times can be conceptualized in different areas related to mental health. The therapy like any other psychotherapy aims at bringing about changes in dysfunctional behaviors, works around interpersonal relationship issues, promotes emotional well-being, and enhances self-esteem. As noted in the studies on fine art forms like music and dance, drama therapy is known to improve quality of life. Over and above these, the participants are presented with an open opportunity to express freely, enact one's own past experiences, keep working through in a graded manner, and improve their confidence. This can be a reliving and resolving experience. This can greatly strengthen their roles in various areas of life.[36]

Besides psychotherapy, drama has been used effectively in creating awareness about mental illnesses. Psychoeducation through drama in the form of street plays can be easy, effective compared to other art forms like dance. The elements of easy communication through dialogues and nonverbal behaviors are known to make it easier for the common people to grasp the reality of the situation. Drama can also be easily incorporated in school mental health programs. It can be used to make teaching more effective. It can be helpful while handling emotional issues in children.[54]

CONCLUSION

Historically music and dance have proven their value in the entertaining mind as well as being important aspect of human lives. Indian forms of music and dance in particular appear to have inbuilt theoretical construct for therapeutics and promotion of mental health. But for them to be used clinically as prescriptions for mental disorders we need more research and gather more evidence clinically as well as through studies. In spite of the fact that it is hard to measure the advantages of these treatments for the mental illnesses. It has been shown that there has been no harm in using these therapies as they are more acceptable to our patients as complementary therapies. They do have proven efficacy in stress management and mental health promotion in children and adolescents. There is an immediate need to put in more efforts by psychiatrists and other mental health professionals in incorporating these therapies in clinical settings, document their experiences—both positive and negative. The need for methodologically sound, both qualitative and quantitative, research studies remains to be taken up by the enthusiastic younger psychiatrists.

REFERENCES

1. Mehta T. Sanskrit Play Production in Ancient India. New Delhi, India: Motilal Banarsidass; 1995. pp. 221-2.
2. Goodman KD. Music therapy. In: Arieti S, Brodie HK (Eds). American Handbook of Psychiatry, 2nd edition. New York: Basic Books Inc; 1981. pp. 564-85.
3. Ghosh M. The Natyasastra: A Treatise on Ancient Indian Dramaturgy and Histrionics, Ascribed to Bharata-Muni, 2nd edition. Calcutta: Granthalaya Private Ltd; 1967.

4. Hanna JL. The power of dance: health and healing. J Altern Complement Med. 1995;1(4):323-31.
5. Lima MM, Vieira AP. Ballroom dance as therapy for the elderly in Brazil. Am J Dance Ther. 2007;29(2):129-42.
6. Alpert PT. The health benefits of dance. Home Health Care Manag Pract. 2011;23(2):155-7.
7. Nizamie SH, Tikka SK. Psychiatry and music. Indian J Psychiatry. 2014;56(2):128-40.
8. Cooke D. The Language of Music. Oxford: Oxford University Press; 1959.
9. Kühlmann AY, de Rooij A, Kroese LF, van Dijk M, Hunink MG, Jeekel J. Meta-analysis evaluating music interventions for anxiety and pain in surgery. Br J Surg. 2018;105:773-83.
10. Chafin S, Roy M, Gerin W, Christenfeld N. Music can facilitate blood pressure recovery from stress. Br J Health Psychol. 2004;9:393-403.
11. Limb CJ. Structural and functional neural correlates of music perception. Anat Rec A Discov Mol Cell Evol Biol. 2006;288:435-46.
12. Rickard NS, Toukhsati SR, Field SE. The effect of music on cognitive performance: insight from neurobiological and animal studies. Behav Cogn Neurosci Rev. 2005;4:235-61.
13. Schellenberg EG. Music and nonmusical abilities. Ann N Y Acad Sci. 2001;930:355-71.
14. Rizzolatti G, Craighero L. The mirror-neuron system. Annu Rev Neurosci. 2004;27:169-92.
15. Karpati FJ, Giacosa C, Foster NE, Penhune VB, Hyde KL. Dance and the brain: a review. Ann N Y Acad Sci. 2015;1337:140-6.
16. Brown S, Martinez MJ, Parsons LM. The neural basis of human dance. Cereb Cortex. 2006;16:1157-67.
17. Malchiodi CA. Expressive therapies: history, theory and practice. In: Malchiodi CA (Ed). Expressive Therapies. New York, NY: Guilford Publications; 2005.
18. National Center for Complementary and Alternative Medicine. (2004). Major domains of complementary and alternative medicine. [online] Available from www.nccam.nih.gov/fcp/classify [Last accessed June, 2021].
19. National Coalition of Creative Arts Therapies Associations. (2004). Dance/movement therapy. [online] Available from www.nccata.org/dance.html [Last accessed June, 2021].
20. Knill P, Barba H, Fuchs M. Minstrels of Soul: Intermodal Expressive Therapy. Toronto: Palmerston Press; 1995.
21. Gladding ST. Counseling as an Art: The Creative Arts in Counseling. Alexandria, VA: American Counseling Association; 1992.
22. Gladding ST, Newsome DW. Art in counseling. In: Malchiodi CA (Ed). Handbook of Art Therapy. New York: Guilford Press; 2003. pp. 243-53.
23. Rose JP, Bartsch HH. Music as Therapy. Basel: Karger Gazette; 2009. pp. 5-7.
24. Chaiklin S, Wengrower H. The Art and Science of Dance/Movement Therapy: Life is Dance. New York: Routledge; 2009.
25. Sundar S. Traditional healing systems and modern music therapy in India. Music Ther Today. 2007;8(3):397-407.
26. Kashyap T. My Body, My Wisdom: A Handbook of Creative Dance Therapy. New Delhi: Penguin Books India; 2005.
27. Kashyap T. Contemporary Dance: Practices, Paradigms and Practitioners. New Delhi: AAYU Publications; 2018.
28. Degmečić D, Požgain I, Filaković P. Music as therapy. Int Rev Aesthetics Sociol Music. 2005;36:287-300.
29. Nizamie SH, Goyal N, Haq MZ, Akhtar S. Central Institute of Psychiatry: a tradition in excellence. Indian J Psychiatry. 2008;50:144-8.
30. López-Muñoz F, Alamo C, Cuenca E, Shen WW, Clervoy P, Rubio G. History of the discovery and clinical introduction of chlorpromazine. Ann Clin Psychiatry. 2005;17(3):113-35.
31. Pierce CM, Schwartz D, Thomas E. Music therapy in a day care center. Dis Nerv Syst. 1964;25:1-4.
32. Meekums B, Karkou V, Nelson EA. Dance movement therapy for depression. Cochrane Database Syst Rev. 2015;(2):CD009895.
33. Pylvänäinen PM, Muotka JS, Lappalainen R. A dance movement therapy group for depressed adult patients in a psychiatric outpatient clinic: effects of the treatment. Front Psychol. 2015; 6:980.
34. Ren J, Xia J. Dance therapy for schizophrenia. Cochrane Database Syst Rev. 2013;(10):CD006868.
35. Lee HJ, Jang SH, Lee SY, Hwang KS. Effectiveness of dance/movement therapy on affect and psychotic symptoms in patients with schizophrenia. Arts Psychother. 2015;45:64-8.
36. Buse Z, Sarikaya Z, Colucci E. The effectiveness of dance-movement therapy (DMT) on reducing symptoms of mental illnesses: a systematic review. 2017. [online] Available from https://www.researchgate.net/project/Dance-Movement-Therapy-Mental-Health [Last accessed June, 2021].
37. Leeder A, Wimmer C. Voices of Pride: Drama Therapy with incarcerated women. Women and Therapy. 2006;29(3):195-213.

38. Karkou V, Meekums B. Dance movement therapy for dementia. Cochrane Database Syst Rev. 2017;(2):CD011022.
39. Bonny JW, Lindberg JC, Pacampara MC. Hip hop dance experience linked to sociocognitive ability. PLoS One. 2017;12(2):e0169947.
40. Aalbers S, Fusar-Poli L, Freeman RE, Spreen M, Ket JC, Vink AC, et al. Music therapy for depression. Cochrane Database Syst Rev. 2017;(11):CD004517.
41. Geretsegger M, Mössler KA, Bieleninik Ł, Chen X, Heldal T, Gold C. Music therapy for people with schizophrenia and schizophrenia-like disorders. Cochrane Database Syst Rev. 2017;(5):CD004025.
42. Geretsegger M, Elefant C, Mössler KA, Gold C. Music therapy for people with autism spectrum disorder. Cochrane Database Syst Rev. 2014;6:CD004381.
43. Zhang F, Liu K, An P, You C, Teng L, Liu Q. Music therapy for attention deficit hyperactivity disorder (ADHD) in children and adolescents. Cochrane Database Syst Rev. 2017;5:CD010032.
44. Cameron H. Long term music therapy for people with intellectual disabilities and the NDIS. Aust J Music Ther. 2017;28:1-15.
45. Paušić J, Grčić V, Kuzmanić B. Dance movement therapy with children and adolescents: a review. Conference paper. 2014. [online] Available from https://www.researchgate.net/publication/270590021_Dance_Movement_Therapy_With_Children_And_Adolescents_A_Review [Last accessed June, 2021].
46. Gordon RL, Fehd HM, McCandliss BD. Does music training enhance literacy skills? A meta-analysis. Front Psychol. 2015;6:1777.
47. Dumont E, Syurina EV, Feron FJ, van Hooren S. Music interventions and child development: a critical review and further directions. Front Psychol. 2017;8:1694.
48. Pavitra KS, Chandrashekar CR, Choudhury P. Creativity and mental health: a profile of writers and musicians. Indian J Psychiatry. 2007;49(1):34-43.
49. Burgess G, Grogan S, Burwitz L. Effects of a 6-week aerobic dance intervention on body image and physical self-perceptions in adolescent girls. Body Image. 2006;3(1):57-66.
50. Swami V, Harris A. Dancing toward positive body image? Examining body-related constructs with ballet and contemporary dancers at different levels. Am J Dance Ther. 2012;34:39-52.
51. Ter Bogt TF, Gabhainn SN, Simons-Morton BG, Ferreira M, Hublet A, Godeau E, et al. Dance is the new metal: adolescent music preferences and substance use across Europe. Subst Use Misuse. 2012;47(2):130-42.
52. Good Therapy. (2015). Drama therapy. [online] Available from https://www.goodtherapy.org/learn-about-therapy/types/drama-therapy [Last accessed June, 2021].
53. Blank BT. (2010). Theater processes therapeutic in drama therapy. The New Social Worker. [online] Available from https://www.socialworker.com/feature-articles/practice/Theater_Processes_Therapeutic_in_Drama_Therapy/ [Last accessed June, 2021].
54. Burkhead J. (2014). Classroom uses drama therapy to help students open up in a safe environment. Well Commons. [online] Available from http://wellcommons.com/groups/bert-nash-community-mental-health-center/2014/mar/27/classroom-uses-drama-therapy-to-help-stu/ [Last accessed June, 2021].

CHAPTER 25

Interface with Anthropology

Siddharth Sarkar, Mahadev Singh Sen

INTRODUCTION

What are we? Where do we come from? What makes us "human" and not animals? It is difficult to make sense of all these queries. Some people answer this question with a biological explanation while others social or spiritual explanation. Anthropologists look at this question with a holistic and integrative point of view. Anthropology (ánthrōpos— "human", lógos—"study") means "the study of the human race, its culture and society, and its physical development".[1] Anthropologists study humans in totality through careful observation with respect to space and time then develop reliable theories. These theories are then compared with results of other scholars and tested in similar situations.

Anthropology is a holistic field which encompasses four major branches, namely (1) biological anthropology, (2) social-cultural anthropology, (3) linguistic anthropology, and (4) archaeological anthropology **(Fig. 1)**. Biological anthropology deals with the evolution of the humankind and includes subfields such as genetics anthropology, paleontology, etc. Cultural anthropology inspects the social and cultural uniqueness of human life including the sociopolitical, medical, and developmental aspects. Archaeological anthropology studies the human behavior and culture usually through material remains such as dresses, tools, houses, etc. Linguistic anthropology focuses on the study of language, symbols, and other features of human communication. It deals with not just sounds and grammar but also the way of looking at the world (for example, Hopi Indians of the American Southwest had no words for past, present, and future in their language thus suggesting that they had different notion of time). Within each branch, there is a subbranch of applied anthropology utilizes knowledge gathered from the anthropological pursuits and enables to solve practical problems.[2]

A field of anthropology is ethnography which deals with "description of a particular culture primarily based on fieldwork (which all anthropologists use for on-location research)".[2] Ethnography involves working within a community and learning their culture, through the informants who offer their own point of view in their own words. Hallmark of ethnographic fieldwork is participant observation which

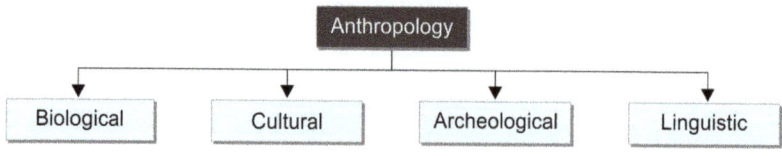

Fig. 1: Branches of anthropology.

is construed as a combination of social participation in a community and personal observation of the community during such participation. Ethnographic approaches have been utilized in the understanding how communities function, and have contributed to an understanding with respect to mental health problems and care seeking.

Anthropology can be understood in terms of ethnocentrism or cultural relativism. Ethnocentrism attempts to understand other cultures with a view that the ways of one's own culture are the only proper one.[2] Cultural relativism considers that different cultures are valid when viewed in objective terms of that own culture. Such an approach attempts to provide a more objective appreciation of cultural aspects, through a nonjudgmental appreciation of the strengths and weaknesses of different cultures and understanding the "why" of phenomena from a neutral posture.

Anthropology as a science has developed over the last one and half century and has significant import on psychiatry. The present chapter explores the interface of anthropology and psychiatry. The various aspects of the relationship of anthropology with psychiatry are briefly enumerated followed by the clinical implications of anthropology. The research approaches of anthropology that can be of use in psychiatry are presented followed by the Indian literature. The chapter provides an overview and refers to other literature in this field where applicable.

RELATIONSHIP OF ANTHROPOLOGY WITH PSYCHIATRY

Psychiatry as a field spreads as much as limited by human thinking, the core of psychiatry being disorders of human thinking. There are many factors which influence the way we approach the human mind. Approaching psychiatry through anthropological means covers both the sociocultural and biological aspects of the human development, from past till present, and also across different populations at a given time. Scientific literature has mainly discussed this interface in terms of:

- Understandings of the human mind, selfhood and extraordinary experiences across different societies. Psychology, psychiatry, and psychoanalysis have contributed to social anthropology and vice versa.
- Using a different approach to study the different understanding approach the relationship between popular and professional recognition of "mental illness" with their roots in the different demographic a socioeconomic aspects of particular societies, with special attention to marginalized groups.

Cultural psychiatrists and psychiatric anthropologists share common pursuit in a variation of disorders across populations with special reference to cultural, ethnic, sociological and structural-institutional features, and the cultural puzzle of significant variations in the course and outcome of disorders transnationally.[3] The branch started emerging from the observations of Obersteiner in 1889 about the mental disorders of different ethnicity which were new to the western civilization. While Jung proposed that "Negroes" lack a historical layer in the brain, Seligman (1924) commented that ethnic minorities have greater suggestibility, proneness to disassociation and extroversion as compared to Europeans. Later some comparative work was also published by Kraepelin between people having mental disorders in Java and Singapore. It was thought at that time that both primitive societies and insanity represented earlier stages of mental evolution. For this reason, ethnic minorities were considered to be laboratories for the study of insanity. It was thought that factors of low self-control and more suggestibility were common between the ethnic minority and the mentally ill.[4,5]

The condition of nostalgia suffered by soldiers during the First World War and drapetomania (the tendency of slaves to run away from owners) urged an initiation of research into this area. It was before the Second World War that the anthropologists and psychiatrists started to identify many issues which required joint efforts ranging from what is normal and what is not, to how these psychosocial factors influence predispose to disease and at the same time increases the functioning of an individual to an optimal level.[6] Earliest work in this field starts from series of paper in 1942, by Ackerknecht who focused on primitive medicine and urged anthropological research on "Indigenous system of medicine". The main focus of the study was that simply calling these primitive techniques of medicine to be superstitions and nonscientific was not a good approach. The focus of this work was the way by which this form of medical practice has influenced the local people and the role of the doctor with the tribes.

Clements, in 1932, has also tried to trace the five different concepts of disease, i.e., (1) sorcery, (2) breach of taboo, (3) object intrusion, (4) spirit intrusion, and (5) soul loss as a regional sociocultural explanation to a disease.[3] Subsequently, Henry and Mead published a series of research on the role of anthropology in psychosomatic medicine. This started an era of interaction between these two broad fields. Jules Henry emphasized that research should be done in the field of culture, personality, and psychosomatic medicine and also urged for a specialized field in this area. Also, Margaret Mead stated the importance of culture in the development of personality of an individual by studying three primitive societies in the Sepik region of Papua New Guinea for 2 years. In her book, *Sex and Temperament in Three Primitive Societies*, she concluded that there was a difference in the socially determined gender roles in different populations which were less attributed to the biological driven sex.

The current literature uses the terms social anthropology, cultural psychiatry, and transcultural psychiatry interchangeably. Though these terms are related, there are finer points of distinction among these. Anthropology is better related to society as a whole and the method employed to study this phenomenon is being within the community so as to gain close and intimate familiarity with a given group of individuals. Psychiatry, on the other hand, is a field of medicine and evidence-based practice lies in its core. Thus, psychiatry relies more on qualitative data and repeatability of facts. According to anthropology, thought process of an individual is attributed to social organization and customs while in psychiatry this is attributed to the psychic mechanisms and underlying psychopathology. **Figure 2** attempts to schematically portray the overall relationship of psychiatry and anthropology.

Due to the involvement of professionals in joint researches of anthropologists and psychiatrists, many issues have come up with regard to the ethnographic context of various populations. For example, the existence of cross-cultural differences the preferred ego-defense mechanisms being used by an individual and on another level different cultural coping strategies being used by various members in a given society.[3,6] Psychiatry, on the other hand, has learned quite a lot from anthropology regarding etiology, clinical features, management, and preventive measures of mental disorders. Some of the salient observations include mental illnesses

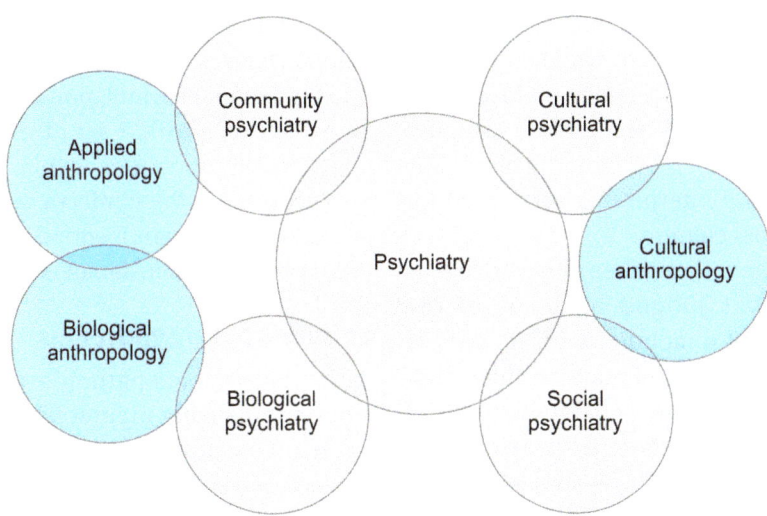

Fig. 2: Relationship between anthropology and psychiatry.

being universal across all human societies. Also, epidemiological variations exist in occurrence and manifestations of mental illnesses, as exemplified by studies such as International Pilot Study of Schizophrenia (IPSS) and Determinants of Outcome of Severe Mental Disorders (DOSMeD). Additionally, culture-specific psychopathological patterns and clusters (in the form of "culture-bound syndromes") are present which are peculiar to certain cultures/societies. Aberrations and adversities of human conditions temporally or geographically may lead to distress which may lead to the occurrence of psychiatric disorders. Lastly, most cultures possess techniques by means of which the mental illnesses are dealt with and some local variations of treatment methods are applicable in the delivery of care.

CLINICAL IMPLICATIONS

Anthropological concerns and views have clinical implications in terms of how psychiatry is practiced. This may include the effect on nosology, clinical assessment, and treatment methods. These are delineated as follows:[7]

Nosology

Anthropology has always accused that psychiatry medicalizes social distress and calls it a mental illness. A lot of sociological and anthropological critiques have challenged this aspect of psychiatric nosology. Labeling the distress into an illness may change the way, it is perceived.[8,9] While psychiatry aims to create illness categories to systematically diagnose and provide suitable medical grounds for providing help, the diagnostic threshold is based upon the social construct of what is construed as an illness. Transplanting the threshold and symptom profile for psychiatric diagnosis of psychiatric illness may not be ideal.[10]

Historically, it was observed in the west that members of particular ethnic minorities were preferentially "psychiatrized". Evidence from the United Kingdom suggests that the threshold of diagnosis for psychosis was lower among those from African heritage. They were more likely to forcefully detained, medicated with antipsychotics and being involuntarily admitted into mental health hospitals. This picture was less intense when compared with the majority white population. This urged a necessity to apply and borrow ideas from the related disciplines of sociology, anthropology, cultural studies, and postmodern critiques of mental health care. The indigenous way of thinking and interpreting accounted for variance across cultures.

There was a time when the psychiatric diagnosis was judged on basis of the relationship of a member with its society and family. But over the years psychiatry has adopted objective and reliable methods of making a diagnosis. Psychiatric assessment is made only on psychosocial reliability and rather there is no biological validity. Thus, the process is influenced by cultural inconsistency and biases in several ways. The latest Diagnostic and Statistical Manual of Mental Disorders, i.e., DSM-5 and the latest version of the International Classification of Diseases, i.e., ICD-11 both have given unprecedented attention to culture. This international psychiatric classification inherits a 19th-century Western model of demarcating diseases by symptoms, etiology, course, and treatment, but proffers scope for a more wider scope for cultural considerations which have an anthropological overlay.[11]

The process of psychiatric diagnosis is subjective in nature. Symptom measures along with a symptom-based classification make it difficult to diagnose a psychiatric illness with very high validity and by excluding other pathologies. Though the interclinician reliability is taken into account, the fact remains that culture frames each psychiatrist's diagnostic assessment differently. These assessments also vary as a patient's reporting of the symptoms change with time and setting as well as they can also change with clinician's experience. Outline for Cultural Formulation (OCF) was included in DSM-IV to make physicians aware of the patient's lived experience. The international consortium of cultural mental health experts revised OCF into the Cultural Formulation Interview (CFI) and this came with a set of new features, i.e., tangible questions, explanations and instructions for the clinician and based on patient and clinician feedback, the CFI was then revised for inclusion in DSM-5.[12]

Culture-bound Syndromes

Pathogenic versus pathoplastic nature of culture in causing mental illness is widely known. Few authors are also now seeing western and eastern syndromes at par with each other and claim that these are similar to each other in many ways especially the milder forms. Culture-bound disorders are psychological disorders or syndromes that are considered specific or closely related to cultural factors and or particular ethnocultural group. The "boundedness" of this syndrome comes from the time when the western civilization interacted with the local colonial civilization and encountered new syndromes which were thought to be nonexistent in the western world.[13,14]

Are culture-bound syndromes restricted to a limited number of cultures by reason of certain psychosocial features? Culture-bound syndromes are usually restricted to a specific setting, and they have a special relationship to that setting. Because culture-bound syndromes are classified on the basis of common etiology (e.g., magic, evil spells, angry ancestors), their clinical pictures may vary. In DSM-IV, the culture-bound syndrome has been defined as "Recurrent, locality-specific patterns of aberrant behavior and troubling experience that may or may not be linked to a particular DSM-IV diagnostic category". Characteristic features being recognition within the society as a deviation from a normal or healthy presentation. The local names, symptoms, course, and social response often influenced by local cultural factors and are limited to specific societies or cultural areas. These were thought to be localized and not globally recognized or spanning different regions, but evidence to the contrary is also emerging.

The DSM-5 has replaced it with the term *Cultural Concepts of Distress* which is defined as "ways that cultural groups and communicate suffering, behavioral problems, or troubling thoughts and emotions". It stresses that all mental distresses are culturally framed and different populations have culturally determined ways of communicating distress, explanations of causality, coping methods, and help-seeking behavior. DSM-5 elaborates on three cultural concepts:

1. *Syndromes:* co-occurring clusters of symptoms and attributions occurring among individuals in specific cultures, community or context.
2. *Idioms of distress:* shared ways of communicating, expressing or sharing the distress.
3. *Explanations:* labels, attributions suggesting causation of symptoms or distress.

The DSM-5 included a clinical interview tool to facilitate comprehensive, person-centered assessments. Only tentative associations were made in ICD-10 between cultural syndromes and recognized psychiatric categories awaiting a stronger evidence base. ICD-10 categorizes culture-bound syndromes in Annexure and lists 12 culture-bound syndromes. It lacks any diagnostic and cultural explanatory guidelines. ICD-10 recognizes a number of culturally uncommon symptom patterns and presentations referred to as culture-specific disorders. ICD-11 is also following the same pattern. Culture-bound syndromes not being easily accommodated in established and international diagnostic categories pose a challenge to anthropologically oriented psychiatrists to research in the field and resolve the diagnostic/clinical confusion affecting many civilizations of the eastern world. Initial description in a particular population or cultural area is required and subsequent association of unique culture-related symptom profile with this community can be made.[15,16]

Effect on Treatment

People have tried to study the role of the local cultural factors in the treatment of mental illnesses. In this area most studied is the ritual typically involving the physical, sensory, and emotional stimulation, and it is also believed to play an important role in the central mechanism of socialization. Studies of emotional memory conclude that evidence that these intense experiences and events are recorded in specific ways that make them more durable. Given the emotionally arousing nature of ritual, memories for material presented in the context of a ritual performed by *shaman/healer* are likely to be enhanced.[17] Each society, prior to globalization and modernization, had developed ways of dealing with certain forms of distress with community-based interventions. Certain members of the society were trained or assumed the responsibility of handling the unknown influences that presumably led to the occurrence of psychiatric symptomatology. The healers had an important position in the society as those suffering from difficult mental (and physical) ailments were brought to their attention. The mechanism through which help was afforded was through community sanctified cures. While sometimes the *cure* would work, and sometimes it did not. Yet, when the intervention did not work, it was construed as the will of the higher forces, absolving them to focus on the next case at hand. With modernization, such traditional practices have remained, though in a muted form where other interventions are too risky or have failed to provide adequate symptomatic improvement. Consideration of such rituals and interventions are of relevance to developing societies like India where traditional methods of healing still hold sway in underserved areas, or for conditions for which modern medicine is not yet popular. Thus, there is policy implication as local needs would be taken into consideration while scaling up treatment services, or being coupled with information dissemination measures.[18]

CONTRIBUTION TO RESEARCH METHODS

Anthropology has contributed to the expansion of the repertoire of research methods in psychiatry. Some of these are enumerated here.

Etic and Emic Approach

Psychiatrist and anthropologist Arthur Kleinman's theory of explanatory models (EMs) suggests that individuals and groups can have vastly different notions of health and disease. The theory also proposed that instead of asking simply about the illness physicians should focus on knowing the patient's answers about "Why", "When", "How", and "What Next" of the disease. With reference to this, application of the etic-emic perspective to mental illness gives useful insights into the cross-cultural research. The standard intercultural approach is the "etic" one and it includes the application of a standardized usually a quantitative (but not always) method of assessing the subject by an internationally accepted classification system which is an appropriately translated and standardized instrument. In brief, the scientifically oriented approach to local situations and interpretations is included under the etic approach. The data obtained is thus standardized and thus comparable to the different parts of the world. In contrast with the etic, the "emic" approach aims at appraising the local phenomena of a community and then describing/conceptualizing the local models of mental illness without imposing western diagnoses **(Figs. 3A and B)**. Data are almost always gathered through open-ended, qualitative and mostly unstructured interviews of local informants. In a simple sense, it is the version of the local people themselves, i.e., how they think. It should be given priority when understanding the perspective of an illness of epical populations like ethnic minorities and also making individualized plans. Recently people have also conceptualized mixed models to apply to this area. But there are very few studies to conclude and translate into clinical practice.[19]

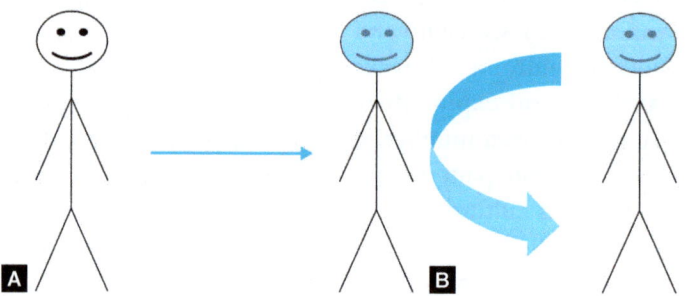

Figs. 3A and B: Schematic representation of: (A) etic approach; (B) emic approach.

Participant Observation

One cannot fully understand other culture by simply observing, one must experience it as well. Participant observation is a type of data collection method taken from anthropology where the aim is to gain a close familiarity with the individuals of the local group/population and eventually through the methods of intensive involvement over an extensive period of time, one gets familiar with the methods and practices of the local cultural environment. Traditionally, participant observation takes many months to years. The researcher has to step out of his/her comfort zone into a world that is new and sometimes challenging; facing physical, sociopolitical, ethical and mental challenges. Usually, a qualitative method of data collection is selected and data may be collected in both qualitative as well as quantitative form. Qualitative data collect information that seeks to describe a topic more than measure it. Anthropological research suggests that just as items on standardized psychological inventories have to be evaluated to assure that they mean the same thing to members of different cultural groups (have "conceptual validity") and that their effect is the same among people in different social contexts (have "technical validity"), experimental manipulations should also be subject to checks for conceptual and technical validity for data collection.[2,19,20] Translating these methods into the knowledge of mental health requires many modifications after ethical consideration and risk-benefit analysis. Participant observation studies in mental health setting may include those where daily functioning is observed closely by residing in a mental health institution, or through residing in a half-way house where individuals who are in the process of recovery stay together **(Fig. 4)**.

INDIAN LITERATURE

If we look at the research done in the context of anthropology and psychiatry in India, there is limited literature. Ganguly et al. in 1995 documented an ethnographic account of people using opium in Rajasthan, India.[21,22] They found that cannabis and opium were often used in a cultural context, as a recreational

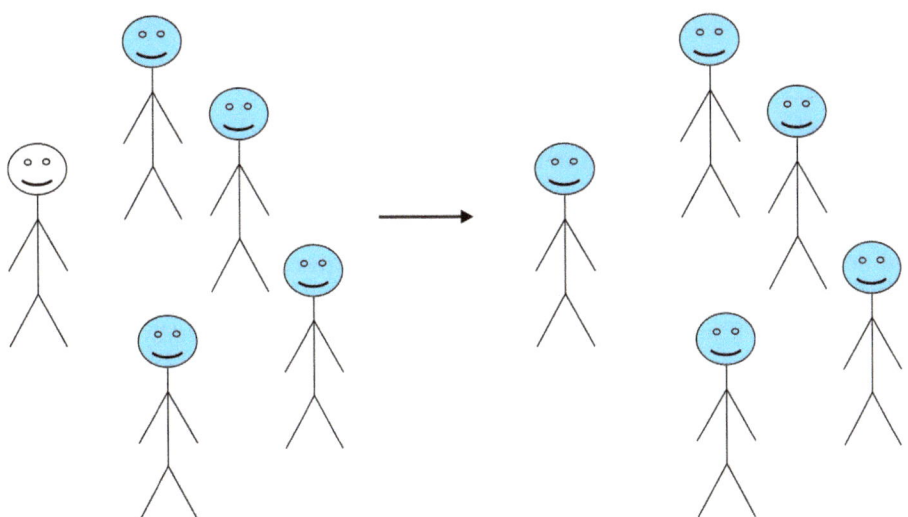

Fig. 4: Participant observation method (the figures show how an individual becomes an almost member of the community to be observed over time and thus gaining close familiarity with the local phenomena).

drug, a social gesture, or a medicine. Ganguly et al. (1995) took accounts of 200 opium using people in three districts of Rajasthan. They employed users of opium interviewed, as the key informant to identify other users of opium. Description of the area, the drug, the settings where they were consumed, the profile of opium users was provided by the authors in depth in their ethnographic account. It was found that "Rajputs" were the highest consumers of opium. The taste of opium developed since childhood as opium was given by mothers to their children as a routine practice. The practice of consumption of opium is considered to be culturally rooted. Use of opium in social gatherings instills the practice among young children. The use of opium in females is driven by their husband's command, or secondary to physical or mental suffering, and gradually some females become dependent on it. Despite belonging to a lower status in the society, the use of opium in women is well-accepted in Rajasthan. Opium was counted as a medicine for pains and aches, cough, and diarrhea by a number of adults in the study area. It was even prescribed by the local doctors in these districts. It was also noted by the authors that opium helps in the expansion of social circle, and better cohesion in a social group. Unless an opium user went on to become grossly deviant such as selling household items for procuring opium or conducting criminal activity, they were considered to be normal. If found, deviant they were taken to psychiatric hospitals for treatment, but rarely, or almost never, to the police. The authors opined that treatment should be targeted toward recent users of opium. They also opined about treating the opium users as patients rather than considering them as a criminal.

Raguram published a report on temple healing, which is a widely practiced phenomenon in India.[23] To conduct this study, the researcher had stayed in the temple for around 2 months and interviewed whoever came to seek help during that time. While interviewing, the author elicited the patients' illness experience as well as caregivers' understanding regarding the illness. A locally adapted semistructured cultural epidemiological interview was formulated, and the approach was emic. Around 31 patients along with their caregivers came to seek help in the temple. The author found that psychotic symptoms (as measured on Brief Psychiatric Symptoms Rating Scale) improved during the stay in the temple despite the absence of any specific healing rituals in the temples. He reported that this improvement which appeared to occur with temple-healing was a result of a nonthreatening and supportive environment present in the temple.

Jain and Jadhav (2009) examined the cultural relevance of community mental health in India.[24] They collected data over 18 months from a community mental health program in Kanpur, Uttar Pradesh. They interviewed clinicians as well as policymakers. The main focus of discussion was on the psychotropic medications. They discussed in their study, about the perspectives of psychiatrists/mental health professionals in understanding and explaining the reasons for the failure of the National Mental Health Programme (NMHP). Facts like doctors and paramedical staff asking less literate population questions which were literally translated into Hindi without taking into consideration the local health and disease model. They concluded that the perspectives differ variedly and the need for changes was emphasized. Also, the authors urged for development of models taking local understanding into account.

Recently, Chavan et al.[25] conducted an ethnographic study to understand the barriers to the treatment process. They based it on the fact that people in the community were hesitant to seek treatment for dependence on alcohol or other drugs. It was seen that a number of patients did not seek treatment for their illness, despite the center being located nearby. The reason for this was found to be the stigma associated with mental illness. There seemed a denial of this problem in the community studied. A six-point questionnaire was developed by the authors to investigate the severity of the problem. After the application of the questionnaire, it was found that those perceiving the problem had no say in making the decision, and those denying the problem were the main hands-on in decision-making. An action plan was chalked out keeping in mind the sociocultural and political ethos of the community, with the help of this study.

FUTURE DIRECTIONS

Development in this field is ongoing and there is a need to further expand the horizons. Designing a nosological system should go through the scrutiny of experts from different related fields and different ethnic-socio-economic groups is a need of the hour. More collaborative researches should be promoted and in addition, a rigorous methodology should be designed using the core principles of both the fields. Local versions of nosology and treatment protocols can be developed rather than applying western concepts adapted for local use.

CONCLUSION

Anthropology is a vast topic and encompasses a wide range of scientific knowledge. There are differences yet many similarities between the two subjects. In past, we have seen that the psychiatry as a branch was criticized for its faulty methods of diagnosing and treating the mental illnesses. This was counterproductive for the marginalized strata of the society. Anthropology has contributed a lot to the field of psychiatry and is continuing to do so right from etiology to symptoms identification and treatment. The various domains like participant observation, emic-etic approach, and transcultural validation are an integral part of the social understanding of mental illness and are gaining recent importance. In India, there is also an emerging trend in contribution to both subjects but in its nascent stage. This knowledge would be helpful in planning treatment interventions as well as changing policies. Together this knowledge allows us to plan and administer the policies for different cultures.

SUMMARY

Anthropology is a holistic way of studying humans as a whole. It junctions the understanding of science and arts and has a bilateral relationship with psychiatry. Right from the Kraepelinian era efforts have been made to understand the nature of the mind by a joint perspective but this joint field has only gained recent importance. Almost all subfields of psychiatry have much in common with anthropology. Sociological phenomena of labeling a person with mental illness, especially from different communities, have somehow evoked a response from the scientific community to reconsider the psychiatric nosology and fit the criteria with an equivalent view toward different cultures. Likewise a need to explore syndromes bounded in specific cultures beyond their boundaries into the western world. More will be discussed in the chapter apart from theoretical influences in terms of how the traditional viewpoints of disease and medicine and research have been influenced by this field. Local beliefs and understandings have always influenced the practice of medicine, research, and further policy planning. Still, a lot of joint efforts are required by both psychiatrists and anthropologist to develop a better understanding of the psychiatric illness, how we manage them and how to plan policies so that those receiving services benefit the most.

REFERENCES

1. Simpson J, Weiner ES. Oxford English Dictionary Online. Oxford: Clarendon Press; Retrieved 1989, 2008.
2. Haviland WA, Prins HE, McBride B. Anthropology: The Human Challenge. Australia: Cengage Learning; 2013.
3. Clements FE. Primitive Concepts of Disease. Berkeley, California: University of California Press; 1932.
4. Skultans V. Anthropology and psychiatry: the uneasy alliance. Transcult Psychiatr Res Rev. 1991;28(1):5-24.
5. Skultans V. Psychiatry through the ethnographic lens. Int J Soc Psychiatry. 2006;52(1):73-83.
6. Dubreuil G, Wittkower ED. Psychiatric anthropology: a historical perspective. Psychiatry. 1976;39(2):130-41.
7. Sapir E. Cultural anthropology and psychiatry. J Abnorm Soc Psychol. 1932;27(3):229-42.
8. Dein S, Bhui KS. At the crossroads of anthropology and epidemiology: current research in cultural psychiatry in the UK. Transcult Psychiatry. 2013;50(6):769-91.
9. Sen MS, Sahoo S, Aggarwal S, Singh SM. Systemic exercise intolerance disease: what's in a name? Asian J Psychiatry. 2016;22:157-8.
10. Singh B. An uncritical encounter between anthropology and psychiatry: AIIMS psychiatrists reading "Affliction". Med Anthropol Theory. 2017;4(3):153.
11. Lock M. DSM-III as a culture-bound construct: commentary on culture-bound syndromes and international disease classifications. Cult Med Psychiatry. 1987;11(1):35-42.
12. Aggarwal NK. Cultural psychiatry, medical anthropology, and the DSM-5 field trials. Med Anthropol. 2013;32(5):393-8.
13. Miranda AO, Fraser LD. Culture-bound syndromes: initial perspectives from individual psychology. J Individ Psychol. 2002;58(4):422-33.
14. Tseng WS. From peculiar psychiatric disorders through culture-bound syndromes to culture-related specific syndromes. Transcult Psychiatry. 2006;43(4):554-76.
15. Balhara YP. Culture-bound syndrome: has it found its right niche? Indian J Psychol Med. 2011;33(2):210-5.
16. Prakash S, Mandal P. Culture-bound syndromes: nosological and management issues. Indian J Psychiatry. 2014;56(1):99.
17. Seligman R, Brown RA. Theory and method at the intersection of anthropology and cultural neuroscience. Soc Cogn Affect Neurosci. 2010;5(2-3):130-7.
18. Leighton AH, Hughes JM. Cultures as a causative of mental disorder. Milbank Q. 2005;83(4).
19. Canino G, Lewis-Fernandez R, Bravo M. Methodological challenges in cross-cultural mental health research. Transcult Psychiatry. 1997;34(2):163-84.
20. Oeye C, Bjelland AK, Skorpen A. Doing participant observation in a psychiatric hospital—research ethics resumed. Soc Sci Med. 2007; 65(11):2296-306.
21. Ganguly KK, Sharma HK, Krishnamachari K. An ethnographic account of opium consumers of Rajasthan (India): socio-medical perspective. Addiction. 1995;90(1):9-12.
22. Seth R, Kotwal A, Ganguly KK. Street and working children of Delhi, India, misusing toluene: an ethnographic exploration. Subst Use Misuse. 2005;40(11):1659-79.
23. Raguram R, Venkateswaran A, Ramakrishna J, Weiss MG. Traditional community resources for mental health: a report of temple healing from India. BMJ. 2002;325(7354):38-40.
24. Jain S, Jadhav S. Pills that swallow policy: clinical ethnography of a Community Mental Health Program in northern India. Transcult Psychiatry. 2009;46(1):60-85.
25. Chavan BS, Patra S, Gupta N, Rozatkar AR. Overcoming barriers to community participation in drug dependence treatment: an ethnography approach. Indian J Soc Psychiatry. 2017;33(1):57-62.

CHAPTER 26

Interface with Social Media

Badr Ratnakaran, Shahul Ameen

INTRODUCTION

In the past about a decade, the use of social media (SM) websites and apps has become immensely popular among the general population. Psychiatrists and those suffering from mental illnesses are no exception. The popularity of SM has, in turn, led to the appearance of various pathological behaviors around their use. In the last few years, a lot of research insights have appeared on what makes SM so attractive to the masses, the physical and mental health consequences of excessive SM use, and the characteristics of various abnormal behaviors related to SM use. SM is being utilized in research as a data collection tool and also as a tool for health education and clinical interventions. Guidelines have appeared to remind health professionals, including psychiatrists, about the ethical ways of SM use. This chapter summarizes the available research in the above areas.

The terms SM and social networking sites (SNSs) have different meanings. SNS refers to any online platform that allows users to create a public profile and interact with other users on that website/app. SM is a broader term and refers to any website that has user-generated content. So, SM includes SNS and also other kinds of websites such as blogs and wikis. However, the terms are often used interchangeably by the scientific community. In this chapter, we merely reproduce the term used by the original researchers.

PSYCHOLOGICAL ASPECTS OF USE

Motivations

Studies have assessed why people use SM and what kind of people use them more. Older adults (30 years and older) grew up without the internet at their disposal. While the younger adults (ages 18–29 years) have grown in an environment where SNS is used as a regular means of communication, the use of SNS in older adults has been related to the openness to new experiences and novelty seeking.[1] College students reported entertainment and convenience as their highest motivations for the use of SNS.[2] A study on Chinese University students found that females used SNS to upload their photos and to update their status, whereas males used SNS to play online games.[3] Extraversion as a personality trait is considered a significant predictor for the motivation to use of SNS, whereas neuroticism is associated with more control of personal information shared in SNS.[4,5]

Facebook has been the most studied of SNS platforms. Majority of studies have shown that people with poor self-esteem spend more time on Facebook.[6-8] This finding has been interpreted by using social compensation theory, where individuals who are introverts, with social anxiety, or who have low self-esteem use SNS to counteract their deficient face-to-face interactions.[9]

Relation to Adolescent Development

One's social life is not fully developed during adolescence. Forming social relationships, developing an identity, and autonomy are important tasks during this period. The use of SM has become widespread among adolescents and has been found to help them in the development of identity and aspirations, along with peer engagement.[10,11] Adolescents use SNS to form friendships and to understand their friends better.[12,13] SM can transform peer relationships in adolescents by altering the frequency and intensity of experiences, modifying the quality of interactions, producing opportunities for compensatory behaviors, and developing new behaviors.[14] The online persona of adolescents on SNS often reflects their offline lives.[15] Interaction with their peers on various SNS platforms can help adolescents in self-exploration and in developing skills related to identity formation, self-disclosure, and creating social support.[16] Thus, in our current digital era, SM can be considered an important tool in the development of adolescents. It is not clear if SM use has any relationship with body image and self-esteem of adolescents.[17] However, cyberbullying, impaired sleep, depression, and anxiety are important negative consequences of SM use in adolescents, which will be discussed later.

Online Disinhibition Effect

Online disinhibition effect (ODE) relates to the lack of inhibition or restraint some people experience while communicating online.[18] Due to this effect, individuals proceed with less caution in divulging personal information online when compared to real life. While online, they show less restriction in demonstrating kindness and generosity and in revealing personal emotions and anxieties. ODE can also bring on undesirable online behaviors, including exploration of pornography and making rude and abusive language, harsh criticisms, incendiary comments, and threats, which the individuals may not be demonstrate in their real life.

Various factors have been identified to influence ODE. The anonymity of one's online persona has a role because the persona provides a safe avenue to express oneself. Due to the invisibility in the SM communication, interactions with peers do not carry any visual or tonal cues of an individual's message. This can lead to a deficit in the expression of empathy while communicating in SM.[19] As SM interactions need not occur in real time, such an asynchronous communication can contribute to ODE. Because an immediate reply is not expected, the individual does not become worried about the repercussions of the response.

IMPACT ON MENTAL HEALTH

Social media-related behaviors influence mental health, often adversely.

Oversharing

Due to the disinhibited nature of the interaction, individuals are prone to sharing too much personal information or inappropriate content in SM. Oversharing can lead to threats to privacy when people other than friends and family have access to one's personal information. Adolescents with low social acceptance or high depression and anxiety scores overshare to cope with psychological distress.[20,21] Individuals with low self-esteem can perceive SM as a low-risk environment to build relationships, leading to versharing.[22] However, such individuals tend to post more negative than positive content, leading to undesirable responses from friends in SM. Other users can perceive oversharing as turning into gossip, as an annoyance, and as attempts to gain attention and increase self-esteem.[20]

Sharenting

Parents tend to post in SM the pictures and updates of their children as they grow. Such practice is known as "sharenting", a word formed by combining "sharing" and "parenting". It is defined as the habitual use of SM to share news, images, etc., of one's children.[23] Parents have been known to share information and images of their children in SM to obtain support, exchange advice about parenting, collect memories, portray themselves as good parents who are proud of their children and keep in touch with their family and friends with regards to their children.[24-27] When parents share details about their children, they inadvertently create an online identity about their children even before they become active online. This causes a conflict in adolescents when their online identities do not match the profile created by their parents in SM about them.[28] Adolescents can feel embarrassed when parents share details about them, making them wish that their parents would exercise more restraint in SM.

Cyberbullying

Cyberbullying has gained prominence during the last decade as SM expanded to users belonging to the pediatric population. It can be defined as harmful behavior that is repeated against an individual or a group of people via the electronic medium.[29] The prevalence of cyberbullying in adolescents ranges from 6.5 to 35.4%. It is considered to be more severe than traditional bullying on the victim, due to its widespread reach in SM, constant accessibility, ease of reproducibility in various SM platforms, lack of face-to-face contact, perceived anonymity, and limited likelihood of an intervention against the perpetrator.[30] Unlike traditional bullying, cyberbullying can occur after school hours and reach audiences beyond one's schoolmates.[31] Cyberbullying is strongly associated with suicide, and its adolescent victims are more prone to depression and anxiety.[31-34] Cyberbullying in adolescents has been associated with emotional problems in females and behavioral problems in males.[35] Adolescent perpetrators of cyberbullying have hyperactivity, aggression, conduct problems, suicidal behavior, and substance use.[36-39] Most victims of cyberbullying do not inform parents or adults, even though family support is a protective factor in cyber perpetration and victimization.[40-42]

Sexting

With the advance of technology, communication through cell phones has expanded from written texts to images, including photos and emojis. The ability to send such images to other people, using smartphones, via SNS, has made sharing images become popular among SM users. Individuals can send each other nude or seminude images of themselves, along with texts of sexual nature. This practice of "sexting" has been of great concern among young adults and adolescents. In a recent review, the prevalence of sexting was 10.2% in adolescents and 53.3% in young adults.[43] Young adults engage in sexting as a part of being sexually active, a safe sex practice, and a risqué behavior.[44] Adolescents have been reported to sext to initiate a relationship or explore their sexuality.[45] Age is considered a positive predictive factor for sexting in adolescents but not young adults.[43] Females are more likely to sext under peer pressure.[46]

Sexting of nude images puts an individual at risk for social blackmail, revenge porn, and cyberbullying. A recent meta-analysis found sexting to have a positive association with depressive and anxiety symptoms among adolescents.[47] The images can also be shared between users without the owner's consent, leading to embarrassment, while adolescents are at risk of sexting with pedophiles.

Body Image

Traditional media outlets of print and television have been known to promote unrealistic expectations of beauty, where women are often depicted thin and with a body shape unattainable for an average person.[48] SM differs from traditional media because it features the users rather than models, uploading their own most ideal and attractive photos to share between themselves.[49] However, SM use in males and preteenage, adolescent, and young females has been associated with body dissatisfaction, drive for thinness, internalization of thin-ideal body image, body surveillance, and self-objectification.[50-56] Individuals also compare their appearances negatively when viewing images of other users in SM, which can also cause a drive for thinness, body image concerns, and self-objectification.[57,58] Viewing SM images that were designed to motivate to exercise and eat healthily and develop an attractive body has also been found to cause a negative mood and body dissatisfaction in females.[59] Such disturbances in body image with relation to SM can also negatively impact food choices and are associated with disordered eating.[60,61] Positive parental influence and a supportive school environment can help to mitigate the negative influence of SM on body image.[62]

Child Sexual Abuse

The number of cases of online child sexual abuse has been increasing steadily over the years.[63] Online sexual exploitation of children has included the use of SM by the perpetrators. The anonymity provided by the internet has allowed the perpetrators to prey on children who use SM. Utilizing the anonymity, they can manipulate children into developing a relationship, with the intention to groom them and later coerce or blackmail them for sexual purposes. The perpetrators can use SM to engage in sexting with children, share nude images, or live stream the abuse of the children with other users. Online sexual abuse has been associated with depression, post-traumatic stress disorder, and suicide attempts.[64] Moreover, children who have been victims of online sexual abuse have been found to score more for post-traumatic stress symptoms when compared to children with offline sexual abuse.[65]

Sleep

With the rapidly growing rate of SM use, individuals find it convenient to engage themselves with their SM platforms in the night while they are free from all work and responsibilities of the day. This has raised concerns about impairment of sleep as the use of SM rises. In adolescents and young adults, the use of SM in nighttime has been associated with delayed onset of bedtime, increased sleep onset latency, decreased duration of sleep, and cognitive impairment.[66-72] The motivations for nighttime use of SM in adolescents and young adults include the perceived risk of being excluded from real-life friends due to missing online conversations in the night.[73,74] Adolescents also fear social disapproval from peers when they are expected to be available online and prompt in responding.[73] The impairment of sleep with SM use in nighttime has also been associated with anxiety, depression, low self-esteem, and poor school satisfaction.[68,69] However, adults who are 75 years and above have been found to have better quality of sleep with night-time use of SM, which has been hypothesized to be due to improved social interactions.[70]

Suicide and Nonsuicidal Self-injury

Social media platforms are used by individuals to express suicidal thoughts and to share information encouraging suicide or nonsuicidal self-injury (NSSI).[75] Cyberbullying can, directly and indirectly, lead to an individual's suicide, known as cyberbullicide.[76] Cyberbullying can increase the risk of suicide and NSSI by increasing the feelings of isolation and hopelessness in adolescents going through multiple stressors in real life.[77] Individuals can form suicide pacts on SM platforms, and these are known as cybersuicide pacts. These are considered an important form of suicide in Japan and Korea.[75,78] Online message boards, chat rooms, and forums catering to a prosuicide or pro-NSSI agenda can promote the spread of information on suicide and create peer-pressure, e.g., to form suicide pacts. In 2008, a Japanese message board had posted a message on suicide by using hydrogen sulfide gas. Subsequently, 220 people attempted suicide using the gas.[79] When content related to suicide becomes more available in SM, a media contagion effect can ensue and lead to an increased risk of suicide in young people.[75] On the other hand, SM has also been used to disseminate information related to suicide prevention and to intervene when individuals expressing suicide thoughts have been identified in SM.[80]

Substance Use

Due to ease of accessibility and increasing reach to a wider audience, SM has become a venue for dispersal of information on various substances of abuse. The alcohol and tobacco industries have used various SM platforms for their marketing strategies to reach a wider audience, including adolescents.[81,82] Compared to traditional forms of media, SM has lesser restrictions on advertisements for alcohol and tobacco products. The alcohol companies push their products via various SM platforms by suggesting specific times to drink and by hosting interactive games and competitions asking users to "like" their brands and to tag themselves in pictures taken while using a particular brand of alcohol.[83] Using SM, e-cigarette companies have propagated the message of vaping as a smoking cessation aid and as an alternative to cigarette smoking.[82] Such campaigns by the alcohol and e-cigarette industry have been found to encourage nonsmokers and young people to use their products.[84,85] Adolescents who use SM have been found to have a high risk for tobacco, alcohol, and cannabis use, with the risk being higher for those who have witnessed SM pictures of their peers in an inebriated state.[86] With the increasing legalization of cannabis, advertisements about cannabis-based products and procannabis messages have made their way to the SM, making it increasingly popular among the youth.[87,88] SM platforms have also been used by drug dealers and recreational drug users for buying and selling drugs.[89]

On the other hand, due to its ability to reach a wider audience, SM can be used for interventions to target substance use disorders. Discussion groups in SM and messages related to quitting tobacco have been found to help in maintaining abstinence and preventing relapse of tobacco use.[90]

PSYCHOPATHOLOGY

Not surprisingly, the popularity of SM has led to the appearance of some unique psychological issues around its use. Research is gradually accumulating on those conditions, though none of them have so far made it to the official lists of psychiatric conditions.

Munchausen by Internet

Munchausen by Internet (MI) is similar to Munchausen syndrome. Here, individuals feign illness in various SM platforms, including forums and chat rooms, to gain the attention and sympathy of other users.[91] With the internet providing a plethora of information on medical conditions, users engaging in MI in SM will describe to other users about exaggerated symptoms of their purported physical ailments. Some cases of possible Munchausen by Proxy by Internet too have been documented. For example, as per one report, using a photo downloaded from a stock photography website, an unmarried female made several posts on an online community for pregnant women, claiming that one of her twin children has repeatedly been suffering from diverse serious physical ailments.[92] Due to the anonymity provided by SM and its asynchronous communication channels, MI sufferers can manipulate their communication and deceive other users.[93] Apart from getting attention and sympathy, the narratives of the MI sufferers have also been linked with sadism when they get enjoyment from their online deception.[91] When other users become aware of the deception, they feel betrayed, and SM avenues like online health forums lose their credibility.[94]

Fear of Missing Out

As individuals post their details, feelings, and updates about the happenings in their life, SM users become curious about the next update or post of other users. This causes a desire to know what other users are doing. This causes a phenomenon of a fear of missing out (FoMO), which is defined as "a pervasive apprehension that one might be having rewarding experience from which one is absent."[95] FoMO has been a concern in young adults and has been considered to be linked with low self-regulation and low satisfaction of basic psychological needs of competence, autonomy, and relatedness.[95,96] FoMO has been associated with problematic SM use and behavior of using SM during conversations in the midst of other people in real life (known as phubbing).[97-99] FoMO has been associated with depression and anxiety along with an impaired quality of sleep by increased presleep arousal due to SM use and delayed sleep onset.[66,100-102]

Jealousy

The presence of positive content in SM can spread happiness through an emotional contagion-like effect.[103,104] Nonetheless, SM users can become jealous or envious when they view positive news or content from other users. The context of jealousy is not only when users negatively compare themselves with others but also when viewing the content of their partners.[105,106] Viewing posts related to purchases of life experiences such as an expensive vacation can elicit more jealousy than materialistic purchases.[107] The envy can become motivating to improve oneself (called benign envy) when the individual has strong emotional ties to the user posting the content.[108] The same study found envy leading to feelings of damaging the position of the user posting the content (called malicious envy), and it was independent of the emotional ties. Envy in relation to SM has also been related to depression in SM users.[105,106]

Addiction

With the increase in popularity of SM, users have been found to use them excessively. Such excessive use, especially of SNS, is related to difficulty in cutting down SM use and experiencing withdrawal symptoms when unable to access SM.[109] Such excessive use of SM has been considered as a type of behavioral addiction.[110] The experience of excessive SM use also appears to be similar to addictive disorders in terms of tolerance, relapse, modification of mood, and salience in relation to cognition and behavior.[111] FoMO has also been considered an important component in addiction to SM.[102,112,113] Decrease in real-life social interaction, relationship problems, and impairment in academic achievement have been considered consequence to SM use, which draws parallels to the consequence of other addictive disorders.[109] Psychiatric distress, maladaptive cognitions, dysfunctional emotional regulation, and preference for online social interaction have been considered important correlates in addiction to SNS.[112] The design of SM apps in smartphones has been considered as a reason for excessive SM use, with endless scrolling, social pressure, social comparisons, social reward, and SM platforms showing what users like as methods used to engage SM users.[114] However, since SM use has now been considered as a way of life, there has been criticism against overpathologizing SM use.[115]

Anxiety and Depression

Social media helps in connecting with people and developing new relationships. This can help in improving social isolation and social connectedness. Along with positive social interactions with other users, SM can help in improving depression and anxiety.[116,117] The use of Facebook over 3 months, along with "psychiatrist as a friend", has shown to improve depressive symptoms in treatment-resistant depression.[118] Because SM provides a space for the expression of one's feelings, it can help sexual minorities to share their experiences and seek social support.[119] This can be a protective factor against depression in them.

On the contrary, negative social interactions, cyberbullying, problematic SNS use or addiction to SNS, and jealousy related to SM have been associated with depression and anxiety in individuals using SM.[116,117] In adolescents, depression and anxiety have been positively correlated with time spent, activity, and addiction to SNS.[120] Constantly surveying other users' profiles and negatively comparing oneself with them, constant surveillance of one's profile, and accepting former partner's invitations have been considered as risk factors.[116,117,119] Higher levels of social anxiety have been correlated with anxious rumination in association with passive Facebook use.[121] Depressive symptoms have been related to an increase in active SM use in terms of content production and interactive communication.[121]

IN THE CLINICAL SCENE

Use by People with Mental Illness

Patients with mental illness have increasingly been using SM with the main purpose to connect with other users, share their illness experience, and seek advice.[122,123] Depressed adolescents use SM to search for content related to entertainment and humor and for content creation. However, they also get involved in negative activities such as risky behaviors, cyberbullying, and comparing negatively with others.[20] SM use in patients with psychosis is helpful in maintaining social connections and improving social isolation.[122] Patients belonging to autism spectrum disorders find SM helpful in maintaining happiness and maintaining social connectedness.[124,125] However, the severity of the mental illness has been considered as a barrier to using SM.[126]

When information posted by the psychiatrist becomes available online, patients can search for their psychiatrist on the internet or various SM platforms. This "therapist-targeted googling" is done by the patient mainly due to the curiosity, when searching for the right therapist, when they try to get to know their therapist and wish to develop a personal relationship, and when they feel the therapist is not going in the right direction.[127]

Use by Psychiatrists

Psychiatrists use SM for personal and professional purposes. SM can be harnessed to spread information about one's practice and academic work.[128] SM can help in networking with peers from the same profession and other disciplines. This can be of help in finding collaborators for academic projects. Various scientific journals have now begun spreading information about published articles through SM for wider dissemination. Psychiatrists can use SM for clinical professional development and also to advocate for changes in public policy on mental illness.

When the patient sends friend requests to the psychiatrist in SM, this blurs the boundaries of the doctor-patient relationship and it has been recommended to continue to preserve the sanctity of the same relationship in SM.[129] Psychiatrists should be aware that when they post their personal information in SM, it is a form of self-disclosure. Thus, discretion should be maintained on how much personal information should be divulged in SM by the psychiatrist and privacy settings of SM platform used should be assessed on how much personal information of the psychiatrist should a potential patient have access to.[130] While posting content online, psychiatrists should continue to maintain confidentiality and professional boundaries with regards to a patient. Psychiatrists should be aware of their online image and keep their professional and personal content separate from each other.[131]

Patient-targeted Googling

With the users posting their content on SM and the Internet, it is easy for the psychiatrist to search for and keep track of the online activities of their patients. This practice, called as "patient-targeted googling", has raised questions about violation of boundaries in the doctor–patient relationship.[132] While searching the internet might provide information on the patient's financial, legal or relationship status, patient-targeted googling is seen as an intrusive behavior from the psychiatrist on the areas that have not been revealed by the patient. The accuracy and clinical relevance of information posted by the patient be unreliable, leading to erroneous assumptions about the patient.[133] Patient-targeted googling should be done only with the motivation to provide effective care and preferably, with the knowledge and consent of the patient.[131]

Role in Research

As medical researchers require more human participants for research, they have now turned to SM to recruit patients for studies. Recruiting via Facebook as shown to help with shorter duration of recruitment, reduced cost and better representation of the sample to be studied.[134,135] It also helps in reaching out to populations that are hard to reach including adolescents, young adults and individuals with sexually transmitted diseases (STDs) and substance use disorders.[136] Online surveys on health topic mental illness can be sent through SM for participants to complete.[137] But as individuals express themselves in SM, their posts include messages and images can reflect their emotions and mental state. Researchers have become interested in using data mining techniques including text and image analysis from the content in SM. Social network analysis has also been used to study symptoms of depression and eating disorders.[80,138,139] Rosenquist et al. in their study, were able to find that depression can be identified through an individual's social network of other users in SM.[140] As health research with regards to the content in SM is being explored, concerns have been raised with regards to privacy and informed to consent for using the user's data.[141]

Use in Interventions

As a part of its evolution, SNS has transformed from general-purpose use, like Facebook, to health-specific SNS, including online forums catering to specific topics related to health, such as smoking cessation and diabetes.[142] SNSs have also been used for public health surveillance of communicable and noncommunicable diseases.[143-145] With the wealth of information available from the content in SM, various interventions using SM to target many health-related behaviors have been used. The health domains that have been targeted include fitness, smoking cessation, sexual health, food safety, and promotion of health.[146] The interventions include providing education, social support, and data sharing to promote social competition. SM has been used to provide psychoeducation to improve mental health literacy on topics such as depression, anxiety, and post-traumatic stress disorder.[147] SM can also be used for posting information on suicide prevention and for tracking suicide notes in SNS and identifying individuals or geographical areas that are at high risk of suicide.[148] Alvarez-Jimenez et al. created an online intervention for patients with first-episode psychosis that included peer-to-peer social networking, individual psychosocial intervention, and interdisciplinary and peer moderation that helped in social connectedness and empowerment.[149]

REFERENCES

1. Correa T, Hinsley AW, de Zúñiga HG. Who interacts on the Web? The intersection of users' personality and social media use. Comput Hum Behav. 2010;26(2):247-53.
2. Alhabash S, Ma M. A tale of four platforms: motivations and uses of Facebook, Twitter, Instagram, and Snapchat among college students? Soc Media Soc. 2017;3(1):205630511769154.
3. Wang JL, Jackson LA, Zhang DJ, Su ZQ. The relationships among the Big Five Personality factors, self-esteem, narcissism, and sensation-seeking to Chinese University students' uses of social networking sites (SNSs). Comput Hum Behav. 2012;28(6):2313-9.
4. Mancinelli E, Bassi G, Salcuni S. Predisposing and motivational factors related to social network sites use: systematic review. JMIR Form Res. 2019;3(2):e12248.
5. Seidman G. Self-presentation and belonging on Facebook: How personality influences social media use and motivations. Pers Individ Differ. 2013;54(3):402-7.
6. Mehdizadeh S. Self-presentation 2.0: narcissism and self-esteem on Facebook. Cyberpsychol Behav Soc Netw. 2010;13(4):357-64.
7. Kalpidou M, Costin D, Morris J. The relationship between Facebook and the well-being of undergraduate college students. Cyberpsychol Behav Soc Netw. 2011;14(4):183-9.
8. Tazghini S, Siedlecki KL. A mixed method approach to examining Facebook use and its relationship to self-esteem. Comput Hum Behav. 2013;29(3):827-32.
9. McKenna KY, Green AS, Gleason ME. Relationship formation on the Internet: What's the big attraction? J Soc Issues. 2002;58(1):9-31.
10. Uhls Y. Media Moms and Digital Dads, 1st edition. Brookline, MA: Routledge; 2015. p. 264.
11. Subrahmanyam K, Šmahel D. Digital youth: The Role of Media in Development. New York, NY, US: Springer Science/Business Media; 2011. p. 236.
12. Anderson M, Jiang J. Teens, Social Media and Technology 2018. Pew Research Center: Internet, Science and Tech. [online] Available from: https://www.pewinternet.org/2018/05/31/teens-social-media-technology-2018/ [Last accessed June, 2021].
13. Borca G, Bina M, Keller PS, Gilbert LR, Begotti T. Internet use and developmental tasks: adolescents' point of view. Comput Hum Behav. 2015;52:49-58.
14. Nesi J, Choukas-Bradley S, Prinstein MJ. Transformation of adolescent peer relations in the social media context: Part 1—a theoretical framework and application to dyadic peer relationships. Clin Child Fam Psychol Rev. 2018; 21(3):267-94.
15. Schwartz HA, Eichstaedt JC, Kern ML, Dziurzynski L, Ramones SM, Agrawal M, et al. Personality,

15. gender, and age in the language of social media: the open-vocabulary approach. PLoS One. 2013;8(9):e73791.
16. Best P, Manktelow R, Taylor B. Online communication, social media and adolescent well-being: a systematic narrative review. Child Youth Serv Rev. 2014;41:27-36.
17. Shah J, Das P, Muthiah N, Milanaik R. New age technology and social media: adolescent psychosocial implications and the need for protective measures. Curr Opin Pediatr. 2019;31(1):148-56.
18. Suler J. The online disinhibition effect. Cyberpsychol Behav. 2004;7(3):321-6.
19. Terry C, Cain J. The emerging issue of digital empathy. Am J Pharm Educ. 2016;80(4):58.
20. Radovic A, Gmelin T, Stein BD, Miller E. Depressed adolescents' positive and negative use of social media. J Adolesc. 2017;55:5-15.
21. Law DM, Shapka JD, Collie RJ. Who might flourish and who might languish? Adolescent social and mental health profiles and their online experiences and behaviors. Hum Behav Emerg Technol. 2019;2(1):82-92.
22. Forest AL, Wood JV. When social networking is not working: individuals with low self-esteem recognize but do not reap the benefits of self-disclosure on Facebook. Psychol Sci. 2012;23(3):295-302.
23. Sharenting definition and meaning. Collins English Dictionary. [online] Available from: https://www.collinsdictionary.com/us/dictionary/english/sharenting [Last accessed June, 2021].
24. Marasli M, Suhendan E, Yilmazturk NH, Cok F. Parents' shares on social networking sites about their children: sharenting. Anthropologist. 2016;24(2):399-406.
25. Blum-Ross A, Livingstone S. Sharenting, parent blogging, and the boundaries of the digital self. Pop Commun. 2017;15(2):110-25.
26. Kumar P, Schoenebeck S. The Modern Day Baby Book: Enacting Good Mothering and Stewarding Privacy on Facebook. New York, USA: ACM Press; 2015.
27. Wagner A, Gasche LA. Sharenting: Making Decisions about Other's Privacy on Social Networking Sites. Darmstadt Technical University, Department of Business Administration, Economics and Law, Institute for Business Studies (BWL); 2018. Report No.: 90477. [online] Available from: https://ideas.repec.org/p/dar/wpaper/90477.html [Last accessed June, 2021].
28. Ouvrein G, Verswijvel K. Sharenting: parental adoration or public humiliation? A focus group study on adolescents' experiences with sharenting against the background of their own impression management. Child Youth Serv Rev. 2019;99:319-27.
29. Tokunaga RS. Following you home from school: a critical review and synthesis of research on cyberbullying victimization. Comput Hum Behav. 2010;26(3):277-87.
30. Sticca F, Perren S. Is cyberbullying worse than traditional bullying? Examining the differential roles of medium, publicity, and anonymity for the perceived severity of bullying. J Youth Adolesc. 2013;42(5):739-50.
31. Juvonen J, Gross EF. Extending the school grounds? Bullying experiences in cyberspace. J Sch Health. 2008;78(9):496-505.
32. Hamm MP, Newton AS, Chisholm A, Shulhan J, Milne A, Sundar P, et al. Prevalence and effect of cyberbullying on children and young people: a scoping review of social media studies. JAMA Pediatr. 2015;169(8):770-7.
33. van Geel M, Vedder P, Tanilon J. Relationship between peer victimization, cyberbullying, and suicide in children and adolescents: a meta-analysis. JAMA Pediatr. 2014;168(5):435-42.
34. Fisher BW, Gardella JH, Teurbe-Tolon AR. Peer cybervictimization among adolescents and the associated internalizing and externalizing problems: a meta-analysis. J Youth Adolesc. 2016;45(9):1727-43.
35. Kim S, Colwell SR, Kata A, Boyle MH, Georgiades K. Cyberbullying victimization and adolescent mental health: evidence of differential effects by sex and mental health problem type. J Youth Adolesc. 2018;47(3):661-72.
36. Schultze-Krumbholz A, Scheithauer H. Social-behavioral correlates of cyberbullying in a German student sample. Z Für Psychol Psychol. 2009;217(4):224-6.
37. Beckman L, Hagquist C, Hellström L. Does the association with psychosomatic health problems differ between cyberbullying and traditional bullying? Emot Behav Difficult. 2012;17(3-4):421-34.
38. Kowalski RM, Limber SP. Psychological, physical, and academic correlates of cyberbullying and traditional bullying. J Adolesc Health. 2013;53(1 Suppl):S13-20.
39. Hinduja S, Patchin JW. Cyberbullying: an exploratory analysis of factors related to offending and victimization. Deviant Behav. 2008;29(2):129-56.

40. Cassidy W, Jackson M, Brown KN. Sticks and stones can break my bones, but how can pixels hurt me? Students' experiences with cyberbullying. Sch Psychol Int. 2009;30(4):383-402.
41. Dooley JJ, Gradinger P, Strohmeier D, Cross D, Spiel C. Cyber-victimisation: the association between help-seeking behaviours and self-reported emotional symptoms in Australia and Austria. J Psychol Couns Sch. 2010;20(2):194-209.
42. Fanti KA, Demetriou AG, Hawa VV. A longitudinal study of cyberbullying: examining risk and protective factors. Eur J Dev Psychol. 2012;9(2):168-81.
43. Klettke B, Hallford DJ, Mellor DJ. Sexting prevalence and correlates: a systematic literature review. Clin Psychol Rev. 2014;34(1):44-53.
44. Levine D. Sexting: a terrifying health risk ... or the new normal for young adults? J Adolesc Health. 2013;52(3):257-8.
45. Lenhart A (2009). Teens and sexting. Pew Research Center: Internet, Science and Tech. [online] Available from: https://www.pewresearch.org/internet/2009/12/15/teens-and-sexting/ [Last accessed June, 2021].
46. Henderson L, Elizabeth M. Sexting and sexual relationships among teens and young adults. McNair Sch Res J. 2011;7(1).
47. Gassó AM, Klettke B, Agustina JR, Montiel I. Sexting, mental health, and victimization among adolescents: a literature review. Int J Environ Res Public Health. 2019;16(13):2364.
48. Grabe S, Ward LM, Hyde JS. The role of the media in body image concerns among women: a meta-analysis of experimental and correlational studies. Psychol Bull. 2008;134(3):460-76.
49. Fardouly J, Vartanian LR. Social media and body image concerns: current research and future directions. Curr Opin Psychol. 2016;9:1-5.
50. Fox J, Rooney MC. The Dark triad and trait self-objectification as predictors of men's use and self-presentation behaviors on social networking sites. Pers Individ Differ. 2015;76:161-5.
51. Tiggemann M, Slater A. NetTweens: The Internet and body image concerns in preteenage girls. J Early Adolesc. 2014;34(5):606-20.
52. Tiggemann M, Slater A. NetGirls: the Internet, Facebook, and body image concern in adolescent girls. Int J Eat Disord. 2013;46(6):630-3.
53. Tiggemann M, Miller J. The Internet and adolescent girls' weight satisfaction and drive for thinness. Sex Roles J Res. 2010;63(1-2):79-90.
54. Mingoia J, Hutchinson AD, Wilson C, Gleaves DH. The relationship between social networking site use and the internalization of a thin ideal in females: a meta-analytic review. Front Psychol. 2017;8:1351.
55. Vandenbosch L, Eggermont S. Understanding sexual objectification: a comprehensive approach toward media exposure and girls' internalization of beauty ideals, self-objectification, and body surveillance. J Commun. 2012;62(5):869-87.
56. Cohen R, Blaszczynski A. Comparative effects of Facebook and conventional media on body image dissatisfaction. J Eat Disord. 2015;3:23.
57. Fardouly J, Diedrichs PC, Vartanian LR, Halliwell E. The mediating role of appearance comparisons in the relationship between media usage and self-objectification in young women. Psychol Women Q. 2015;39(4):447-57.
58. Fardouly J, Vartanian LR. Negative comparisons about one's appearance mediate the relationship between Facebook usage and body image concerns. Body Image. 2015;12:82-8.
59. Tiggemann M, Zaccardo M. Exercise to be fit, not skinny: the effect of fitspiration imagery on women's body image. Body Image. 2015;15:61-7.
60. Rounsefell K, Gibson S, McLean S, Blair M, Molenaar A, Brennan L, et al. Social media, body image and food choices in healthy young adults: a mixed methods systematic review. Nutr Diet. 2020;77(1):19-40.
61. Holland G, Tiggemann M. A systematic review of the impact of the use of social networking sites on body image and disordered eating outcomes. Body Image. 2016;17:100-10.
62. Burnette CB, Kwitowski MA, Mazzeo SE. I don't need people to tell me I'm pretty on social media: a qualitative study of social media and body image in early adolescent girls. Body Image. 2017;23:114-25.
63. Bentley H, Burrows A, Hafizi M, Kumari P, Mussen N, O'Hagan O, et al. (2020). How safe are our children? [online] Available from: https://learning.nspcc.org.uk/research-resources/how-safe-are-our-children/ [Last accessed June, 2021].
64. Say GN, Babadağı Z, Karabekiroğlu K, Yüce M, Akbaş S. Abuse characteristics and psychiatric consequences associated with online sexual abuse. Cyberpsychol Behav Soc Netw. 2015;18(6):333-6.
65. Hamilton-Giachritsis C, Hanson E, Whittle H, Beech A. (2017). Impact of online and offline child sexual abuse: everyone deserves to be happy and safe. [online] Available from: https://learning.nspcc.org.uk/research-resources/2017/

impact-online-offline-child-sexual-abuse/ [Last accessed June, 2021].
66. Scott H, Woods HC. Fear of missing out and sleep: cognitive behavioural factors in adolescents' nighttime social media use. J Adolesc. 2018;68:61-5.
67. Scott H, Biello SM, Woods HC. Social media use and adolescent sleep patterns: cross-sectional findings from the UK millennium cohort study. BMJ Open. 2019;9(9):e031161.
68. Woods HC, Scott H. #Sleepyteens: social media use in adolescence is associated with poor sleep quality, anxiety, depression and low self-esteem. J Adolesc. 2016;51:41-9.
69. Vernon L, Barber BL, Modecki KL. Adolescent problematic social networking and school experiences: the mediating effects of sleep disruptions and sleep quality. Cyberpsychol Behav Soc Netw. 2015;18(7):386-92.
70. Exelmans L, Scott H. Social media use and sleep quality among adults: the role of gender, age and social media checking habit. PsyArXiv; 2019. [online] Available from: https://osf.io/eqxdh [Last accessed June, 2021].
71. Levenson JC, Shensa A, Sidani JE, Colditz JB, Primack BA. Social media use before bed and sleep disturbance among young adults in the United States: a nationally representative study. Sleep. 2017;40(9):zsx113.
72. Xanidis N, Brignell CM. The association between the use of social network sites, sleep quality and cognitive function during the day. Comput Hum Behav. 2016;55:121-6.
73. Scott H, Biello SM, Woods HC. Identifying drivers for bedtime social media use despite sleep costs: the adolescent perspective. Sleep Health. 2019;5(6):539-45.
74. Vorderer P, Krömer N, Schneider FM. Permanently online—permanently connected: explorations into university students' use of social media and mobile smart devices. Comput Hum Behav. 2016;63:694-703.
75. Luxton DD, June JD, Fairall JM. Social media and suicide: a public health perspective. Am J Public Health. 2012;102(Suppl 2):S195-200.
76. Hinduja S, Patchin JW. Bullying Beyond the Schoolyard: Preventing and Responding to Cyberbullying. Thousand Oaks, California: Corwin Press; 2014. p. 339.
77. Hinduja S, Patchin JW. High-Tech Cruelty. Educ Leadership. 2011;68(5):48-52.
78. Rajagopal S. Suicide pacts and the internet. BMJ. 2004;329(7478):1298-9.
79. Morii D, Miyagatani Y, Nakamae N, Murao M, Taniyama K. Japanese experience of hydrogen sulfide: the suicide craze in 2008. J Occup Med Toxicol. 2010;5:28.
80. Robinson J, Cox G, Bailey E, Hetrick S, Rodrigues M, Fisher S, et al. Social media and suicide prevention: a systematic review. Early Interv Psychiatry. 2016;10(2):103-21.
81. Moreno MA, Whitehill JM. Influence of social media on alcohol use in adolescents and young adults. Alcohol Res. 2014;36(1):91-100.
82. McCausland K, Maycock B, Leaver T, Jancey J. The messages presented in electronic cigarette-related social media promotions and discussion: scoping review. J Med Internet Res. 2019;21(2):e11953.
83. Nicholls J. Everyday, everywhere: alcohol marketing and social media—current trends. Alcohol Alcohol. 2012;47(4):486-93.
84. Westgate EC, Holliday J. Identity, influence, and intervention: the roles of social media in alcohol use. Curr Opin Psychol. 2016;9:27-32.
85. Roditis M, Delucchi K, Cash D, Halpern-Felsher B. Adolescents' perceptions of health risks, social risks, and benefits differ across tobacco products. J Adolesc Health. 2016;58(5):558-66.
86. Center of Addiction and Substance Use. National Survey of American Attitudes on Substance Abuse XVII: Teens. New York, NY: Columbia University; 2012. [online] Available from: https://www.centeronaddiction.org/addiction-research/reports/national-survey-american-attitudes-substance-abuse-teens-2012 [Last accessed June, 2021].
87. Cavazos-Rehg PA, Krauss M, Fisher SL, Salyer P, Grucza RA, Bierut LJ. Twitter chatter about marijuana. J Adolesc Health. 2015;56(2):139-45.
88. Daniulaityte R, Nahhas RW, Wijeratne S, Carlson RG, Lamy FR, Martins SS, et al. Time for dabs: analyzing Twitter data on marijuana concentrates across the US. Drug Alcohol Depend. 2015;155:307-11.
89. Demant J, Bakken SA, Oksanen A, Gunnlaugsson H. Drug dealing on Facebook, Snapchat and Instagram: a qualitative analysis of novel drug markets in the Nordic countries. Drug Alcohol Rev. 2019;38(4):377-85.
90. Naslund JA, Kim SJ, Aschbrenner KA, McCulloch LJ, Brunette MF, Dallery J, et al. Systematic review of social media interventions for smoking cessation. Addict Behav. 2017;73:81-93.
91. Feldman MD. Munchausen by Internet: detecting factitious illness and crisis on the Internet. South Med J. 2000;93(7):669-72.
92. McCulloch V, Feldman MD. Munchausen by proxy by Internet. Child Abuse Negl. 2011;35(11):965-6.

93. Pulman A, Taylor J. Munchausen by Internet: current research and future directions. J Med Internet Res. 2012;14(4):e115.
94. Uridge L, Rodan D. A Moderator's Dilemma: Munchausen Syndrome by Internet. Adelaide, Australia: Australian and New Zealand Communication Association; 2012. p. 12.
95. Przybylski AK, Murayama K, DeHaan CR, Gladwell V. Motivational, emotional, and behavioral correlates of fear of missing out. Comput Hum Behav. 2013;29(4):1841-8.
96. Alt D, Boniel-Nissim M. Links between adolescents' deep and surface learning approaches, problematic internet use, and fear of missing out (FoMO). Internet Interv. 2018;13:30-9.
97. Coskun S, Karayagız Muslu G. Investigation of problematic mobile phones use and fear of missing out (FoMO) level in adolescents. Community Ment Health J. 2019;55(6):1004-14.
98. Wolniewicz CA, Tiamiyu MF, Weeks JW, Elhai JD. Problematic smartphone use and relations with negative affect, fear of missing out, and fear of negative and positive evaluation. Psychiatry Res. 2018;262:618-23.
99. Franchina V, Vanden Abeele M, van Rooij AJ, Lo Coco G, De Marez L. Fear of missing out as a predictor of problematic social media use and phubbing behavior among Flemish adolescents. Int J Environ Res Public Health. 2018;15(10):2319.
100. Elhai JD, Yang H, Fang J, Bai X, Hall BJ. Depression and anxiety symptoms are related to problematic smartphone use severity in Chinese young adults: fear of missing out as a mediator. Addict Behav. 2020;101:105962.
101. Dempsey AE, O'Brien KD, Tiamiyu MF, Elhai JD. Fear of missing out (FoMO) and rumination mediate relations between social anxiety and problematic Facebook use. Addict Behav Rep. 2019;9:100150.
102. Oberst U, Wegmann E, Stodt B, Brand M, Chamarro A. Negative consequences from heavy social networking in adolescents: the mediating role of fear of missing out. J Adolesc. 2017;55:51-60.
103. Coviello L, Sohn Y, Kramer AD, Marlow C, Franceschetti M, Christakis NA, et al. Detecting emotional contagion in massive social networks. PLoS One. 2014;9(3):e90315.
104. Kramer AD, Guillory JE, Hancock JT. Experimental evidence of massive-scale emotional contagion through social networks. Proc Natl Acad Sci. 2014;111(24):8788-90.
105. Pera A. Psychopathological processes involved in social comparison, depression, and envy on Facebook. Front Psychol. 2018;9:22.
106. Tandoc EC, Ferrucci P, Duffy M. Facebook use, envy, and depression among college students: is facebooking depressing? Comput Hum Behav. 2015;43:139-46.
107. Lin R, van de Ven N, Utz S. What triggers envy on social network sites? A comparison between shared experiential and material purchases. Comput Hum Behav. 2018;85:271-81.
108. Lin R, Utz S. The emotional responses of browsing Facebook: happiness, envy, and the role of tie strength. Comput Hum Behav. 2015;52:29-38.
109. Kuss DJ, Griffiths MD. Online social networking and addiction—a review of the psychological literature. Int J Environ Res Public Health. 2011;8(9):3528-52.
110. Kuss DJ, Griffiths MD. Social networking sites and addiction: ten lessons learned. Int J Environ Res Public Health. 2017;14(3):311.
111. Griffiths M. A 'components' model of addiction within a biopsychosocial framework. J Subst Use. 2005;10(4):191-7.
112. Pontes HM, Taylor M, Stavropoulos V. Beyond "Facebook addiction": the role of cognitive-related factors and psychiatric distress in social networking site addiction. Cyberpsychol Behav Soc Netw. 2018;21(4):240-7.
113. Stead H, Bibby PA. Personality, fear of missing out and problematic internet use and their relationship to subjective well-being. Comput Hum Behav. 2017;76:534-40.
114. Montag C, Lachmann B, Herrlich M, Zweig K. Addictive features of social media/messenger platforms and Freemium games against the background of psychological and economic theories. Int J Environ Res Public Health. 2019;16(14):2612.
115. Billieux J, Schimmenti A, Khazaal Y, Maurage P, Heeren A. Are we overpathologizing everyday life? A tenable blueprint for behavioral addiction research. J Behav Addict. 2015;4(3):119-23.
116. Seabrook EM, Kern ML, Rickard NS. Social networking sites, depression, and anxiety: a systematic review. JMIR Ment Health. 2016;3(4):e50.
117. Baker DA, Algorta GP. The relationship between online social networking and depression: a systematic review of quantitative studies. Cyberpsychol Behav Soc Netw. 2016;19(11):638-48.

118. Mota Pereira J. Facebook enhances antidepressant pharmacotherapy effects. Sci World J. 2014;2014:892048.
119. Escobar-Viera CG, Whitfield DL, Wessel CB, Shensa A, Sidani JE, Brown AL, et al. For better or for worse? A systematic review of the evidence on social media use and depression among lesbian, gay, and bisexual minorities. JMIR Ment Health. 2018;5(3):e10496.
120. Keles B, McCrae N, Grealish A. A systematic review: the influence of social media on depression, anxiety and psychological distress in adolescents. Int J Adolesc Youth. 2019;25(4):1-15.
121. Shaw AM, Timpano KR, Tran TB, Joormann J. Correlates of Facebook usage patterns: the relationship between passive Facebook use, social anxiety symptoms, and brooding. Comput Hum Behav. 2015;48:575-80.
122. Highton-Williamson E, Priebe S, Giacco D. Online social networking in people with psychosis: a systematic review. Int J Soc Psychiatry. 2015;61(1):92-101.
123. Naslund JA, Grande SW, Aschbrenner KA, Elwyn G. Naturally occurring peer support through social media: the experiences of individuals with severe mental illness using YouTube. PLoS One. 2014;9(10):e110171.
124. Ward DM, Dill-Shackleford KE, Mazurek MO. Social media use and happiness in adults with autism spectrum disorder. Cyberpsychol Behav Soc Netw. 2018;21(3):205-9.
125. Van Schalkwyk GI, Marin CE, Ortiz M, Rolison M, Qayyum Z, McPartland JC, et al. Social media use, friendship quality, and the moderating role of anxiety in adolescents with autism spectrum disorder. J Autism Dev Disord. 2017;47(9):2805-13.
126. Abu Rahal Z, Vadas L, Manor I, Bloch B, Avital A. Use of information and communication technologies among individuals with and without serious mental illness. Psychiatry Res. 2018;266:160-7.
127. Eichenberg C, Sawyer A. Do patients look up their therapists online? An exploratory study among patients in psychotherapy. JMIR Ment Health. 2016;3(2):e22.
128. Liu HY, Beresin EV, Chisolm MS. Social media skills for professional development in psychiatry and medicine. Psychiatr Clin North Am. 2019;42(3):483-92.
129. Sabin JE, Harland JC. Professional ethics for digital age psychiatry: boundaries, privacy, and communication. Curr Psychiatry Rep. 2017;19(9):55.
130. Petrow S. (2014). When psychiatrists are on Facebook, their patients can get a case of TMI (The Washington Post). [online] Available from: https://www.washingtonpost.com/national/health-science/when-psychiatrists-are-on-facebook-their-patients-can-get-a-case-of-tmi/2014/08/25/ed31e522-110a-11e4-9285-4243a40ddc97_story.html [Last accessed June, 2021].
131. Frankish K, Ryan C, Harris A. Psychiatry and online social media: potential, pitfalls and ethical guidelines for psychiatrists and trainees. Australas Psychiatry. 2012;20(3):181-7.
132. Clinton BK, Silverman BC, Brendel DH. Patient-targeted googling: the ethics of searching online for patient information. Harv Rev Psychiatry. 2010;18(2):103-12.
133. Thabrew H, Sawyer A, Eischenberg C. Patient-targeted googling by New Zealand mental health professionals: a new field of ethical consideration in the Internet age. Telemed J E Health. 2018;24(10):818-24.
134. Amon KL, Campbell AJ, Hawke C, Steinbeck K. Facebook as a recruitment tool for adolescent health research: a systematic review. Acad Pediatr. 2014;14(5):439-47.e4.
135. Whitaker C, Stevelink S, Fear N. The use of Facebook in recruiting participants for health research purposes: a systematic review. J Med Internet Res. 2017;19(8):e290.
136. Capurro D, Cole K, Echavarría MI, Joe J, Neogi T, Turner AM. The use of social networking sites for public health practice and research: a systematic review. J Med Internet Res. 2014;16(3):e79.
137. Wongkoblap A, Vadillo MA, Curcin V. Researching mental health disorders in the era of social media: systematic review. J Med Internet Res. 2017;19(6):e228.
138. Xu R, Zhang Q. Understanding online health groups for depression: social network and linguistic perspectives. J Med Internet Res. 2016;18(3):e63.
139. Wang T, Brede M, Ianni A, Mentzakis E. Detecting and characterizing eating-disorder communities on social media. Proceedings of the Tenth ACM International Conference on Web Search and Data Mining. New York, NY, USA: ACM; 2017. pp. 91-100. [online] Available from: https://dl.acm.org/doi/10.1145/3018661.3018706 [Last accessed June, 2021].
140. Rosenquist J, Fowler J, Christakis N. Social network determinants of depression. Mol Psychiatry. 2011;16(3).

141. Golder S, Ahmed S, Norman G, Booth A. Attitudes toward the ethics of research using social media: a systematic review. J Med Internet Res. 2017;19(6):e195.
142. Korda H, Itani Z. Harnessing social media for health promotion and behavior change. Health Promot Pract. 2013;14(1):15-23.
143. Eysenbach G. Infodemiology and infoveillance: framework for an emerging set of public health informatics methods to analyze search, communication and publication behavior on the Internet. J Med Internet Res. 2009;11(1):e11.
144. Salathé M, Freifeld CC, Mekaru SR, Tomasulo AF, Brownstein JS. Influenza A (H7N9) and the importance of digital epidemiology. N Engl J Med. 2013;369(5):401-4.
145. Weitzman ER, Kelemen S, Quinn M, Eggleston EM, Mandl KD. Participatory surveillance of hypoglycemia and harms in an online social network. JAMA Intern Med. 2013;173(5):345-51.
146. Laranjo L, Arguel A, Neves AL, Gallagher AM, Kaplan R, Mortimer N, et al. The influence of social networking sites on health behavior change: a systematic review and meta-analysis. J Am Med Inform Assoc. 2015;22(1):243-56.
147. Brijnath B, Protheroe J, Mahtani KR, Antoniades J. Do web-based mental health literacy interventions improve the mental health literacy of adult consumers? Results from a systematic review. J Med Internet Res. 2016;18(6):e165.
148. Christensen H, Batterham PJ, O'Dea B. E-health interventions for suicide prevention. Int J Environ Res Public Health. 2014;11(8):8193-212.
149. Alvarez-Jimenez M, Bendall S, Lederman R, Wadley G, Chinnery G, Vargas S, et al. On the HORYZON: moderated online social therapy for long-term recovery in first episode psychosis. Schizophr Res. 2013;143(1):143-9.

Index

Page numbers followed by *b* refer to box, *f* refer to figure, and *t* refer to table

A

Academic stress 253
Acne excoriée 106*f*
Acotiamide 82
Acquired immunodeficiency
    syndrome 258
Activity observation network 273
Addictive disorders 303
Additional psychiatric disorder
    250
Adrenocorticotropic hormone 91,
    109
Alcohol 257
Alleviate sickness symptoms 195
Alopecia areata 103, 108
Alpha-synuclein 30
Alzheimer's disease 30, 119
Amantadine 25
Amateur tango dancers 273
Amnesia 267
Analytical psychology 212
Ankylosing spondylitis 60
Anorectal pain 75
Anthropology 286, 287, 289, 289*f*,
    290, 295
    branches of 286*f*
    field of 286
Antibiotics 81
Antidepressants 51, 54, 82, 116
Antiepileptics 52
Antiphospholipid syndrome 90
Antipsychiatry 147, 162, 166, 168
Antipsychotics 51, 54, 117
Antiretroviral therapy 96
Antituberculosis treatment 96
Anxiety 27, 29, 43, 114, 237, 241,
    303
    disorder 25, 32, 33, 55, 92, 254
        generalized 24, 29, 32
    high level of 130
Apathy 31, 32
Appropriate facial expression, lack
    of 250
Archaeological anthropology 286

Archetypal psychology 212
Arousal reduction training 84
Arrhythmias 119
Art therapy 208
    evidence base of 213
    scope of 215
    task force on 216
Arthur Kleinman's theory 292
Artificial intelligence 242
Asexuality spectrum 127
Asthma 215
Astrological influences 195
Atopic dermatitis 108, 109
Attachment theory 257
Attention deficit hyperactivity
        disorder 26, 36, 56, 249,
        250
Autism 9, 104
    spectrum disorder 26, 36, 249,
        250, 279
Autoimmune
    diseases 90
    disorders 47
    encephalitis 34
    encephalomyelitis 24
    thyroiditis 90
Autonomic dysfunction 77
Autonomic nervous system 3, 75,
    124
Autoscopy 233

B

Bacterial mutations 184
Bacteriotherapy 81
Bahujan Hitaye, Bahujan Sukhaye
    136
Bender Gestalt test 212
Benzodiazepines 20, 53
Bethanechol 82
Biological anthropology 286
Biology 9
Bipolar disorder 9, 24, 35, 55, 114,
    191, 196
Blood tests 150

Body
    dysmorphic disorder 102
    mass index 95
Bolitho test 224
Borderline personality disorder 27
Brain 248, 273
    decade of 168
    gut
        interactions 75
        psychotherapies 83
    relevance of 182
Breastfeeding 53
Briquet's syndrome 78

C

Cancer 215
Cardiology 112
Cardiovascular disease 112, 113,
    116, 117
Catecholamine 109
Central nervous system 3, 19, 72,
    99
Centrally mediated abdominal
    pain syndrome 74
Cerebrospinal fluid 12
Cerebrovascular disorders 31
Child sexual abuse 300
Child's cognitive development 252
Childhood psychiatric disorders
    279
Cholesterol 119
Chronic fatigue syndrome 3, 62
Civil law 22
    cases 218
Clozapine 51, 54
Coercion 187
Cognitive behavioral therapy 24,
    44, 84, 113, 200, 215, 242
Communication system 209
Complex-partial seizures 196
Conduct disorders 251
Confusion assessment method 21
Congestive cardiac failure 119
Contemporary dance 276
Contraception 49

Index

Convolutional neural network 243
Cornelia de Lange syndrome 104
Coronary artery disease 20, 112, 118
Coronary bypass graft surgery 119
Coronary heart disease 113
   Stockholm women's intervention trial for 118
Corticosteroids 96
Corticotropin-releasing hormone 109
Cortisol 109
COVID-19 6, 57, 240
   pandemic 242
Criminal law 222
Cultural mental health 290
Culture bound syndromes 170, 289, 290
Culture specific disorders 291
Curricular stress 253
Cushing's disease 91
Cushing's syndrome 91
Cycloserine 90

D

Dance
   and music 282
      therapy 272
   classes 281
   components 275
   movement therapy 277, 278
      effectiveness of 278
   music 274
      and mind 272
   performer-choreographer 272
   therapy 275, 279, 281
      field of 275
      role of 277
Daydreaming 233
Deep brain stimulation 29
Delirium 19, 20
   differential diagnosis of 21t
   risk factors for 20t
   tremens 19
Delusional disorders 101
Dementia 9, 22, 30
   etiology of 22t
   psychological symptoms of 23
   treatment for 278
Depression 29, 31, 33, 43, 55, 113, 118, 119, 191, 197, 199, 201, 241, 254, 267, 277, 279, 303
   incidence of 198
   management of 55
   mild 29
   moderate 29
   moderate-to-severe 277
   perimenopausal 48
   severe 29
   severity of 198
   symptoms 278
Dermatillomania 105
Dermatitis
   artefacta 103, 104f
   para-artefacta syndrome 106
Dermatological disorders 100, 107
Dermatological obsessive-compulsive disorders 102
Dermatology 99, 100t
   interface of 100
Dermatomyositis 60
Dextromethorphan 25
Dhat syndrome 128
Diabetes mellitus 20, 89, 95, 118, 276
Digital phenotyping 241
Disability benefits 181
Disaccharides 78
Disgust 273
Distress
   cultural concepts of 291
   idioms of 170, 291
District Mental Health Programme 221
Divergence, phase of 168
Divine wrath 195
Domestic Violence
   Act 221
   female victims of 278
Dopamine 12
   dysregulation syndrome 30
Double-blind randomized controlled trials 271
Down syndrome 183
Dozing 233
Drama therapy 282, 283
Drapetomania 288
Draw-a-man test 212
Drug hypersensitivity syndrome 106, 106f
Dualism, theory of 73
Dysbiosis 76
Dysmetria, cognitive 35
Dysmorphic facies 250
Dyspareunia 128
Dyspepsia, functional 74

E

Eating disorders 56, 104, 254-257
Ebstein's anomaly 52
Efavirenz 90
Electra complex 178
Electroconvulsive therapy 24, 150, 266, 267
Electroencephalogram 26, 241
Electronic health records 242
Emotional resilience 252
Emotions, active expression of 279
Empirical adequacy 184
Endocrine disorders 91, 130
Enteric nervous system 3
Epigastric pain syndrome 74
Epilepsy 25, 26, 26t, 27
Epistemic injustice 146
Erectile dysfunction 125, 130
Escherichia coli 81
Ethnographic fieldwork, hallmark of 286
Euphoria 25
Exfoliative cheilitis 106f
Extrasensory perception 229
Eye movement desensitization 162

F

Facial expressions 271
Factitious dermatitis 103
Feelings 274
Fermentable oligosaccharides 78
Fitness 305
Follicular-stimulating hormone 48
Food safety 305
Foramen magnum 19
Forensic psychiatry 218
Freud's psychoanalysis 160
Functional abdominal pain 74
Functional gastrointestinal disorders 4, 72, 72b, 73, 85
   assessment of 79
   management of 81
   pathophysiology of 75

G

Gamma-aminobutyric acid 11, 21
Gastroenterology 3, 72
Gastrointestinal system 4
Gender identity 123
Gestalt therapist 212
Glutamate 11
Gouty arthritis 60
Grandiose delusions 193
Guru-chela paradigm 179
Gut
   brain interaction, disorders of 72

microbiome 76
psychopharmacology 81
Gynecological oncology 57

H

Habit and impulse disorders 103
Haloperidol 117
Hanuman complex 179
Hashimoto's thyroiditis 96
Health Insurance Portability and Accountability Act 243
Health Promotion Using Life Skills in Adolescent Program 260
Health, promotion of 305
Heart disease 115, 118
Hepatitis
 B virus 95
 C virus 95
Hermaphroditism 178
Hindu Marriage Act 224
Hodgkin lymphoma 183
Holism, principle of 73
Hospital anxiety and depression scale 61
Human behavior 265
Human communication systems 209
Human immunodeficiency virus 47, 90, 215
Human mind 287
Hyperparathyroidism 92
Hyperprolactinemia 130
Hypertension 89, 119
 arterial 131
Hypnotherapy 84
Hypothalamic-pituitary-adrenal axis 114
 dysfunction 48

I

Ideographs 209
Immune dysfunction 77
Impulse control disorders 30
Indian Education System 248, 249f
Indian Journal of Social Psychiatry 170
Indian Psychiatry Society 151, 269
Induced abortion 49
Infectious diseases 90
Infertility 48
 psychological effects of 49
Inflammatory diseases 90
Influence 187
Information technology 239
Insanity plea 225

Insomnia 43
Institutional neurosis 168
Intellectual disability, prevalence of 249
Intensive care units 20
Internal psychokinesis 232
International Association on Political Use of Psychiatry 5
International Classification of Diseases 4
International Journal of Social Psychiatry 170
Interpersonal therapy 113
Irritability 43
Irritable bowel syndrome 73
Ischemic heart diseases 89
Isolation, feelings of 237

J

Jacobson's progressive muscle relaxation training 84
Joint researches 288
Judicial psychiatry 151
Judiciary, role of 226

K

Kidney diseases, chronic 89
Kinesthetic reaction 210
Kleine-Levin syndrome 34, 178

L

Lactobacillus plantarum 81
Language and speech disorder 249
Law regulating psychiatry profession 220
Legal system 189
Lesch-Nyhan syndrome 104
Levator ani syndrome 75
Levodopa 25
Lewy bodies 30
Limbic encephalitis 96
Linguistic anthropology 286
Lip-lick cheilitis 102f
Lipoprotein, high-density 118
Literature, types of 231
Lorazepam 54
Lower depressive symptoms 198
Luteinizing hormone 48
Lyme disease 90
Lysergic acid diethylamide 11

M

Magnetic resonance
 imaging 25
 spectroscopy 12

Major depressive disorder 23, 24, 50, 113
Major histocompatibility complex 10
Major psychiatric disorders 90
Male erectile disorders 128
Mania 31, 33
Marriage and divorce 224
Martha Mitchell effect 146
Matchbox sign 101
McDonald criteria 23
Media, traditional forms of 301
Medical Council Act 222
Medical
 illness 276
 insanity 225
 issues 95
Medication adherence 191, 197
Mefloquine 90
Menarche 43
Menopause 48
Menstrual cycle 43
Mental disorders 181, 288
 care for 195
 severe 289
 statistical manual of 290
Mental disturbances 267
Mental health 149, 154, 215, 239, 240, 270, 283
 action plan 144
 care 139t
  act 220, 221
  implementation of 219
  services 220, 221
 conditions 266
 education 254
 hospitals 289
 impact on 298
 issues 254, 256
  risk factor for 253
 legislation 219, 220, 221
 problems 255, 281
 professionals 266, 269, 270, 283
  portrayal of 266
 promotion of 283
 scope of 248
 symptoms 214
 themes, realistic portrayals of 268
Mental illness 18, 57, 129, 191, 193, 218, 219, 223, 226, 227, 254, 274, 280, 283, 288, 295, 303
 absence of 248
 depiction of 266
 development of 241
 music therapy for 279

representation of 269
severe 1, 95, 129, 196
symptoms of 191
treatment for 275
types of 276
Mental Retardation and Multiple Disabilities Act 221
Mental stress
  acute 115
  chronic 115
Metabolic syndrome 112, 118
Microbiota-gut-brain axis 77
Midface toddler excoriation syndrome 104
Migration 149
Mind
  philosophy of 181, 182
  theory of 183
Mini-mental state examination 22
Mirtazapine 25, 54
Monoamine oxidase inhibitors 117
Monosaccharides 78
Monozygotic twins 232
Mood
  disorder 27, 36
  disturbances 254, 256
  stabilizers 52, 54
Multiple sclerosis 23, 24, 90
Murphy argues 184
Muscle tension, electromyographic biofeedback for 84
Music
  advantages of 275
  and dance 276, 280
  therapy 274, 275, 279, 281
Myocardial infarction, acute 113
Mythology 174, 175
  and mind 175
  and therapy 179

N

Narcissistic personality disorder 178
Narcotic Drugs and Psychotropic Substances Act 222, 256
National Institute of Mental Health and Neurosciences 93
National Mental Health Programme 221, 259, 294
Near-death experiences 231, 233
Necrotic deep ulcers 101f
Neostigmine 82
Neurodevelopmental disorders 104, 248
Neurodiversity theory 188

Neuroimmunocutaneous system 93
Neuroimmunopathogenesis 9
Neurological disorders 23
Neurological soft signs 34, 34t, 35
Neurological system 248
Neurology 2, 18
Neuropsychiatry 18, 19, 89
Neurosyphilis 90
Neurotic excoriations 102f
Neuroticism 78
Neutral posture 287
Nitric oxide 124
N-methyl-D-aspartate 11 acid 23
Noncommunicable diseases 89, 221
Nonreductive physicalism 186
Nonsteroidal anti-inflammatory drugs 67
Nonverbal communication 208
Nonverbal language 209
Norepinephrine reuptake inhibitor 25
North American Psychiatry, growth of 160
Nosological system 295
Nosology 289

O

Obsessive-compulsive disorder 3, 9, 24, 33, 36, 55, 91, 102, 119, 191, 199, 242, 267
Obstetrics and gynecology 2, 42
Oedipus complex 178
Official classification systems 184
Olanzapine 54
Onychotillomania 102f
Orbitofrontal cortex 33
Orgasmic disorders 128
Osteoarthritis 60
Out-of-body experiences 232, 233
Oxidative stress 12

P

Pain 94
Palliative care 94
Panic disorder 29, 177
Paralysis agitans 28
Paranormal phenomena 229, 233, 234
  types of 231
Parapsychology 229, 230
Parkinson's disease 28, 29t, 31t
Paroxetine 24

Paroxysmal supraventricular tachycardia 119
Pathological laughter and crying scale 32
Pediatric autoimmune neuropsychiatric disorders 3, 63, 91
Pentazocine addiction 101f
Perinatal psychiatric illness 45
Personal data protection bill 243
Personality disorder 27, 104
Pharmacological management 44, 67
Phenomenology 181, 183
Philosophy 6, 181
Phonological awareness skills 280
Physical
  disability 216
  exercise 276
  fitness 272
Political psychology 144
Polycystic ovarian syndrome 57
Polymyositis 60
Polyols 78
Poor neonatal adaptation syndrome 52
Positive and negative syndrome scale 277
Positive emotions 278
Positron emission tomography scanner 273
Postencephalitis syndromes 90
Postpartum bipolar disorder 47
Postpartum blues 45, 47
Postpartum depression 45, 47
  effects of 46
  management of 46
Postpartum mood disorder 47t
Postpartum psychosis 46, 47
  management of 47
Postprandial distress syndrome 74
Poststroke depression 31
Post-traumatic stress
  diagnosis scale 256
  disorder 33, 120, 130, 149, 160, 209, 241
Post-war victims, well-being of 275
Prebiotics 81
Pregnancy 47, 57
  loss of 49
Premenstrual dysphoric disorder 43, 44b
Priapism 178
Probiotics 81
Problematic behaviors 280
Proctalgia 75
  chronic 75
  fugax 75

Prokinetics 82
Prolactin 109
Protection of Children from Sexual Offenses 256
Protection of Human Rights Act 221
Proximity 210*f*
Prurigo nodularis 105*f*
Pseudobulbar affect 25, 32
Pseudoseizures 27, 28*t*
Psoriasis 131
  area severity index 108
Psoriatic arthritis 60
Psychiatric
  advanced directives, use of 188
  anthropologists 287
  assessment 290
  categories 234
  comorbidity 78
  conditions 182
  curriculum 216
  diagnosis 290
  disorders 24*t*, 26, 26*t*, 29, 29*t*, 42, 63, 92, 100, 101, 107, 118, 254, 277
    brain plasticity basis for 11
    causal association of 64
    management of 66
    neurobiology of 36
    neurological aspects of 34
    neurotransmitter basis for 11
    nonpharmacological management of 68
    pharmacological management of 67
    primary 90
    somatic treatment for 69
    treatment of 54
  evaluation 64
  illness 296
    diagnosis of 289
  implications 100, 107
  issues 92
  medications, cardiac side effects of 116
  morbidity 64*b*
    epidemiology of 61
  nosology, aspect of 289
  phenotypes 184
  research, internal stages of 185
  researchers 185
    moral responsibilities of 184
  side effects of cardiac drugs 116
  symptoms 277
    rating scale 294
    treatment of 187
Psychiatrist
  assisting judiciary system 222
  role of 95, 222
Psychiatry 1, 18, 62, 88, 100*t*, 136, 159, 162, 166, 169*t*, 181, 184, 186, 229, 265, 269, 276, 282, 287, 289*f*, 295
  and law 219
  interface 220*f*
  central institute of 276
  deals 229
  field of 295
  global initiative on 5
  interface of 100
  philosophy of 181-183
  practice of 138
  sociology of 166
Psychoactive substance use 25
Psychocardiology 89
Psychodermatology 93
Psychodrama 282
Psychoeducation 83
Psychogenic nonepileptic seizures 27
Psychogynecology 89
Psychokinesis 232
  kind of 232
Psychological issues 68, 258
Psychonephrology 89, 94
Psycho-oncology 89, 92
Psycho-ophthalmology 89
Psychopathology 193, 196
Psychopharmacology, basic principles of 68*b*
Psychosis 25, 27, 29, 32, 33
Psychosocial factors 77, 112
Psychosomatic diseases 130
Psychotherapy 283
Psychotic symptoms 277, 294
Psychotropic drugs 27
  effects of 27*t*
Psychotropics 50, 51
  medication 53
Pyridostigmine 82

Q

Quarantine 187
Quasi-legal instruments 220
Quetiapine 54
Quinidine 25

R

Racial attitudes 239
Racial disparity 266
Randomized controlled trials 213
Rashtriya Bal Swasthya Karyakram 260
Relaxation therapy 84
Religiosity 192
  impact of 198
Religious assistance, acceptance of 196
Renal disease, end-stage 95
Repetitive transcranial magnetic stimulation 29
Reproductive medicine 42
Rheumatic diseases 3
Rheumatoid arthritis 3, 60, 90, 131
Rheumatological diseases 60, 61, 63, 64, 64*b*, 65*b*, 66
Rheumatology 3, 60
  interface of 62
Rorschach's inkblot test 212

S

Schizophrenia 9, 11, 35, 54, 95, 115, 191, 193-197, 241, 267, 277, 279
  awareness association 267
  disorders 279
  negative symptoms of 12
  proportion of 195
  treatment of 54
School health systems, part of 259
School mental health 260
  programs 280
  promotion of 259*f*
Science, philosophy of 181
Scientific Foundation for Dance Therapy 276
Scleroderma 60
Sedatives 54
Selective serotonin reuptake inhibitors 12, 24, 44, 114, 117
Self-awareness mode 272
Sensationalize violence and substance use 266
Serotonin 11
Sertraline 24, 54
  antidepressant heart attack randomized trial 113
Sex education, role of 250, 253, 254, 256
Sexting 299
Sexual abuse 256
Sexual assaults 257
Sexual behavior 123
  high-risk 254
Sexual disorders 122
Sexual dysfunction 63, 115, 128, 130, 131
  primary 131
  secondary 131
  tertiary 131

Sexual functioning 129, 130
Sexual health 305
Sexual identity 123, 126*t*
Sexual orientation 123
    components of 126*f*
Sexual response cycle 123
    neurobiology of 124
Sexuality 4, 122, 125
    Michael storms model of 127*f*
    spectrum concept of 125
Sexually transmitted diseases 256, 304
    screening for 258
Sheehan's syndrome 47
Shell shock 159
Sjögren's syndrome 60, 131
Skin-picking disorder 105
Sleep 300
    disorders 30, 31*t*, 56
Small intestinal bacterial overgrowth 76
Social
    and political philosophy 188
    and psychiatry 181
    anthropology 287
    anxiety, levels of 303
    blackmail 299
    cultural anthropology 286
    epidemiology 166
    gesture 294
    hygiene 189
    media 269, 297, 303
        impact of 252
        use of 297
    medicine 167
    networking sites 297
    psychiatry and psychiatric epidemiology 170
    skills 249, 279
    smile, lack of 250
Sociocultural intervention 212
Socioemotional theory 257
Sociology 6, 166, 169*t*, 290

Somatoform disorders 102
Specific learning disorder 249, 251, 254, 259*f*
Spirit 195
    intrusion 195
Split attraction model 128*f*
Stevens-Johnson syndrome 106
Strengthens cardiovascular health 272
Streptococcal infection 3, 63, 91
Streptococcus pyogenes infection 91
Stress 254
    impact of 63
    reduction 272
Subpoena 226
Substance abuse 254, 256
    disorders 101
Substance use 301
    disorder 56, 267
Suicidal behavior 191, 198, 200, 254, 256
Suicidal ideation 199, 267
    presence of 255
Suicide 27, 167, 301
    attempts 201
Synbiotics 81
Synchronicity 235
Systemic lupus erythematosus 3, 60, 90

T

Teachers, training of 251
Telepathy 231
Temporal lobe epilepsy 26
Testamentary capacity 223
Testosterone 125
Thematic apperception test 212
Tic disorders 103
Tort law 224
Tourette syndrome 119
Toxic epidermal necrolysis 106
Transcendental meditation 84

Transcranial magnetic stimulation 150
Transcultural psychiatry 288
Traumatic brain injury 32, 34*t*, 92
Trichotillomania 102*t*, 103, 103*f*, 105
Tricyclic antidepressant 24, 51

V

Vaginal dryness 131
Vaginismus 128
Valve replacement 120
Valvular heart disease 119
Verbal language 209
Vietnam war and psychiatry 161
Visceral hypersensitivity 76
Visual communication, characteristics of 209
Visual language 209
    components of 211
Vitiligo 108

W

War and psychological warfare, psychological costs of 148
Watching television 239
Weakness 267
Wernicke's encephalopathy 34
Working memory 209
World Association of Social Psychiatry 171
World Health Organization 144

Y

Yudhishthir syndrome 178

Z

Ziplock sign 101
Zippy's friends program 260
Zolpidem 53
Zopiclone 53

EU GSPR Authorised Reprsentative
Logos Europe, 9 rue Nicolas Poussin
1700, La Rochelle, France
Phone: +33 (0) 6 67 93 73 78
E-mail: contact@logoseurope.eu

www.ingramcontent.com/pod-product-compliance
Ingram Content Group UK Ltd.
Pitfield, Milton Keynes, MK11 3LW, UK
UKHW050429150426
5217IPUK00019B/1307